Digital Healthcare and Artificial Intelligence

Digital technologies are essential to future-proof our health service. With an ageing population and the landscape of the post-pandemic world making increasing demands on an already-stretched human workforce, maximising the potential of a digital future is necessary. This book introduces the concepts and underpinning technology behind recent developments to give a snapshot of the state of the art in the field of digital health and provides information for clinicians at all levels of experience. The reader will gain insight into digital health in general, with clinical, technical and industrial insights providing context to the theory.

Key Features

■ Defines the value that Artificial Intelligence (AI) brings to healthcare, resulting in improved clinical diagnosis and decision-making

■ Enables not just imaging staff but other healthcare practitioners to extract the best ways of working with AI using the underpinning knowledge from this text

AI in Clinical Practice

AI and Precision Medicine in Infectious Disease Management
Jen-Tsung Chen

The Impact of Artificial Intelligence in Radiology
Adam Eltorai, Ian Pan, and Henry H Guo

Digital Healthcare and Artificial Intelligence: A Primer for Clinicians and Students
Edited by Clare Rainey, Sonyia McFadden, and Jonathan McConnell

For more information about the series, please visit https://www.routledge.com/AI-in-Clinical-Practice/book-series/AICLINICAL

Digital Healthcare and Artificial Intelligence
A Primer for Clinicians and Students

Edited by
Clare Rainey, Sonyia McFadden,
and Jonathan McConnell

CRC Press
Taylor & Francis Group
Boca Raton London New York

CRC Press is an imprint of the
Taylor & Francis Group, an **Informa** business

Designed cover image: Shutterstock: Image Id: 2353878985

First edition published 2026
by CRC Press
2385 NW Executive Center Drive, Suite 320, Boca Raton FL 33431

and by CRC Press
4 Park Square, Milton Park, Abingdon, Oxon, OX14 4RN

CRC Press is an imprint of Taylor & Francis Group, LLC

ISBN: 9781032709925 (hbk)
ISBN: 9781032709895 (pbk)
ISBN: 9781032709956 (ebk)

DOI: 10.1201/9781032709956

Typeset in Palatino
by KnowledgeWorks Global Ltd.

Contents

Foreword by Susan C. Shelmerdine

As a medical doctor, academic, AI enthusiast, and advocate for critical thinking, I view the rise of AI in medical imaging as both an exciting frontier and one of profound challenge. These technologies bring promise and hope – but also disruption. They are already reshaping how we work, our roles, our clinical pathways, and raising new questions about patient safety, accountability, equity, and what it truly means to be human in the healthcare system.

One thing however is certain: AI is here to stay.

It has been said that "AI won't replace radiologists – but radiologists who use AI will replace those who don't". In healthcare, however, where the risks are high and the stakes personal, the real issue isn't using or not using AI – but using it wisely. Intelligent implementation, rooted in clinical expertise and critical thought, is what will make the difference between helpful tools and harmful distractions.

In an era where we are seeing "AI-first" thinking, we must remember that healthcare is – and must remain – "human-first". So, the real question is how do we best to prepare ourselves to lead its integration in a way that enhances, not erodes, our clinical judgement, compassion, and connection with patients.

That begins with understanding – understanding what AI is and isn't, what it can do, and where it falls short. Without this foundation, we risk becoming passive users of systems we don't fully trust or control. Worse, we risk being sidelined altogether as decisions increasingly become made by those without clinical insight.

As imaging professionals, we are uniquely positioned to shape how AI supports our field – if we choose to step into that role. This book is a timely and essential step in that direction. It offers an accessible yet rigorous introduction to AI, grounded in both the technical foundation and the lived realities of clinical practice written by those who are on the frontlines. The authors explore everything from the evolution of automation to real-world examples of AI in workflow, patient perspectives, and critical issues like representation. Throughout, they centre the human role – recognizing that AI doesn't exist in a vacuum but within the daily decisions and relationships that define patient care.

I congratulate the authors on this important contribution. Their work helps uncover a complex and often intimidating topic. I hope it serves as a valuable companion on your way to shaping the future of imaging.

Susan C. Shelmerdine
RCR Roentgen Professor 2025
Royal College of Radiologists
London, U.K.

Associate Professor of Radiology
UCL Great Ormond Street Institute of Child Health,
London, U.K.

Consultant Paediatric Radiologist
Department of Clinical Radiology
Great Ormond Street Hospital for Children NHS Foundation Trust,
London, U.K.

Foreword by Raymond Bond

This is a fantastic book for healthcare professionals or researchers who want to further understand and explore the use of AI in healthcare. The book provides accessible and excellent background material to introduce the reader to the history and nomenclature of AI. Given that we are very likely living in an AI summer, this book can enable readers to engage in the wider conversation on the use of AI in healthcare. This book can help healthcare professionals develop their "AI literacy". Developing AI literacy is fundamental because the world needs domain experts to critically appraise AI technologies to ensure patient safety and to help calibrate the right level of user trust. I don't think there is a need for users to understand all the math behind AI technologies, but there is a need to understand the principles behind AI technologies. In general, I imagine that a greater understanding of how something works may influence how it is responsibly adopted, improved, integrated, and used.

It is brilliant to see that this book introduces the reader to statistics and metrics that are used to evaluate AI systems. That chapter is important to allow readers to understand the performance of AI systems as well as for readers who want to engage with the scientific literature that describe studies that evaluate AI algorithms in healthcare. The statistical metrics are presented using clear examples. The book even discusses an AI course and curriculum. The book not only educates the reader about AI and statistics but also covers details related to human–computer interaction, cognitive biases, as well as professional and ethical issues. The book discusses principles related to person-centred practice. This is critical, given that the patient should be at the centre of clinical decision-making and the use of AI. You will learn a lot about contemporary issues. This includes concepts such as automation bias (a user overtrusting AI recommendations) and algorithmic aversion (a user's disposition to not trust AI technologies). Other key issues include the concern of healthcare inequalities and algorithmic fairness/bias (where an AI algorithm may not perform as well for all demographic groups [creating disparities]). There is a chapter dedicated to equity which presents the different types of fairness and provides examples.

The reader will be able to explore the use of AI across a number of healthcare domains, including radiology, where topics such as radiomics are discussed as well as the use of AI to reconstruct images. There is also a chapter related to AI in onco-radiology which discusses the concept of "off-view" AI, and the chapter related to AI in histopathology discusses concepts such as "digital weather" (which I understand is the idea of continuous software updates) and drift (where the performance of an AI system may change over time). There is also a chapter related to the application of AI in ophthalmology which makes mention of important issues such as "health data poverty", which in my understanding is when there is a lack of data from all populations which could negatively affect certain demographic groups that are underrepresented. Data poverty is a key issue that needs addressed given that many AI algorithms learn from the data that are provided. There is also a chapter on the use of AI in dermatology, which does point out a key concept known as a predetermined change control plan.[1] I understand that this is in relation to the potential need to safely update AI systems post-market, for example, to improve the performance of the AI.

Whilst this book provides great educational material on AI and includes several chapters on the application of AI in different healthcare domains, there is also a key chapter related to AI sustainability. AI sustainability is an important issue given the amount of energy required to train AI algorithms. This chapter presents an AI sustainability checklist in healthcare and presents the idea of a dashboard to help measure/manage energy usage. Finally, a fantastic addition to the book includes detailed and insightful case studies on the use of technology and AI in healthcare. I highly recommend this book, and I really enjoyed reading the draft that was provided to me.

Raymond Bond,
Professor of Human Computer Systems, Ulster University, Northern Ireland, UK

NOTE

1. https://www.fda.gov/regulatory-information/search-fda-guidance-documents/marketing-submission-recommendations-predetermined-change-control-plan-artificial-intelligence

Preface

AI is continuing to reshape the landscape of healthcare and service delivery. Regardless of your role, technical background, or connection to healthcare, the impact of AI will touch your work. As AI continues to rapidly evolve across multidisciplinary healthcare, it is fair to say that understanding AI is no longer optional; it is essential.

This book is designed to serve as a practical, cross-disciplinary introduction to AI in healthcare. It was written for all healthcare professionals, trainees, and students, regardless of their background or technical expertise. It is anticipated that this book will also be of interest to data analysts, computer scientists developing AI tools, industry representatives, administrators, educators, researchers, and policy leaders, to name but a few. Understanding the application of AI in healthcare is essential not just for keeping pace with change, but to enable us to shape how that change unfolds.

This book does not require any prior knowledge of computer science. Instead, it offers a general introduction with a practical and balanced exploration of how AI is being applied across clinical, operational, and research settings. A series of case studies at the end of the book identify how these changes impact real-world healthcare delivery.

This book aims to demystify AI by highlighting real applications, benefits, limitations, and ethical implications in clinical practice. From research and diagnostic tools to predictive analytics, from virtual health assistants to increased automation of administrative tasks, AI is already shaping clinical workflows and patient outcomes. The integration of AI into healthcare is incredibly complex and carries many well-documented challenges, e.g. the risk of bias, transparency and trust, data privacy, sustainability, and the lack of human empathy, and this book addresses each of these.

Our goal is to provide a broad overview of the use of AI in healthcare across the multidisciplinary team. We offer a thoughtful guide to inform the reader of the range of applications currently in clinical use to help navigate this rapidly evolving field. We believe that a cross-disciplinary understanding bridging clinical insight with technological innovation will offer a healthcare system that is more efficient, equitable, and compassionate.

We invite you to approach this book not just with curiosity but with critical engagement. You should be thinking not only about what AI can do but what it should and could do and where else can it be applied. Regardless of your background, your perspective is vital in shaping the inception of ideas and how these tools are researched, developed, and deployed. The future of AI in healthcare is not just about computers and machines; it is about us, the people involved, the safeguarding of the practical implications of the systems used, and the digitally responsible future we collectively choose to build.

This book explores both the present and the future applications of AI in healthcare. It looks at what is currently working, what is emerging, and what is aspirational. The future is being shaped today, and we all have a role to play. We hope this book sparks new ideas of where you can utilize AI in your respective disciplines in the future.

Editors' Biographies

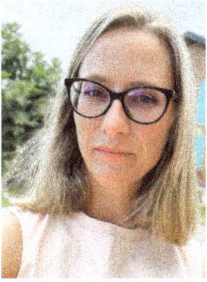

Dr Clare Rainey is a lecturer in the discipline of radiography within the School of Medicine at University College Cork, in Ireland. Clare previously held positions at Ulster University, including course director of the undergraduate diagnostic radiography programme, and prior to this, in the NHS, where she worked for 11 years as a clinical radiographer.

Clare obtained her PhD from Ulster University in AI for radiographic image interpretation, with a focus on the impact of AI on human cognitive processes, including decision-making and the impact of user interfaces on trust and automation bias. She has published extensively in well-known, international journals in the fields of AI, human–computer interaction, technology-enabled education and leadership and has contributed to a number of textbooks in the field of AI.

Clare supervises master's and PhD students across a range of topics and disciplines, including research into technology use in diverse clinical settings and user interface design. She works with colleagues in medicine, computer science/data analytics and, of course, radiography. Through this she supports and promotes open research principles by mentoring students to publish research and sharing open access data sets.

Clare is chair of the Society of Radiographers AI advisory board and is an associate editor of the *Journal of Medical Imaging and Radiation Sciences.*

Clare is driven by a passion for exploring how technology can be used responsibly to reduce health disparities both nationally and globally to secure parity of care for all and is committed to the future visibility of radiographer research in AI and other emerging technologies.

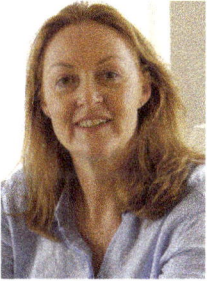

Dr Sonyia McFadden is a registered diagnostic radiographer and currently a senior lecturer in diagnostic radiography and imaging at Ulster University in Northern Ireland. She completed her MSc in 2000, investigating radiation exposure in interventional cardiology, and her PhD in 2010, investigating radiation dose optimisation in paediatric interventional cardiology. Sonyia was awarded the International Society of Radiographers and Radiological Technologists Dosewise International Radiographer of the Year (2014), a Fellowship of the College of Radiographers by Portfolio (2016), and a Gold Medal Award from the Society and College of Radiographers (2021).

Sonyia previously held the position of research director of the Institute of Nursing and Health Research in the Faculty of Life and Health Sciences at Ulster University and is the past chair of the Society of Radiographers AI Advisory Board in the UK.

Currently Sonyia is on the editorial board of the international journal *Cardiovascular Imaging Asia*. She has over 20 years' clinical experience in general radiography/interventional cardiology and 24 years' teaching and research experience in an academic setting.

Sonyia has several areas of ongoing research, publishes/presents widely, and supervises and assesses PhD students locally, nationally, and internationally. She is passionate about education, training, and research in all aspects of medical imaging and strives to advance the field of research in medical imaging through shared knowledge.

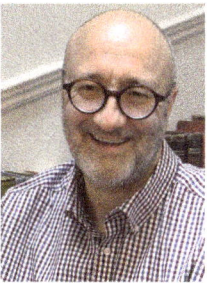

Dr Jonathan McConnell is a registered diagnostic radiographer. He is currently a visiting professor at Ulster University in Northern Ireland. He completed his MSc in 1999, investigating radiographer reporting consensus of role extension between the reporters and their managers. Jonathan completed his PhD at Monash University, Australia, in 2015, asking whether role development by radiographer interpretation could reposition the profession in Australia. Having a mixed clinical and academic career, he led the radiographer reporting team at NHS Greater Glasgow and Clyde as a consultant-grade radiographer between 2013 and 2022, receiving the national team award for Scotland in 2016, and was awarded Fellowship by Portfolio of the College of Radiographers in 2019.

Jonathan has served in multiple roles in the UK and internationally, including advisory positions to the New Zealand Registration Board and the education committee for the State of Victoria Registration Board, as a radiographer (role development and advanced practice) to NHS Education for Scotland, the Scottish Radiology Transformation

Programme, the College of Radiographers Consultant Radiographers Advisory Group, the Diagnostic Imaging Advisory Group, and the Assessment and Accreditation Board. He contributed to the CoR Education and Career Framework development between 2020 and 2022 as a consultant radiographer and frequently reviews articles from a range of peer-reviewed journals and has been an editorial board member and now an international advisory group member for the *Radiography* journal since 2005. Currently he acts as a fitness-to-practice registrant panel member for the UK Health and Care Professions Council and is a member of the National Institute for Health and Care Research, Radiographer Research Incubator steering group.

Jonathan has several areas of ongoing research, publishes/presents widely, and supervises and assesses PhD students. He is passionate about education, training, and research in all aspects of medical imaging and enthusiastically advances the field of research in medical imaging.

List of Contributors

Lisa A. Adams

Patrick Brennan
DetectedX and University of Sydney, Australia

Keno K. Bressem
Institute for Cardiovascular Radiology and
  Nuclear Medicine, German Heart Center
  Munich, TUM University Hospital,
  Technical University of Munich, Munich,
  Germany

Tamsin Browne
Paediatrician, Cambridge, UK, Founder of Hear
  Glue Ear

Felix Busch
School of Medicine and Health, Department of
  Diagnostic and Interventional Radiology,
  Klinikum rechts der Isar, TUM University
  Hospital, Technical University of Munich,
  Munich, Germany

Siddhant Dogra
New York University, New York City, NY, USA

Florence X. Doo
University of Maryland School of Medicine,
  Baltimore, MD, USA and University of
  Maryland-Institute for Health Computing
  (UM-IHC), North Bethesda, MD, USA

Ziba Gandomkar
DetectedX and University of Sydney, Australia

Avneet Gill
Ulster University, Belfast, Northern Ireland, UK ·

Willem Grootjans
Leiden University Medical Centre

Ramsey Hafer
Thomas Jefferson University, Sidney Kimmel
  Medical College, Philadelphia, USA

Pearse Keane
Moorfields Eye Hospital, London, UK

Christopher McKee
Better Medicine, UK

Rohan Misra
Moorfields Eye Hospital, London, UK

Fahad Mohammed
NHS, Oxford University Hospitals, UK

Bhuvanesh Mural
University of Maryland – College Park, USA

Derrik Nghiem
Oakland University William Beaumont School
  of Medicine, Rochester, Michigan, USA

Vanessa Otti
Barts Health NHS Trust, Moorfields Eye
  Hospital, London, UK

Jordan Perchik
University of Alabama, USA

Alicja Jasinska-Piadlo
Royal Victoria Hospital, Northern Ireland, UK

Mary Rickard
DetectedX and University of Sydney, Australia

Mertcan Sevgi
University College London, UK

Milda Shams
Senior Marketing Manager, Oxipit, Vilnius,
  Lithuania

Vijay Sharma
Liverpool University Hospitals NHS
  Foundation Trust UK

Moayyad Suleiman
DetectedX and University of Sydney, Australia

Holly Toner
Senior AI Architect, Kainos, Belfast, Northern
  Ireland

Kaushik Venkatesh
Bringham and Women's Hospital/Harvard
  Medical School, Boston, MA, USA

Siegfried Wagner
University College London, Moorfields Eye
  Hospital, UK

1 Introduction and Learning Objectives

Clare Rainey

1.1 INTRODUCTION

With the new age in healthcare upon us, accompanied by a new generation of digitally literate clinicians, we need to be aware of the potential pitfalls in the way we interact with computers. We may encounter a balance between both overreliance and undue caution, both potentially exacerbated by a lack of understanding of the functionality and limitations of our current state of technology. However, we also need to have our eyes on the future – what is yet to be achieved, and when will the technology match, and even outperform, our expectations?

To make the most of what the future has to offer, we need to *all* have a seat at the table, to have the knowledge and confidence to give our professional perspectives and engage in meaningful conversations between developers and clinicians. Developers are pushing the boundaries of what technology is capable of, but only clinicians know what will benefit them, as end-users of these systems, and ultimately make a difference to patients.

This book aims to introduce the concepts and underpinning technology behind recent developments – to give a snapshot of the 'state of the art' in the field of digital health and provide a suitable level of information for clinicians and those interested in the development of advanced technologies from all backgrounds and levels of experience. The reader will gain insight into digital health in general, with clinical, technical and industry insights providing context to the theory. *Our digital future is here; are you ready?*

1.2 HISTORY OF COMPUTING IN MEDICAL SETTINGS – *COMPUTING BASICS – NOT MAGIC, MATHS!*

There has been an exponential increase in computing capabilities in recent years. The way in which computers are used to accomplish tasks is impressive – they are doing things faster than humans, sometimes with greater accuracy and without inherent human weaknesses and biases. This can be difficult for the non-expert end-user to rationalise – it can seem unintelligible at times. An understanding of the functionality of these systems is essential to be able to interact with advanced technologies in a responsible manner, to give the computer credit where due, to recognise the strengths and weaknesses of the system, and to understand its fragility and capabilities in *each situation*. This knowledge will allow the user to interact with the system as it should – realising that the outputs are not a result of magic, *just maths*!

According to the Oxford English Dictionary, the word 'computer' was first used in the early 1600s. Whilst not the first reference to the word, we have evidence of its use in common parlance from Samuel Pepys, in his diaries from June/July 1660, where he refers to the 'computing' of the ship's pay:

> *All the morning with the Captain, computing how much the thirty ships that come with the King from Scheveling their pay comes to for a month (because the King promised to give them all a month's pay), and it comes to L6,538, and the Charles particularly L777. (Page 2,* Diary of Samuel Pepys, June/July 1660*). [1]*

This is somewhat contradictory to the use of the word in our common vernacular, where the word is more commonly considered in reference to a 'thing' rather than a 'person' or action. This may motivate us to seek further clarity by looking to the etymology of the word – in the world before widespread use of the complex mechanics and electronics which we associate with the word today, what was 'computing' referring to?

The word 'computer' has its roots in the Latin word 'putare', meaning variously 'to think', 'to reckon' and 'to prune'. The link between meanings here is difficult to fathom, but there is a suggestion that it indicates an 'ordering' or 'making right' in both horticulture and cognition. The addition of the prefix 'com', meaning 'with', leans further into our modern use of the word [2]. By its most basic definition, a computing machine analyses and sorts information or data. In the National Archaeological Museum in Athens, Greece, sits the Antikythera Mechanism (Figure 1.1). This 'computer', found by divers in 1902, dates to the 2nd century BC, during the Hellenistic period in ancient Greek history [3]. This machine was constructed of a series of bronze toothed gears and dials, which are proposed to have been used to predict the position of structures in the cosmos, including

DOI: 10.1201/9781032709956-1

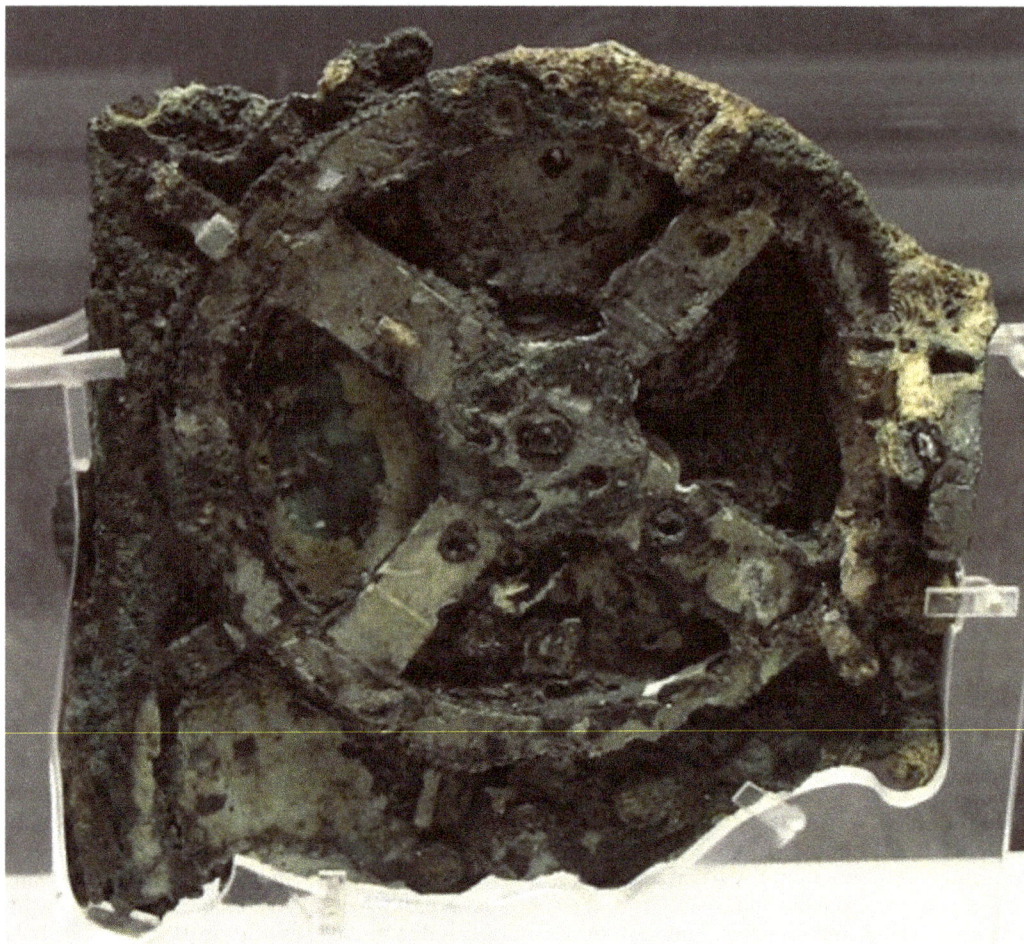

Figure 1.1   Antikythera Mechanism available at zeeweez, CC BY 2.0, via flickr.

the sun, moon and planets visible at that time. This machine was essentially a 'calculating machine' and provides evidence of early success in mechanising complex mathematics, saving time and reducing human input to accomplish a specific task.

Even at this time in history, over 2000 years ago, the evidence points to acknowledgement that there were certain tasks well suited to, and optimised, by mechanisation. This is not so different from today, where computer systems have been developed to allow for efficiencies in our day-to-day lives.

From Ancient Greece to more recent times, there is a lack of evidence to demonstrate continuous technological development. A boost in computing innovation occurred around the turn of the 19th century, as mathematicians began to investigate ways to further mechanise complicated calculations. In the 1820s and '30s, Charles Babbage developed and published plans for the building of machines which performed complex calculations. In 1822, Babbage published a description of the first iteration of his 'difference engine'. This was a complex machine with precise engineering of at least 2000 parts (Figure 1.2). These various specific gears and cogs were used together to compute and print mathematical calculations, such as astronomical, tide and logarithm tables. Although this was not fully built at the time, with government funding for the construction of the machine withdrawn in 1832, it provided a springboard for further technological development. In fact, this further development led to the so-called 'analytical engine' in 1824, which has many similarities with modern computers of today. The analytical engine had storage capacity and conditional branching capabilities, based on Boolean logic, i.e., the ability to control the flow of the calculations based on conditions, e.g., 'if' a condition is met, 'then' another action is prompted [4]. When translating the paper on the analytical engine, Ada Lovelace recognised further computational capabilities of the machine and developed a set of instructions for the use of the system in the calculation of Bernoulli

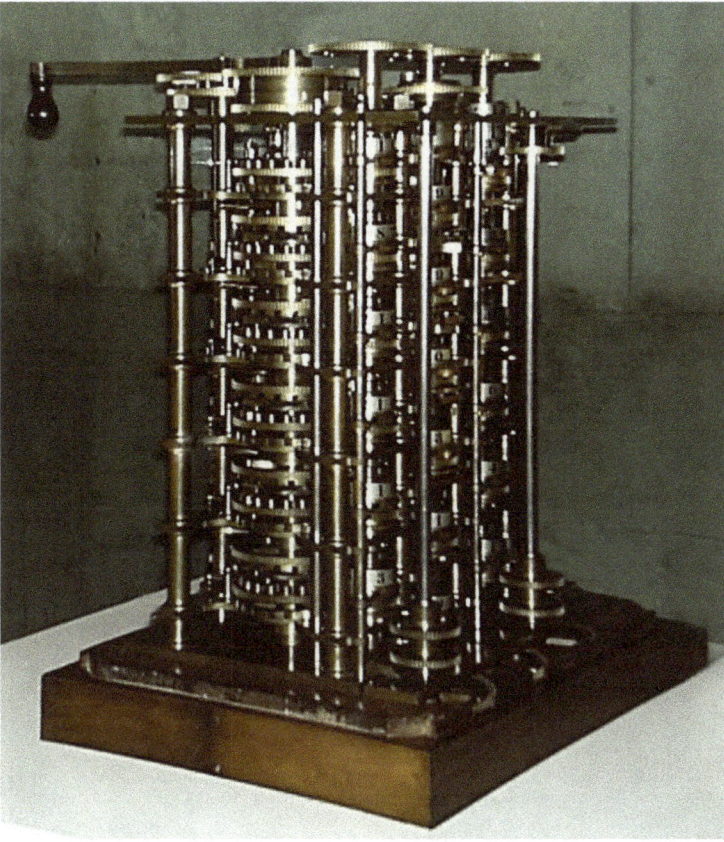

Figure 1.2 Charles Babbage's Difference Engine 1 (1832), displayed in the Science Museum, London. Reproduced under Creative Commons license – Sebastian Wallroth/Wikimedia Commons/Public Domain https://commons.wikimedia.org/wiki/File:Babbages_difference_engine_1832.jpg.

numbers (numbers which appear frequently in mathematical calculations and are useful for numerical analysis) [4]. She became, therefore, arguably the first 'computer programmer'. A full-scale analytical engine was never constructed.

Development continued with Belfast-born brothers James and William Thompson's differential analyser. William Thompson, a.k.a. Lord Kelvin, is perhaps better known for his work on electromagnetism, thermodynamics and the development of the international system of absolute temperature, a measure which bears his name, the 'Kelvin'. The differential analyser was constructed based on the wheel-and-disc integrator, invented by James Thompson (1876), and is considered to be the first general-purpose computer [5]. The function of this device was to integrate and solve linear differential equations. Further development of these analogue computers resulted in the development of tide prediction machines (Figure 1.3) [6]. A version of this was in use at the Port of Liverpool until the 1960s. These machines were used during the World Wars to predict optimal times for amphibious attacks [7]. Prior to the mechanisation of this task, the complex calculations required to calculate the tides at a given location took an excessive length of time, and the requirement for speed was usually at the expense of accuracy.

Furtherance of the work on the differential analyser, using Thompson's wheel-and-disc system, resulted in the first large-scale analogue computer, built by Vannevar Bush at the Massachusetts Institute of Technology (MIT) in 1931 [8]. Versions of this were soon in use around the world, despite being physically difficult to manually reconfigure between tasks (mallets at the ready!). The original wheel-and-disc technology was eventually replaced by electronic devices, eliminating the need for physical 'resetting' by a mechanic [4, 8].

A shift in technological development came about at around this time with work by Alan Turing – a name synonymous with the thinking behind the philosophy of computing. Turing postulated that in order for a computer to be 'intelligent', it should be able to perform tasks with behaviours

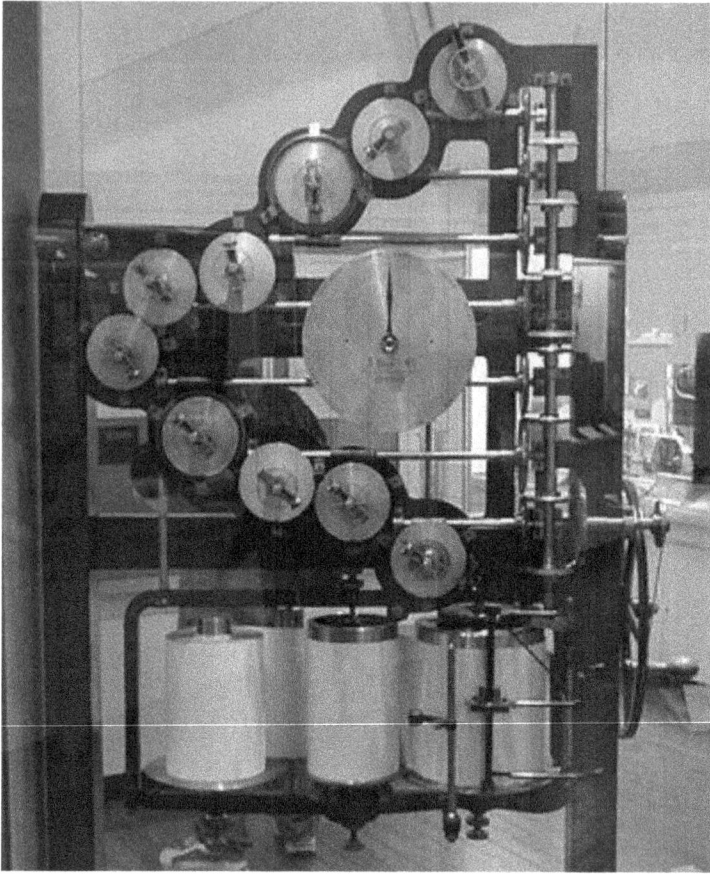

Figure 1.3 William Thompson's Tide Predicting Machine (1872). Located in the Science Museum, London.

equivalent to those of a human, and the human using the technology would be unable to distinguish the source of the intelligence – i.e., the human would be unable to distinguish between human and machine intelligence – otherwise known as the 'Turing Test'. This seemed like a challenge at the time, but with recent developments in technology, this is becoming – or in some cases, has become – a reality. There are problems, however, with how 'human intelligence' is defined, with some robust arguments suggesting that for an AI model to have human intelligence for a certain task, it should have to exhibit and prove the same assessments we would pose to a human to enable them to safely perform the tasks. Take medicine, for example. For a doctor or other healthcare professional to practise, they need to pass several key competencies to achieve the eventual goal of autonomy in their field. Whilst AI has been able to 'pass' many aspects of medical competency assessments, for example, the radiology exams (albeit barely) [9], we know that this is only one aspect of being a proficient clinician. Other human factors, such as advanced practical skills, are currently not possible using AI alone.

Whilst the passing of the Turing Test may be something considered to aspire to, there may be situations where an awareness of the source of advice is beneficial. One example is in the use of chatbots in mental healthcare, where strict ethical design principles should be adhered to and where it may be undesirable for the user to incorrectly believe they are conversing with a human [10]. Many clinicians may be confident in their ability to distinguish human from machine; however, this may not always be the case. Gaube et al. [11] presented diagnostic 'advice' to internal/emergency medicine physicians ($n = 127$) and radiologists ($n = 138$). This advice was labelled as being from either a human or from an AI source. They found that the radiologists, overall, rated the AI advice as lower quality than that of the human. This seems intuitive and even reasonable; however, in this study, all the advice was human generated, despite participants being told otherwise! This indicates that there may be a tendency towards algorithmic aversion in this population of clinical experts who may have a preconceived bias. (See also Chapter 5.)

The notion of technology singularity (i.e., the stage of technological development from which there is no point of return) has caused much media hype, and the rise of the supercomputer (essentially the fastest highest-performing machines at a point in time) in our lifetime has been predicted as far back as the 1950s. The ability of a computer to improve itself without human oversight further feeds into the theoretical concept of singularity plus the potential and imperceptible impact on humankind [12]. The need to steer and manage AI and ensure the human is in the loop is of paramount importance to safeguard the future working alongside our AI colleagues and, hopefully, friends!

1.3 THE ERA OF COMPUTERS IN MEDICINE

Historical retrospection allows us to see that there are tasks for which automation is suited. These tasks may be complex (normally requiring a substantial volume of human input and data), repeatable, or both. Automating suitable tasks allows humans to do what they are uniquely good at. Computer processing is fast, with large memory capacity, and computers may be less prone to errors than humans. This may be particularly notable when humans are fatigued or subject to situational distraction. Humans, however, are creative; they can think around a problem and conclude or make decisions using multiple, sometimes unexplainable, data points. They may use intuition and previous experience to help formulate a solution to a problem. Sometimes the way a human reaches a decision can be difficult to quantify and translate to another human or programme into a computer. A human can adapt their communication style to situations: i.e., when to talk and when to allow silence when to enforce a point or when to deliver information more gently. These 'soft skills' are vitally important in medicine. Medicine and associated fields are so much more than 'information'; however, data is a vitally important factor in patient management – the doctor or healthcare professional gathers data (e.g., patient history, symptoms), requests more data (e.g., imaging, pathology lab tests), processes and analyses this data and decides on an outcome or patient journey (Figure 1.4).

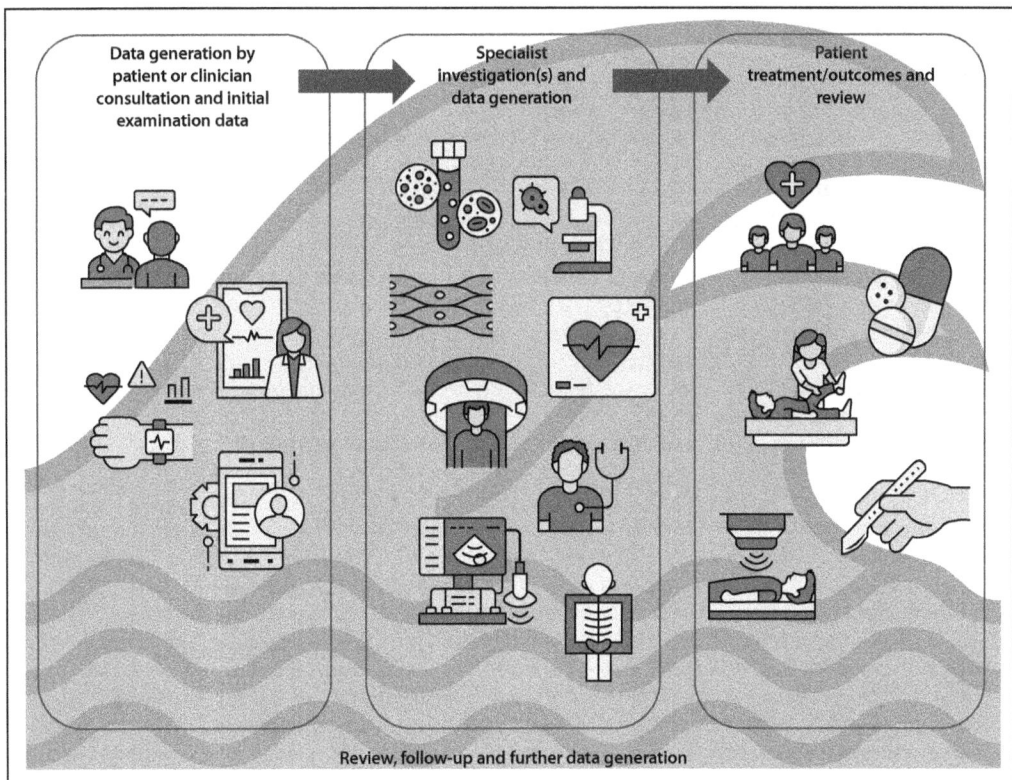

Figure 1.4 Patient data generation in healthcare – a simplified infographic.

This is an oversimplification and does not include other significant data sources such as the size-able volume of data generated by home monitoring systems/wearable devices, yet it highlights the vast amount of data obtained through a single patient presentation [13]. Looking to the future, this volume of data is projected to increase as there are more medical investigations and tests available, greater access to home monitoring technologies, better access to healthcare and more sophisticated diagnostic tests generating more data than ever before. This potential tsunami of data needs to be managed, and the most useful information extracted from it to assist the clinician and therefore to benefit the patient. How, therefore, is this data to be managed and synthesised by humans? For the most part, it cannot be – not fully, anyway, and certainly not with current healthcare resources and in a timely enough manner to benefit the patient.

1.4 DATA GENERATION IN HEALTHCARE SETTINGS

In general, data production is increasing each year. It is estimated that 90% of data globally has been generated in the past two years [14]. The 'average hospital' generates approximately 50 petabytes per year [15] – in other words, 1,048,576 gigabytes or 1,125,899,906,842,624 bytes [16]! It is important to note that this figure was generated in 2019, and one must wonder, with the increase in AI development and use in the intervening years, if this is somewhat conservative. Healthcare data make up 30% of all data globally; however, only 3% of these data are being used for the furtherance of care [17, 18]. Data management is a huge issue in healthcare, with much of a clinician's time spent simply on administrative and data-management tasks. A study conducted in 2020, across 16 US states, found that a third of clinicians' time was spent doing administrative tasks, while the typical allocation for these tasks is four hours per week [19, 20]. This study found that inputting data into the electronic health record (EHR) amounted to 20.7% of the working week alone. The impact of this data-management burden is being felt by clinicians – the *Elsevier: Clinician of the Future* report found that, of the 1691 doctors and 1108 nurses surveyed, 69% agreed that 'the volume of patient data is overwhelming' (p. 54) [21]. With a finite number of hours in the day, where does this time for data management come from? With stretched workforces, additional staffing resources are not the answer. To take the example of radiology, as a particularly data-heavy specialism, the Royal College of Radiologists census predicts that by 2028 there will be a 40% shortfall in the number of clinical radiology consultants [22]. This is coupled with increased demand for radiology services. The British Medical Association (BMA) reports that, whilst the number of doctors working in the National Health Service (NHS) has increased, this is not sufficient to meet demand. The BMA also notes that many current vacancies are being filled because of international rather than national recruitment streams [23]. If this is the solution to the immediate problem, one must consider the balance from a global, rather than a national, standpoint, and it may give pause for thought of the impact of this on existing global health disparity.

Clearly, AI and advanced computing would be perfectly placed to deal with many forms of patient and other health data. However, there are issues with the use of AI in healthcare which we need to be aware of, and some of these challenges are raised in the following chapters of this book. As mentioned in the previous section, there may be issues with mistrust of AI-generated data. At times this is despite its impressive performance. The flip side to this is an overreliance on AI feedback, at the expense of one's own judgement. This can be called 'automation bias' and is discussed in full in Chapter 5 of this book. The user of the technology needs to be made aware of the features of the feedback and should be able to readily interrogate the system to access data, such as failure analysis data, performance in a specific area and forms of explainability, if desired [24]. (See also Chapter 3.)

1.5 USES OF ADVANCED COMPUTING IN MEDICAL APPLICATIONS

Much of the attention in the media and public sphere has centred on AI for decision support. Rule-based systems for clinical decision support were among the first used in practice, including the CASNET model for glaucoma diagnosis [25], MYCIN for antibiotic prescribing (early 1970s) [26] and DXplain, an electronic medical textbook and differential diagnosis automation system (version 1, 1986) [27], to name a few. These 'expert systems' made use of a series of rules, devised by human experts and embedded in a 'decision tree' type model. Early computer-assisted diagnosis (CAD) systems, such as those used in mammography, came into use in the 1980s [28]. Whilst these systems are basic by today's standards, they proved to be useful in the tasks they were developed for. For instance, whilst mammography CAD systems had an inherently high false positive rate, when used to assist the radiologist in their detection of breast calcification, a significant improvement in diagnostic accuracy was noted [29]. Users became accustomed to what the system could and could not do – what to rely on it for and where to exercise caution. These systems were largely interpretable –

they were programmed by human domain experts, the users were also usually domain experts, and when the machine output was not as expected, the clinician could understand why. Whilst the user did not have ultimate trust in the system, they had appropriate trust (i.e., they were realistic in their expectations and used it where they knew it could help).

Modern AI systems used in clinical decision support exhibit far more impressive performance than these rule-based systems. These systems are trained in a different way to the previous rule-based systems in that they are presented with a large number of labelled examples. The system will then 'teach itself' the best configuration of system 'weightings' to reach an acceptable accuracy. The exact way in which this is accomplished is not always clear to the user, or indeed, the developer. This is sometimes referred to as the AI 'black box' and is explained more fully in Chapter 3. These advanced systems are more accurate; however, by nature, they are less interpretable. For instance, a recent study by Eisemann et al. [30] found that an AI model used for cancer detection on screening mammography assisted the radiologist in the detection of 17.5% more cancers than human interpretation alone. However, as mentioned, traditional rules-based systems also provided increased diagnostic accuracy and detection rates when used alongside the clinician. The Eisemann study reported that recall rates (i.e., follow-up for repeat mammograms and biopsies) fell following the use of the AI model, and furthermore, the false positive rate was actually lower in the AI group than the control group of human interpretation only – representing current practice. This is in contrast to the older systems where high false positive rates were a notable problem. Due to the decreased interpretability of these modern AI models, trust may become an issue, particularly in the high-stakes healthcare environment [31]. Forms of explainability have been proposed, such as heatmaps, regions of interest indication and textual descriptions, to allow the human user to gain some understanding of why the model made the decision it did. However, as you will read in Chapter 5 of this book, careful consideration should be made of these forms of 'explainable AI' also [32] (Figure 1.5).

Diagnostics are not the only area that AI is being used in healthcare today. Applications relating to workflow efficiencies, such as natural language processing for transcription of reports and searching of patient data and automation of billing and appointment making can make the patient

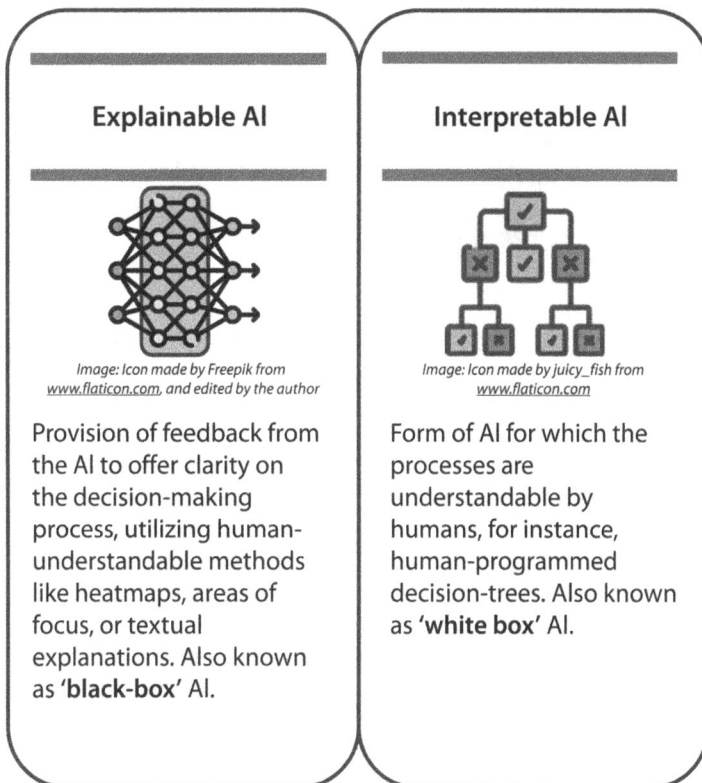

Explainable AI

Image: Icon made by Freepik from www.flaticon.com, and edited by the author

Provision of feedback from the AI to offer clarity on the decision-making process, utilizing human-understandable methods like heatmaps, areas of focus, or textual explanations. Also known as **'black-box'** AI.

Interpretable AI

Image: Icon made by juicy_fish from www.flaticon.com

Form of AI for which the processes are understandable by humans, for instance, human-programmed decision-trees. Also known as **'white box'** AI.

Figure 1.5 Distinction between explainable and interpretable AI.

journey more efficient, saving the health system money and ensuring the best care for the patient. Predictive analytics can monitor health data and identify patients at risk of disease progression, such as in sepsis monitoring. A systematic review by Bignami et al. [33] found that there was some promise for AI in clinical management and patient outcome (mortality), but notes that important issues remain, such as high false positive rates. AI-enabled genomic sequencing can be used in oncology to tailor treatments to allow maximum treatment efficacy for the patient by creation of 'digital twins'. (For an example in pancreatic cancer survival rate prediction, see Osipov et al. [34]). With the pace of development of new technologies, such as generative AI and agentic AI making inroads into healthcare, it is vitally important that all healthcare professionals and leaders remain abreast of the most recent developments and the areas of clinical practice and patient care they are likely to impact.

1.6 VALUES-BASED AI

As technology has so rapidly advanced, world leaders have had to try and keep pace with developments and ensure that the direction of development and the permitted use is in line with human-centric principles. In 2021, the United Nations Educational, Scientific and Cultural Organization (UNESCO) published the first global standards recommendations on AI, which was subsequently adopted by all member states [35]. They produced ten 'core principles' on how to ensure a 'human rights approach to AI', based around four key values (Figure 1.6). These values and principles should form the basis for any decisions made by any actor in the AI space – from inception of an innovation to development and practical use. Included in these are recommendations to ensure the safety and security of the users of AI and the need for domain experts to continue to challenge AI to ensure the systems are working within the boundaries of its intended use.

To ensure that AI systems entering the market meet reliable safety standards, regulatory approval is essential – especially in healthcare. In the European Economic Area (including the UK), this typically involves obtaining a Conformité Européenne (CE) mark under the Medical Device Directive. In the

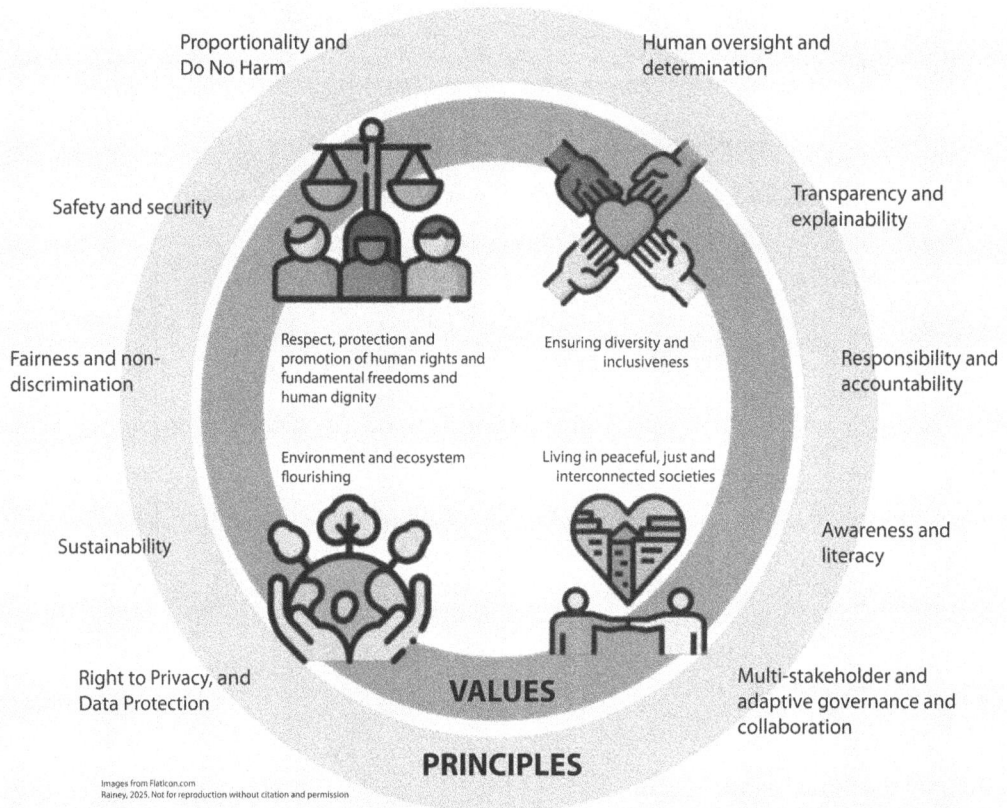

Figure 1.6 UNESCO Values and Principles of Ethical AI [35].

8

United States, approval is granted by the Food and Drug Administration (FDA). For further reading, see Fink and Akra [36], Warraich et al. [37] and EMA [38].

1.7 ENVIRONMENTAL IMPACT OF ADVANCED TECHNOLOGIES AND AI

While professional publications rightly focus on the performance and capabilities of AI, there is growing awareness of the environmental impact associated with its use. For instance, a single generative AI search is estimated to generate from 4 to 10 times more carbon than that of a simple search query [39, 40]. The accuracy of this data, however, is debated, as developers currently do not publish the environmental impact of their models. A viewpoint presented by Saenko in a 2023 *Scientific American* article highlights some of the practical considerations surrounding the efficient use of advanced AI models and their net environmental impact. She discusses the challenges with acquiring accurate data around the actual energy cost of an AI model, reminding the reader that each step in the 'development and use' cycle requires some energy expenditure – from the physical construction of the technology to the energy required for each use. That said, with greater model complexity comes greater quality of output, which in turn may reduce the number of steps required to achieve the required response from a lesser form of technology [39]. For additional reading in the context of healthcare, see, for example, Ueda et al. [41], who outline various practical ways in which the development and use of AI can be made more sustainable. This is further addressed in detail by Drs Nghiem, Dogra and Doo, who discuss the implications of AI in healthcare for the environment and outline some measures to ensure environmental sustainability in Chapter 14 of this book.

1.8 EVIDENCE-BASED USE OF CLINICAL AI AND EDUCATION

Responsible use of technology will become more important as technologies continue to evolve. Between 2022 and 2023, there was a 133.7% increase in the number of AI publications in health, in various fields from ophthalmology to cardiology and gastroenterology [42]. This indicates the pace of development of AI in medicine. The volume of information indicates a period of rapid change in the field. Clinicians are busy and, whilst AI offers the 'gift of time', they still must be able to knowledgeably critique any development to be able to engage with it responsibly for the benefit of the patient. However, numerous surveys investigating the perception of the readiness of the healthcare professions for a future with AI find that, whilst clinicians are excited about the future with AI, further education and training should be provided to keep pace with technology developments (in radiography: Rainey et al. [43]; in radiology: Huisman et al. [44]; in medicine: Rampton et al. [45]). In Chapter 6 of this book, Dr J Perchik presents a blueprint for a very successful education programme in AI for radiology residents at the University of Alabama, a proforma which could be further rolled out into other fields of healthcare education. As mentioned, it can be challenging for clinicians to keep up with the rapid developments in the field, particularly when faced with other demands on their time, as previously discussed. However, gaining a basic understanding of the underlying theory can help reduce feelings of intimidation and encourage ongoing professional development and learning.

This book may help with this by presenting an overview of the use of advanced technologies and AI in various areas of medicine, from histopathology to radiology, and present real-life case studies on how AI is impacting the patient journey. It is hoped that the reader will use the book for an introduction to the field of healthcare AI and develop a thirst for further learning. The case studies presented are intended to spark reflection on how AI and advanced technologies could enhance individual areas of clinical practice, while also helping to ease some of the fear and hesitation often associated with adopting these innovations. Whilst the mainstream media will continue to express opinion, it is hoped that with reliable education and critical awareness, the clinician will be able to filter this information and be able to utilise technologies with confidence. It is hoped that the non-clinical readership will appreciate the unique challenges and requirements of healthcare AI and gain an understanding of the technological applications which will be useful and desired by both those working in healthcare and the members of the public. Case Study D, by Drs Busch, Adams and Bressem, presents the findings of a large international patient survey which shines light on the unique perceptions of those for whom, ultimately, healthcare AI impacts most greatly. Further to this, Chapter 2 provides valuable direction on how to ensure that person-centred care can be maintained in the era of AI.

1.9 CONCLUSION AND FINAL COMMENTS

It is hoped that this primer will generate self-reflection and a desire for enquiry. The background and examples presented here are good for a moment in time, but it is predicted that the rapidity of development in this field will continue, and all healthcare professionals have a responsibility to have a critical awareness of all technologies they are using in the same way that they would with a new treatment or drug being introduced into clinical practice. The inception of any ideas on new developments should include every actor in the AI space – beginning and ending with patients.

While healthcare AI development may be a lengthier process than in other disciplines, it is essential that all steps are followed to ensure acceptance and usefulness of any clinical AI tool produced and to ensure that we are upholding our obligations to the patient and service user. However, it should be recognised that only through education and awareness can we engage in useful discussion – clinicians should be aware of the potential of advanced technologies but also what cannot be achieved and indeed the pitfalls of their use through an awareness of areas of fragility. It is our hope that the reader will engage with this book, not only in areas applicable to their practice, but also gain an understanding of the wider landscape, to allow this to generate thought, reflection and interdisciplinary discussion, collaboration and sharing of good practice to allow for meaningful advancement in the field. As we have reflected on the mathematical and engineering achievements of the Ancient Greeks – exemplified by the Antikythera Mechanism – and considered the 'summers' and 'winters' of technological progress and stagnation that followed, it prompts us to wonder: where might technology take us in the years ahead? Fundamentally, we should know for certain that, done well, technology advancement which is directed and managed by human oversight shows great promise, and we owe it to our future to get it right today to allow a firm foundation for the future.

REFERENCES

1. The Diary of Samuel Pepys, Jun/Jul 1660 Translator: Mynors Bright, Editor: Wheatley. Available at: http://public-library.uk/ebooks/89/33.pdf [accessed 01 March 2025]
2. Reviriego, P., Merino-Gomez, E., Lombardi, F. (2022) Latin and Greek in Computing: Ancient Words in a New World. Computer. Available at: https://ieeexplore-ieee-org.ucc.idm.oclc.org/stamp/stamp.jsp?tp=&arnumber=9789305&tag=1&tag=1 [accessed 01 March 2025]
3. Freeth, T., Higgon, D., Dacanalis, A. et al. (2021) A Model of the Cosmos in the Ancient Greek Antikythera Mechanism. Sci Rep. 11:5821. https://doi.org/10.1038/s41598-021-84310-w
4. Copeland, B.J. (2020) The Modern History of Computing. (Winter 2020 Edition), Edward N. Zalta (ed.). The Stanford Encyclopedia of Philosophy. Available at: https://plato.stanford.edu/archives/win2020/entries/computing-history/ [accessed 01 March 2025]
5. Thomson, J. (1876) An Integrating Machine having a new Kinematic Principle. Proc R Soc. 24:164–170 https://doi.org/10.1098/rspl.1875.0033. Reprinted in Thomson J. (1912). Joseph Larmor & James Thomson (ed.). Collected Papers in Physics and Engineering by James Thomson. Cambridge University Press. pp. xvii, 452–7. ISBN 0-404-06422-1.
6. Marsh, A. (2024) Lord Kelvin and His Analog Computer. Available at https://spectrum.ieee.org/tide-predictions [accessed 02 June 2025]
7. 'The Shipyard'. (2022) Tide Predictors: The Surprising Analog Computers that Helped win WW2. Available at: https://www.theshipyardblog.com/tide-predictors-the-analog-computers-that-helped-win-wwii/. [accessed 02 June 2025]
8. Lundberg, K.H. (2005) Vannevar Bush's Differential Analyzer. Available at: https://www.mit.edu/~klund/analyzer/ [accessed 28 May 2025]
9. Shelmerdine, S.C., Martin, H., Shirodkar, K. et al (2022) Can Artificial Intelligence Pass the Fellowship of the Royal College of Radiologists Examination? Multi-Reader Diagnostic Accuracy Study. BMJ. 379:e072826. https://doi.org/10.1136/bmj-2022-072826
10. Cameron, G., Cameron, D., Megaw, G. et al. (2018) Best Practices for Designing Chatbots in Mental Healthcare – A Case Study on iHelpr. In R. Bond, M. Mulvenna, J. Wallace, & M. Black (Eds.), Proceedings of the 32nd International BCS Human Computer Interaction Conference (HCI-2018). BCS Learning & Development Ltd. https://doi.org/10.14236/ewic/HCI2018.129
11. Gaube, S., Suresh, H., Raue, M. et al. (2021) Do as AI Say: Susceptibility in Deployment of Clinical Decision-Aids. NPJ Digit Med. 4(1):31. https://doi.org/10.1038/s41746-021-00385-9
12. Mucci, T. (2024) What Is the Technological Singularity? Available at: https://www.ibm.com/think/topics/technological-singularity [accessed 02 June 2025]
13. Khatiwada, P., Yang, B., Lin, J.C. et al. (2024) Patient-Generated Health Data (PGHD): Understanding, Requirements, Challenges, and Existing Techniques for Data Security and Privacy. J Pers Med. 14(3):282. https://doi.org/10.3390/jpm14030282
14. Duarte, F. (2025) Amount of Data Created Daily. Available at https://explodingtopics.com/blog/data-generated-per-day [accessed 02 June 2025]
15. Moore, J. (2024) How to Harness the Power of Health Data to Improve Patient Outcomes. Available at: https://www.weforum.org/stories/2024/01/how-to-harness-health-data-to-improve-patient-outcomes-wef24/ [accessed 08 June 2025]
16. BusinessTech Weekly. (2025) What Is a Petabyte? Definition, Uses and Its Role in Data Storage. Available at https://www.businesstechweekly.com/operational-efficiency/cloud-computing/what-is-a-petabyte/ [accessed 08 June 2025]
17. Hughes, L., Rodgers, L., Joiner, S. et al. (2025) Patient Data Could Power the NHS. Much of It Is Still Stuck on Paper. The Financial Times. Available at: https://www.ft.com/content/63a99def-87ae-4c66-bf21-b80029677612?accessToken=zwAGNgUcxaQ4kc9jqZ3vh65MZtO_IbgAKWd2Eg.MEYCIQCPUWcgNRpkop00pTLx0xGLQo_kJpaMwNr5raoPFntEiAIhALvk92TXIFkRT_Tvc6wXgcG5OUcDxeyy-DMyGOwLvhsm&sharetype=gift&token=1a043ed2-ee78-4722-ba67-db0166f63a37 [accessed 20 May 2025]

18. Capital Markets. The Healthcare Data Explosion. N.D. Available at: https://www.rbccm.com/en/gib/healthcare/episode/the_healthcare_data_explosion#content-panel. [accessed 02 June 2025]
19. Toscano, F., O'Donnell, E., Broderick, J.E. et al. (2020) How Physicians Spend Their Work Time: An Ecological Momentary Assessment. J Gen Intern Med. 35:3166–3172. https://doi.org/10.1007/s11606-020-06087-4
20. White, B. (2025) How much schedules 'admin time' vs. patient-facing time do primary care physicians need? FPM Journal Blog. Available at: https://www.aafp.org/pubs/fpm/blogs/inpractice/entry/scheduling-admin-time.html#r3 [accessed 02 June 2025]
21. Goodchild, L., Mulligan, A., Shearing Greem, E. et al. (2022) Elsevier Clinician of the Future Report 2022. Available at: https://www.elsevier.com/connect/clinician-of-the-future [accessed 02 June 2025]
22. The Royal College of Radiologists. (2024) Clinical Radiology Workforce Census. Available at: https://www.rcr.ac.uk/news-policy/policy-reports-initiatives/clinical-radiology-census-reports/ [accessed 02 June 2025]
23. The British Medical Association. (2025) Medical staffing in the NHS. Available at: https://www.bma.org.uk/advice-and-support/nhs-delivery-and-workforce/workforce/medical-staffing-in-the-nhs [accessed 02 June 2025]
24. Gill, A., Rainey, C., McLaughlin, L. et al. (2025) Artificial Intelligence User Interface Preferences in Radiology: A Scoping Review. J Med Imaging Radiat Sci. 56(3):1–9. https://doi.org/10.1016/j.jmir.2025.101866
25. Weiss, S.M., Kulikowski, C.A., Amarel, S. et al. (1978) A Model-Based Method for Computer-Aided Medical Decision-Making. Artificial Intelligence. 11(1–2):145–172. https://doi.org/10.1016/0004-3702(78)90015-2
26. Shortliffe, E.H. (1976) Computer-Based Medical Consultations: MYCIN. American Elsevier Publishing Co., Inc.
27. The Massachusetts General Hospital Laboratory of Computer Science. (2017) DXplain. Available at: https://www.mghlcs.org/projects/dxplain [accessed 02 June 2025]
28. Chan, H.P., Doi, K., Galhotra, S. et al. (1987) Image Feature Analysis and Computer-Aided Diagnosis in Digital Radiography. I. Automated Detection of Microcalcifications in Mammography. Med Phys. 14(4):538–548. https://doi.org/10.1118/1.596065
29. Chan, H.P., Doi, K., Vyborny, C.J. et al. (1990) Improvement in radiologists' Detection of Clustered Microcalcifications on Mammograms: The Potential of Computer-Aided Diagnosis. Invest Radiol. 25: 1102–1110.
30. Eisemann, N., Bunk, S., Mukama, T. et al. (2025) Nationwide Real-World Implementation of AI for Cancer Detection in Population-Based Mammography Screening. Nature Medicine. 7:1–8. https://doi.org/10.1038/s41591-024-03408-6
31. Rainey, C., Bond, R., McConnell, J. et al. (2024) Reporting radiographers' Interaction with Artificial Intelligence—How Do Different Forms of AI Feedback Impact Trust and Decision Switching? PLOS Digital Health. 3(8). https://doi.org/10.1371/journal.pdig.0000560
32. Rainey, C., Bond, R., McConnell, J. et al (2025) The Impact of AI Feedback on the Accuracy of Diagnosis, Decision Switching and Trust in Radiography. PLoS One. 20(5):e0322051. https://doi.org/10.1371/journal.pone.0322051
33. Bignami, E.G., Berdini, M., Panizzi, M. et al. (2025) Artificial Intelligence in Sepsis Management: An Overview for Clinicians. J Clin Med. 14(1):286. https://doi.org/10.3390/jcm14010286
34. Osipov, A., Nikolic, O., Gertych, A. et al. (2024) The Molecular Twin Artificial-Intelligence Platform Integrates Multi-Omic Data to Predict Outcomes for Pancreatic Adenocarcinoma Patients. Nat Cancer. 5(2):299–314. https://doi.org/10.1038/s43018-023-00697-7
35. UNESCO (2023) Recommendation on the Ethics of Artificial Intelligence. Available at: https://www.unesco.org/en/articles/recommendation-ethics-artificial-intelligence [accessed 06 May 2025]
36. Fink, M., Akra, B. (2023) Comparison of the International Regulations for Medical Devices–USA Versus Europe, Injury. 54(5). https://doi.org/10.1016/j.injury.2023.110908.
37. Warraich, H.J., Tazbaz, T., Califf, R.M. (2025) FDA Perspective on the Regulation of Artificial Intelligence in Health Care and Biomedicine. JAMA. 333(3):241–247. https://doi.org/10.1001/jama.2024.21451
38. European Medicines Agency (EMA). (2025) Medical Devices. Available at: https://www.ema.europa.eu/en/human-regulatory-overview/medical-devices [accessed 17 June 2025]
39. Saenko, K. (2023) A Computer Scientist Breaks Down Generative AI's Hefty Carbon Footprint. Available at: https://www.scientificamerican.com/article/a-computer-scientist-breaks-down-generative-ais-hefty-carbon-footprint/ [accessed 17 June 2025]
40. Nazir, A. (2024) Energy Hungry AI: What's the Hidden Cost of Your GenAI Search? Available at: https://www.ndtv.com/ai/ai-climate-ai-energy-ai-emissions-energy-hungry-ai-whats-the-hidden-cost-of-your-genai-search-6041452 [accessed 17 June 2025]
41. Ueda, D., Walston, S.L., Fujita, S. et al. (2024) Climate Change and Artificial Intelligence in Healthcare: Review and Recommendations Towards a Sustainable Future. Diagn Interv Imaging. 105(11):453–459. https://doi.org/10.1016/j.diii.2024.06.002
42. Fairhurst, V., Marcum, C.S., Haun, C. et al. (2024) Artificial Intelligence in Healthcare: 2023 Year in Review. JMIRx Med. 5:e65151. https://doi.org/10.2196/65151
43. Rainey, C., O'Regan, T., Matthew, J. et al. (2021) Beauty Is in the AI of the Beholder: Are We Ready for the Clinical Integration of Artificial Intelligence in Radiography? An Exploratory Analysis of Perceived AI Knowledge, Skills, Confidence, and Education Perspectives of UK Radiographers. Frontiers in Digital Health. 3:739327. https://doi.org/10.3389/fdgth.2021.739327
44. Huisman, M., Ranschaert, E., Parker, W. et al. (2021) An International Survey on AI in Radiology in 1,041 Radiologists and Radiology Residents Part 1: Fear of Replacement, Knowledge, and Attitude. Eur Radiol. 31:7058–7066. https://doi.org/10.1007/s00330-021-07781-5
45. Rampton, V., Mittelman, M., Goldhahn, J. (2020) Implications of Artificial Intelligence for Medical Education. Lancet Digit Health. 2(3):e111–e112. https://doi.org/10.1016/S2589-7500(20)30023-6

2 Person/Patient-Centred Practice with AI

The Patient, the Practitioner and the Use of Technology to Enable Better Patient Care

Sonyia McFadden and Jonathan McConnell

2.1 INTRODUCTION

Person-centred practice (PCP) and person-centred care (PCC) recognise that each person is an expert in their own life and promotes collaboration between healthcare professionals and patients for tailoring service delivery to meet the individual's specific needs. Much has been written about PCP and PCC in the discipline of nursing and in more recent years in the field of radiography [1–7]. AI is now having a significant impact on how we care for our patients, and further research is required on how AI impacts the delivery of PCP.

This chapter has two objectives:

1. To develop an understanding of PCP when using AI in healthcare, specifically using radiographic practice as an illustration.

2. To explore the significance of PCP in healthcare settings and discuss the integration of AI whilst focusing on an individual's needs and preferences.

The fundamental principles of PCP illustrated in Figure 2.1 and described over include the following:

Respect: PCP accentuates respect as a core principle that involves recognising the inherent worth and dignity of every individual. Healthcare professionals treat patients with empathy, courtesy and compassion, acknowledging their autonomy and choices for a patient's decision-making in their own care.

Dignity: PCP emphasises the importance of preserving the individual's self-worth and maintaining their privacy, confidentiality, and integrity. Healthcare providers create an environment to uphold a patient's dignity for treatment with sensitivity and discretion, without discrimination or judgement.

Involvement in decision-making: PCP promotes shared decision-making between healthcare professionals and patients, whereby patients have the right to be actively involved in decisions

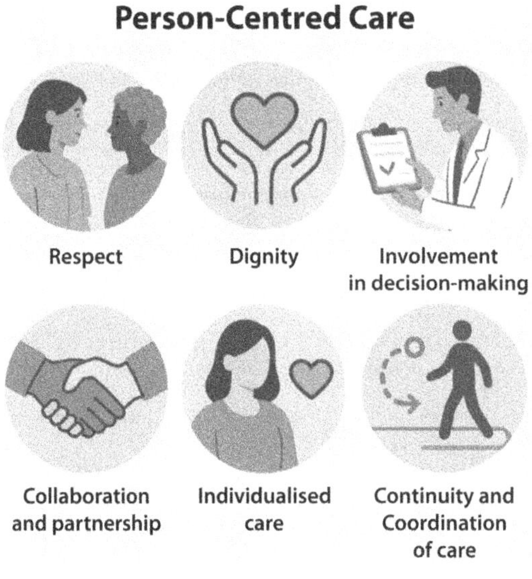

Person-Centred Care

Respect Dignity Involvement in decision-making

Collaboration and partnership Individualised care Continuity and Coordination of care

Figure 2.1 Fundamental principles of PCP.

DOI: 10.1201/9781032709956-2

about their care, treatment options and goals. Through information giving, support and guidance patients make informed choices consistent with their values and preferences.

Collaboration and partnership: PCP emphasises collaboration and partnership between healthcare professionals, patients and their families or support networks. Through open and honest communication, active listening and mutual respect, healthcare professionals and patients can achieve personal health needs, set realistic goals and create values and priorities-based care plans.

Individualised care: PCP recognises that each person has their own set of needs, preferences and circumstances. Healthcare professionals strive to provide individualised care that accounts for individual physical, emotional, social and cultural contexts via tailored care plans.

Continuity and coordination of care: PCP extends beyond individual encounters to encompass the continuity and coordination of care for seamless transitions between different healthcare settings. It involves patients in care transitions and ensures information sharing between healthcare providers to enhance well-being and avoid fragmented care.

Healthcare staff need to ensure that AI tools assist rather than replace these fundamental principles.

2.2 PERSON-CENTRED PRACTICE FRAMEWORK

This chapter is underpinned by the person-centred practice framework (PCPF; McCance & McCormack), which was originally established in the field of nursing but can be applied across the full healthcare spectrum [8]. The framework itself consists of four main domains listed below and illustrated in Figure 2.2:

i. The prerequisites (e.g. staff attributes like being professionally competent, good interpersonal skills, committed to the role, clear beliefs and values and knowing self)

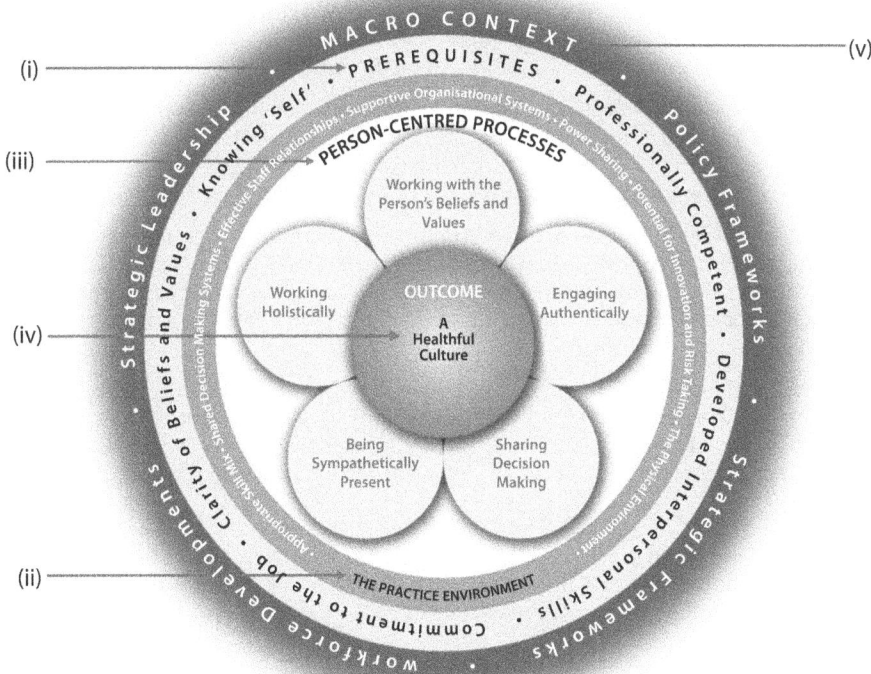

Figure 2.2 The Person-centred practice framework (McCance & McCormack) [8].

ii. The practice environment (e.g. healthcare context including the people, processes and structures – this includes the physical environment, an appropriate skill mix, shared decision-making and power, good staff relationships, supportive organisational systems and potential for innovation)
iii. The person-centred processes (e.g. ways of engagement amongst all persons working with individual beliefs and values, engaging authentically, being sympathetically present and working holistically to enable shared decision-making across patients and teams)
iv. The outcome (a healthful culture where innovative practice is supported, decisions are shared, there is collaboration in relationships and leadership is transformational), ensuring the best experience for both those involved in giving care and those who receive care

These four domains are all interrelated and sit within the broader macro context (v), which is controlled by political and strategic factors that influence practice and culture.

2.3 THE ROLE OF RADIOGRAPHERS DELIVERING PCP WHEN USING AI IN HEALTHCARE

2.3.1 Prerequisites for Delivering PCP

Radiographers play a crucial role in healthcare as specialised healthcare professionals who perform and interpret medical imaging procedures. They are trained to develop all the essential prerequisites (i) to perform their roles, working closely with other members of the healthcare team to provide accurate and timely diagnostic information to aid patient care and treatment decisions. However, authors have recently reported that some staff feel ill-prepared for the implementation of AI and not only lack the appropriate skill mix but also the confidence to communicate AI decisions to relevant stakeholders [9, 10]. Further work suggests there is a lack of education and training on AI in educational curricula [11–15], whilst other authors identify a fear of staff deskilling and loss of professional identity [16–20]. As AI continues to evolve, ongoing education is essential to ensure staff remain *professionally competent*. Via direct interactions with patients, radiographers are often the first point of contact during the imaging process. Hence, a PCP approach enhances the patient experience to improve outcomes. Radiographers practising PCP are

- responsible for performing imaging examinations on patients as prescribed by examination referrers. They ensure that the imaging equipment is applied correctly and use ionising radiation safely to obtain high-quality images. Radiographers may also administer contrast agents for certain imaging procedures to enhance the visibility of specific structures.

- skilled in operating various types of imaging equipment, such as X-ray machines, CT scanners, MRI scanners, and ultrasound machines. Their technical operational understanding enables effective use of equipment to obtain accurate images while ensuring the safety of staff, patients and themselves during imaging procedures.

- responsible for providing direct care and support to patients undergoing imaging procedures by explaining the imaging processes, addressing any concerns or anxieties whilst ensuring their comfort and safety. Radiographers maintain a PCP approach by considering the unique needs and preferences of each patient, respecting their dignity and involving them in the decision-making process during imaging procedures.

- able to analyse and interpret images to play a role in image analysis and initial assessment. They review the images they have obtained to ensure technical quality, identify any abnormalities or artefacts and communicate relevant findings to radiologists or other physicians. This collaborative approach ensures accurate and timely reporting/action on imaging results.

2.3.2 The Practice Environment

Having well-trained staff with the appropriate skill mix enables effective power sharing across service delivery. Organisational leaders and managers must fully consider the implications AI will have on their service delivery and implement supportive systems within the physical environment to ensure it is accepted into practice.

Implications for the radiology department may include the following:

Improved accuracy and efficiency: AI algorithms can analyse large volumes of medical data quickly and accurately, potentially reducing human error, improving diagnostic accuracy and providing quantitative measurements that lead to more precise and reliable diagnoses. This can lead to reduced waiting times for patients, faster diagnoses and improved workflow across departments. AI algorithms can also detect subtle abnormalities and patterns in medical data that may be difficult for humans to otherwise identify.

Enhanced workflow and productivity: AI tools can automate routine and time-consuming tasks. By eliminating these tasks, healthcare staff can focus more on critical decision-making and complex cases.

Faster turnaround time: AI algorithms can analyse medical data in real time. This enables waiting-time reduction for patients, prompt diagnosis and treatment planning, and consequently improves patient care and outcomes, particularly in emergency situations.

Decision support and second opinions: AI systems can serve as valuable decision support tools through provision of additional information and insights to aid *shared clinical decision-making*. Second opinions and multidisciplinary collaboration is rapidly facilitated, leading to improved patient management.

Overall enhanced efficiency and increased productivity: AI has the potential to streamline health service workflows (Figure 2.3) by automating various tasks and processes, leading to reduced waiting times, improved resource allocation and enhanced patient experiences.

AI powered triage: AI-powered triage systems can automatically analyse and prioritise test results based on the urgency and clinical relevance of the cases. By quickly identifying critical or high-priority cases, healthcare staff can allocate their attention and resources efficiently to reduce waiting times for patients requiring urgent care, ensuring timely diagnosis and treatment. Workflows can be optimised by automating administrative tasks (e.g. data entry, appointment scheduling and report generation to reduce time spent on these repetitive tasks). Historical data, patient records, and resource utilisation patterns can be used to make predictions and forecasts for enhanced departmental resources, such as equipment and staff, and appointment scheduling. By using predictive analytics, service bottlenecks are reduced, AI algorithms can optimise appointment scheduling using criteria like patient preferences, staff availability and equipment capacity.

Despite the myriad advantages that AI offers, it also presents challenges in healthcare delivery from a PCP position. These include the following:

Data quality and bias: AI algorithms require large amounts of high-quality data for training and validation. The availability of diverse and accurately labelled datasets can be challenging because, if the training data are biased or not representative of the population, biased AI models will impact the accuracy and fairness of the results to influence patient-care decisions. (See also Chapters 3 and 5.)

Integration into clinical workflows: Integrating AI systems into the existing clinical workflows can be complex. Ensuring seamless integration and interoperability with existing infrastructure is crucial to maximise the benefits of AI.

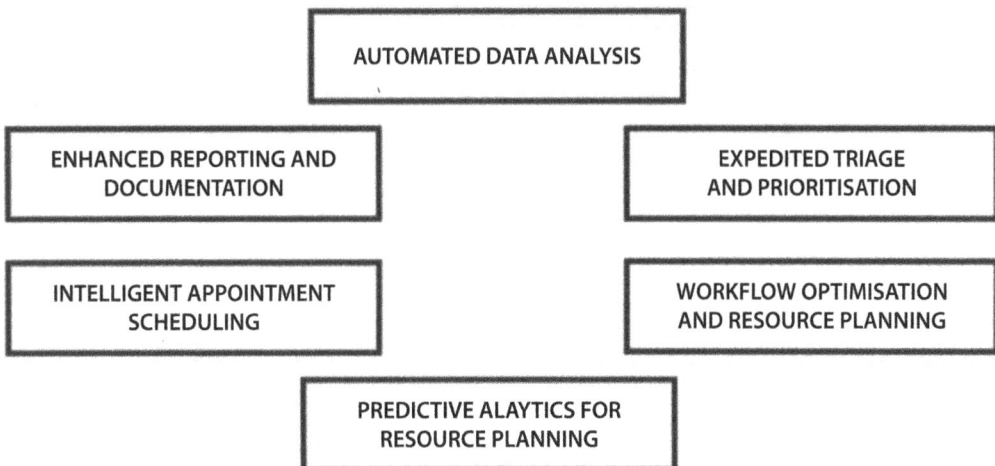

AUTOMATED DATA ANALYSIS

ENHANCED REPORTING AND DOCUMENTATION

EXPEDITED TRIAGE AND PRIORITISATION

INTELLIGENT APPOINTMENT SCHEDULING

WORKFLOW OPTIMISATION AND RESOURCE PLANNING

PREDICTIVE ALAYTICS FOR RESOURCE PLANNING

Figure 2.3 Workflow enhancements made available with AI.

Legal and ethical considerations: The use of AI in healthcare raises legal and ethical considerations regarding patient privacy, data security and liability. Regulations and policies need to be established to address these concerns and ensure the responsible and ethical use of AI technologies.

Continuous learning and validation: AI models need continuous training and validation to stay current with advancements in healthcare (often driven by AI benefits) and to ensure their ongoing accuracy and performance. This requires dedicated efforts and resources for maintenance, monitoring and retraining of AI systems.

Radiography staff need to learn to work seamlessly with their 'AI colleagues' and organisational support must be made available to facilitate effective relationships that enable shared decision-making. One solution recommended by Stogiannos et al. [16] would include the innovative practice of role development for radiographers to train AI champions within departments to lead on AI integration, training, cascading of information and overall management. Transparency in AI is essential to get acceptance from all stakeholders. Patients and staff need to know when and where AI is being used in their practice, with an understanding of the advantages, risks and limitations.

2.3.3 Person-Centred Processes

The use of AI tools may alter the patient interaction and staff/team dynamics in the department. Rather than having more time with the patient, clinicians might find the converse is true and their contact time is reduced if this freed time merely enables them to focus on other tasks (e.g. if AI has reported the scan, triaged the patient already or referred them on to the next part of the treatment pathway, they may not have the same contact with the clinician that they would normally have). Radiographers as a first line of contact can compensate for this change in patient pathway and improve the patient experience through the following:

Communication and empathy: Through a sympathetic and empathetic approach radiographers address patient concerns, providing clear instructions and maintain open lines of dialogue. Through *authentic engagement* and active listening patients feel respected, heard and involved in their own care.

Informed consent: Obtaining informed consent from patients before any imaging procedure is a vital role of radiographers through providing information about the examination, its benefits, risks and alternatives, allowing patients to make *informed decisions* based on their individual circumstances. Radiographers ensure that patients understand the procedure and can ask questions or express any concerns.

Privacy and dignity: Radiographers respect patients' privacy and dignity during imaging procedures to create a comfortable, respectful and confidential experience. Through sensitivity towards patient cultural *beliefs and values*, religious or personal preferences, a positive experience is achieved by adjusting their professional approach accordingly.

Individualised care: Each patient has unique needs, such as age, mobility and physical or cognitive abilities to tailor the imaging procedure accordingly. Radiographers strive to provide a personalised experience that is responsive to the patient requirements and preferences.

Working holistically: All healthcare workers and patients/families/carers/communities experience healthcare together, whether they are giving it or receiving it. Radiographers can use the PCPF as a philosophy that places *people* at the centre of the healthcare system. AI tools enable this holistic approach more than ever as staff and patients can work across teams, departments, disciplines and hospitals to deliver the best outcome for all.

2.3.4 A 'Healthful' Culture

Several authors have identified the concerns of both clinicians and patients on the use of AI in clinical practice [21–26]. A lack of trust, transparency and ethical and legal responsibility have all been identified as potential concerns [27–32] Considering the benefits of AI in practice, this reticence needs to be overcome by further education for all. Alongside delivering the best care and outcome for the patient, staff should be supported to work in their respective roles and maximise their potential.

AI can contribute to the desired outcome of a healthful culture where collaborative relationships enable shared decision-making amongst staff and patients. This will be made possible through the responsible use of AI where both staff and patients are informed on the potential advantages of AI

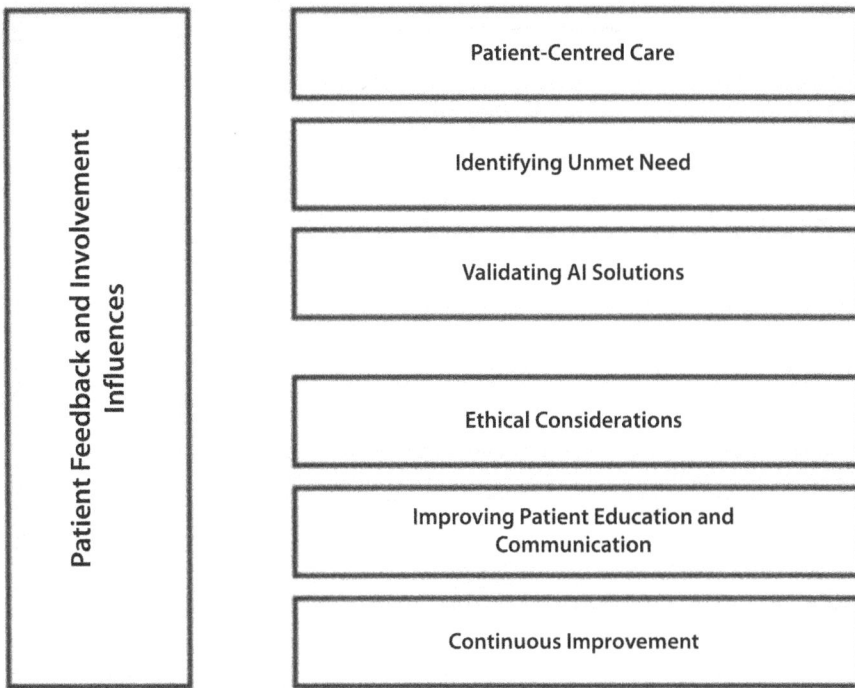

Figure 2.4 Using patient feedback to enhance AI implementation.

use whilst any pitfalls are explainable and transparent. Seeking patient feedback and involving them in decision-making processes are crucial aspects of PCP and AI implementation. Patient perspectives can enhance AI implementation as indicated in Figure 2.4.

Patient feedback and involvement empower healthcare professionals to provide PCP by actively seeking and considering patient perspectives. This way staff can understand patients' unique needs, preferences and concerns to tailor their approach, communication and treatment plans accordingly.

2.3.5 The Macro Context

Many policies and strategies have been developed globally which recommend PCP/PCC, integrated health services and the advantages of using AI [33–36]. The European AI Act, which came into force on August 1, 2024, introduced requirements for manufacturers and developers of AI medical devices [37, 38]. Article 4 of the Act states that from February 2025, healthcare providers in the EU must ensure that AI literacy is developed across all staff with role specific training in place. By August 2027, deployers of medical high-risk AI tools need to adhere to Article 26, which identifies that human oversight needs to be maintained with regular auditing and reporting of any incidents, whilst Article 50 stipulates the need for transparency for all users [37].

2.4 ETHICAL CONSIDERATIONS OF AI FROM A PCP PERSPECTIVE

When using AI in healthcare, several ethical considerations should be considered to ensure responsible and ethical implementation from a PCP position. Key ethical considerations are seen in Figure 2.5 and discussed below:

Data privacy and security: Protecting patient data privacy and ensuring data security are paramount when using AI in healthcare. Strict protocols and measures must be in place to safeguard patient information, including secure data storage, data encryption, access controls and compliance with applicable privacy regulations.

Transparency: It is essential to be transparent about the use of AI in healthcare. Patients should be informed about how AI algorithms are being used to assist in their diagnosis or treatment planning. Staff should provide clear explanations of the capabilities and limitations of AI systems, allowing patients to make informed decisions and understand the role of AI in their care.

```
┌─────────────────────────────────────────────────────────┐
│              DATA PRIVACY AND SECURITY                    │
└─────────────────────────────────────────────────────────┘

┌───────────────────────────┐   ┌───────────────────────────┐
│       TRANSPARENCY        │   │     BIAS AND FAIRNESS     │
└───────────────────────────┘   └───────────────────────────┘

┌───────────────────────────┐   ┌───────────────────────────┐
│      ACCOUNTABILITY       │   │ CONTINUAL MONITORING AND  │
│                           │   │        EVALUATION         │
└───────────────────────────┘   └───────────────────────────┘

┌───────────────────────────┐   ┌───────────────────────────┐
│     PATIENT CONSENT       │   │   ETHICAL GOVERNANCE &    │
│                           │   │   REGULATORY COMPLIANCE   │
└───────────────────────────┘   └───────────────────────────┘
```

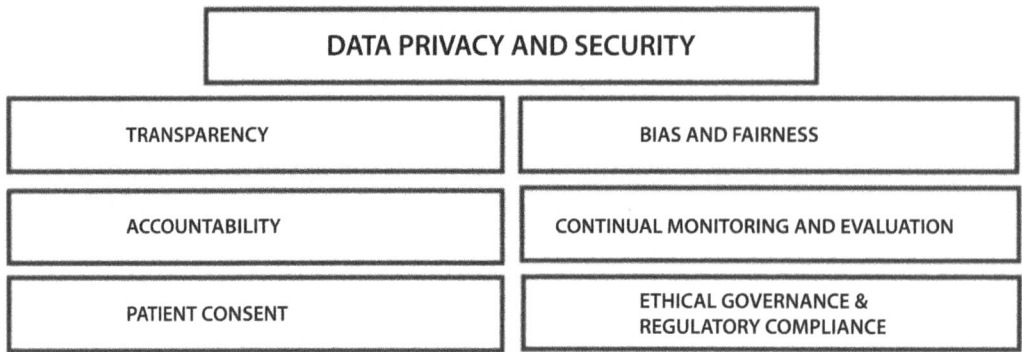

Figure 2.5 Key ethical AI considerations and their impact on PCP.

Accountability: Accountability is crucial when utilising AI in healthcare as clear lines of responsibility should be established to ensure that the decisions made by AI systems are traceable and accountable. Healthcare organisations and their staff must take responsibility for the outcomes of AI-assisted assessments and treatment decisions.

Patient Consent: Patients should be informed about how AI is utilised, including how their data will be used and the potential impact on their diagnosis or treatment. Informed consent ensures that patients have the autonomy to make decisions regarding their healthcare and data privacy.

Bias and fairness: AI algorithms in healthcare should be developed and validated with attention to potential biases. Biases can arise from biased training data or algorithmic design, leading to inaccurate or unfair results. Efforts should be made to ensure the fairness and equity of AI systems, mitigating biases and addressing any disparities in healthcare outcomes.

Continual monitoring and evaluation: Ongoing monitoring and evaluation of AI systems is crucial to identify any ethical issues, biases or unintended consequences that may arise. Regular assessments should be conducted to ensure that AI algorithms are performing as intended with adjustments or improvements made based on the outcomes of these evaluations.

Ethical governance and regulatory compliance: Establishing ethical governance frameworks and adhering to relevant regulations and guidelines are essential requirements of the use of AI in healthcare practices. Policies and procedures that address the ethical considerations of using AI should be developed for compliance with local, national and international regulations regarding data privacy, patient consent and ethical use of AI.

2.5 BENEFITS AND CHALLENGES OF INTEGRATING AI IN RADIOGRAPHY

AI applications in PCP-based healthcare offer several advantages that can enhance efficiency, accuracy and patient outcomes. Sample key benefits include the following:

Early detection and diagnosis: AI can assist in the early detection and diagnosis of diseases and conditions. By analysing medical data and comparing to a vast database of prior cases, AI systems can identify potential abnormalities that might be missed by human observers. Early detection allows for timely interventions and treatment, which can significantly improve patient outcomes.

Quantitative analysis and measurement: AI algorithms can provide automated and precise measurements of anatomical structures or abnormalities in medical data such as images, or results such as electrocardiograph traces. This quantitative analysis can assist in tracking disease progression, evaluating treatment response and facilitating more accurate treatment planning.

Personalised medicine: Through AI analysis of a patient's medical images, clinical data and genetic information, treatment plans and interventions can be tailored to the individual's specific needs. A personalised approach improves the precision and effectiveness of treatments to minimise unnecessary procedures and optimise patient outcomes.

Healthcare from a PCP perspective also faces several challenges and concerns related to patient privacy, data security, and potential biases, which are discussed in greater depth elsewhere in the book. Key challenges include the following:

Data quality and quantity: AI algorithms require large amounts of high-quality, labelled data to train and validate subsequent models effectively. However, obtaining diverse and accurately labelled datasets can be challenging as obtaining representative and comprehensive data is crucial to avoid biased or inaccurate AI models.

Bias and fairness: AI algorithms are susceptible to biases that may be present in the training data. If the training data is biased or not representative of the population, the AI models can produce inaccurate or unfair results, leading to disparities in healthcare. Efforts should be made to mitigate biases and ensure fairness, diversity, and inclusivity in the development and validation of AI models.

Patient privacy and data security: AI implementation in healthcare involves the use of sensitive patient data. Protecting patient privacy and ensuring data security are paramount and require robust measures to safeguard patient data. This includes secure storage, data encryption, access controls and adherence to privacy regulations. (See Chapter 3.)

Ethical considerations: The ethical implications of AI in radiography must be carefully addressed. This includes obtaining informed consent from patients for the use of their data in AI research, ensuring transparency in how AI algorithms are developed and used, and maintaining patient autonomy and confidentiality throughout the process.

Informed consent and communication: Patient-centred care necessitates clear and effective communication amongst healthcare professionals, AI systems and patients. Practitioners should explain the use of AI in their processes to patients, addressing any concerns or questions they may have. Obtaining informed consent is crucial, as patients should be aware of how their data are used and the potential impact of AI on their care.

Integration and workflow challenges: Integrating AI systems into the existing radiography workflow and clinical infrastructure can be complex. Seamless integration with picture archiving and communication systems (PACS), for example, and electronic health records (EHR) is crucial for effective implementation. Ensuring compatibility, interoperability and user-friendly interfaces is essential to maximise the benefits of AI in radiography. (See Chapter 5.)

Continuous learning and validation: AI models require ongoing maintenance, monitoring and retraining to stay current and maintain accuracy. Establishing mechanisms for continuous learning and validation of AI algorithms is necessary to ensure their reliability and effectiveness over time. Regular assessments of AI algorithms and their impact on patient outcomes, patient satisfaction and healthcare provider experience help identify potential biases, limitations or areas for improvement.

Balancing technology with patient-centred practice: While AI brings undeniable benefits, it is crucial to balance technology-driven approaches with patient-centred care. This means ensuring that the use of AI does not compromise the core principles of PCP, such as respect, dignity and involvement in decision-making. It requires integrating AI tools in a way that supports and enhances the patient's experience rather than replacing the human element of care.

Personalisation and individualised care: Despite the advantages of AI, each patient is unique and may have specific needs that cannot be fully addressed by technology alone. Healthcare staff must continue to consider individual preferences, cultural backgrounds and physical or emotional states when providing care. It is the personalised interaction and adaptation of AI in the patient care context that maintain PCP.

2.6 THE CURRENT IMPACT OF AI ON PCP

While AI can bring significant advancements and efficiencies to practices, it is essential to maintain a balance between technology-driven approaches and PCP. In the UK we now live in an era when patients can log in to a National Health Service app and access their medical data, scan results, blood tests, etc [39]. They have instant access to the results of diagnostic tests but in some situations these results may be accessed before the patient has even spoken to the health professional. Whilst our quest for efficiency is fulfilled, our ability to deliver PCP is hindered. Are we sympathetically present, engaging authentically or working holistically when the patient who is sitting at home alone gets a potentially life changing result with a bad prognosis from an app? If it was your loved one or someone you care about, would you not like these results communicated in a more compassionate manner?

If the patient doesn't fully understand the diagnostic report, they are now in a position where they can use freely available generative AI (GenAI) models (e.g. Google Gemini, ChatGPT) and get the full report summarised in lay language [40–42]. These GenAI models lack the emotional intelligence that humans have and will simply state the facts generated from the data provided. They are unable to tailor their outputs to allow for subjective emotional understanding (unless prompted to do so). In addition to this, we then run into the problem of AI hallucination and factual inaccuracies, which may not only exacerbate the patient distress but lead to an increased workload for the clinician in the long term when they have to address these additional concerns.

2.7 CONCLUSION

The use of AI in healthcare has made considerable strides in recent years and shows no signs of slowing down. Our patients and clinicians of the future will be much more AI literate than our current generation. Generation Z (born between mid-1990s and 2010s) grew up in a world where Wi-Fi and mobile devices enabled 24/7 access to the internet, hence leading to the descriptor of 'digital natives.' Comparably, generation Alpha (born between 2010 and 2024) grew up immersed in AI-powered devices, voice assistants and an unprecedented technological knowledge. Hence, they will adapt to new technology faster than any previous generation and when they enter the workforce, they will expect AI technology to be the norm.

It is imperative that the foundations are laid now for the patients and clinicians of the future. Inevitably health service delivery will change as AI technology continues to advance, and we continually find new ways to do things. As we navigate this period of innovation in the imaging department, we must remember to keep the patient at the centre of everything we do. AI tools offer great potential for the future; however, we must strive to ensure that ethical vigilance is maintained alongside a basic commitment to the individual needs of everyone in our care.

REFERENCES

1. McCormack, B. and McCance, TV. (2025) Development of a Framework for Person-Centred Nursing. J Adv Nurs. 56(5):472–479. https://doi.org/10.1111/j.1365-2648.2006.04042.x
2. O'Donnell, D. and Cook, N. (2025) Exploring Person-Centred Practice. Nurs Stand. 40(3):67–74. https://doi.org/10.7748/ns.2025.e12341
3. Kelsall-Knight, L. and Stevens, R. (2024) Exploring the Implementation of Person-Centred Care in Nursing Practice. Nurs Stand. 39(1):70–75. https://doi.org/10.7748/ns.2023.e12190
4. Hyde, E. and Hardy, M. (2021) Patient Centred Care in Diagnostic Radiography (Part 1): Perceptions of Service Users and Service Deliverers. Radiography (Lond). 27(1):8–13. https://doi.org/10.1016/j.radi.2020.04.015
5. Hyde, E. and Hardy, M. (2021) Patient Centred Care in Diagnostic Radiography (Part 2): A Qualitative Study of the Perceptions of Service Users and Service Deliverers. Radiography (Lond). 27(2):322–331. https://doi.org/10.1016/j.radi.2020.09.008.
6. Hyde, E. and Hardy, M. (2021) Patient Centred Care in Diagnostic Radiography (Part 3): Perceptions of Student Radiographers and Radiography Academics. Radiography (Lond). 27(3):803–810. https://doi.org/10.1016/j.radi.2020.12.013
7. Hardy, M. and Harvey, H. (2020) Artificial Intelligence in Diagnostic Imaging: Impact on the Radiography Profession. Br J Radiol. 93(1108):20190840. https://doi.org/10.1259/bjr.20190840
8. McCance, T. and McCormack, B. (2021) The Person-Centred Practice Framework. In McCormack B, McCance T, Bulley C, Brown D, McMillan A & Martin S (Editors) *Fundamentals of Person-Centred Healthcare Practice*, pp. 23–32. Oxford, Wiley-Blackwell
9. Rainey, C., O'Regan, T., Matthew, J. et al. (2022) UK Reporting radiographers' Perceptions of AI in Radiographic Image Interpretation – Current Perspectives and Future Developments. Radiography (Lond). 28(4):881–888. https://doi.org/10.1016/j.radi.2022.06.006
10. Rainey, C., O'Regan, T., Matthew, J. et al. (2022) An Insight into the Current Perceptions of UK Radiographers on the Future Impact of AI on the Profession: A Cross-Sectional Survey. J Med Imaging Radiat Sci. 53(2022):347–361. https://doi.org/10.1016/j.jmir.2022.05.010
11. Doherty, G., Mc Laughlin, L., Hughes, C. et al. (2024) Radiographer Education and Learning in Artificial Intelligence (REAL-AI): A Survey of Radiographers, Radiologists, and Students' Knowledge of and Attitude to Education on AI. Radiography. 30(Suppl 2):79–87 . https://doi.org/10.1016/j.radi.2024.10.010
12. Doherty, G., Hughes, C., McConnell, J. et al. (2025) Integrating AI into Medical Imaging Curricula: Insights from UK HEIs. Radiography. 31(3):102957. https://doi.org/10.1016/j.radi.2025.102957
13. Morrow, E., Zidaru, T., Ross, F. et al. (2023) Artificial Intelligence Technologies and Compassion in Healthcare: A Systematic Scoping Review. Front Psychol. 13:971044. https://doi.org/10.3389/fpsyg.2022.971044
14. Busch, F., Hoffmann, L., Truhn, D. et al. (2024) Global Cross-Sectional Student Survey on AI in Medical, Dental, and Veterinary Education and Practice at 192 Faculties. BMC Med Educ. 24(1):1066. https://doi.org/10.1186/s12909-024-06035-4

15. Rainey, C., O'Regan, T., Matthew, J. et al. (2021) Beauty Is in the AI of the Beholder: Are We Ready for the Clinical Integration of Artificial Intelligence in Radiography? An Exploratory Analysis of Perceived AI Knowledge, Skills, Confidence, and Education Perspectives of UK Radiographers. Front Digit Health. 3:739327. https://doi.org/10.3389/fdgth.2021.739327

16. Stogiannos, N., Walsh, G., Ohene-Botwe, B. et al. (2025) R-AI-Diographers: A European Survey on Perceived Impact of AI on Professional Identity, Careers, and radiographers' Roles. Insights Imaging. 16:43. https://doi.org/10.1186/s13244-025-01918-6

17. Busch, F., Hoffmann, L., Xu, L. et al. (2025) Multinational Attitudes Toward AI in Health Care and Diagnostics Among Hospital Patients. JAMA Netw Open. 8(6):e2514452. https://doi.org/10.1001/jamanetworkopen.2025.14452

18. Wong, S.H., Al-Hasani, H. and Alam, Z. (2019) Artificial Intelligence in Radiology: How Will We Be Affected? Eur Radiol. 29:141–143. https://doi.org/10.1007/s00330-018-5644-3

19. Ryan, M.L., O'Donovan, T. and McNulty, J.P. (2021) Artificial Intelligence: The Opinions of Radiographers and Radiation Therapists in Ireland. Radiography. 27(suppl. 1):74–82. https://doi.org/10.1016/j.radi.2021.07.022

20. Huisman, M., Ranschaert, E., Parker, W. et al. (2021) An International Survey on AI in Radiology in 1,041 Radiologists and Radiology Residents Part 1: Fear of Replacement, Knowledge, and Attitude. Eur Radiol. 31(9):7058–7066. https://doi.org/10.1007/s00330-021-07781-5

21. Kühne, S., Jacobsen, J., Legewie, N. et al. (2025) Attitudes Toward AI Usage in Patient Health Care: Evidence from a Population Survey Vignette Experiment. J Med Internet Res. 27:e70179. https://doi.org/10.2196/70179

22. Beets, B., Newman, T.P., Howell, E.L. et al. (2023) Surveying Public Perceptions of Artificial Intelligence in Health Care in the United States. Syst Rev. 25:e40337. https://doi.org/10.2196/40337

23. Kauttonen, J., Rousi, R., Alamäki, A.J. (2025) Trust and Acceptance Challenges in the Adoption of AI Applications in Health Care: Quantitative Survey Analysis. Internet Res. 27:e65567. https://doi.org/10.2196/65567

24. Abuzaid, M.M., Elshami, W., Tekin, H. et al. (2022) Assessment of the Willingness of Radiologists and Radiographers to Accept the Integration of Artificial Intelligence into Radiology Practice. Acad Radiol. 29(1):87–94. https://doi.org/10.1016/j.acra.2020.09.014

25. Chen, Y., Stavropoulou, C., Narasinkan, R. et al. (2021) Professionals' Responses to the Introduction of AI Innovations in Radiology and their Implications for Future Adoption: A Qualitative Study. BMC Health Serv Res. 21(1):813. https://doi.org/10.1186/s12913-021-06861-y

26. Osnat, B. (2025) Patient Perspectives on Artificial Intelligence in Healthcare: A Global Scoping Review of Benefits, Ethical Concerns, and Implementation Strategies. Int J Med Inform. 203:106007. https://doi.org/10.1016/j.ijmedinf.2025.106007.

27. Ploug, T., Sundby, A., Moeslund, T.B. et al. (2021) Population Preferences for Performance and Explainability of Artificial Intelligence in Health Care: Choice-Based Conjoint Survey. Med Internet Res. 23(12):e26611. https://doi.org/10.2196/26611

28. Kitamura, F.C., Marques, O. (2021) Trustworthiness of Artificial Intelligence Models in Radiology and the Role of Explainability. J Am Coll Radiol. 18(8):1160–1162. https://doi.org/10.1016/j.jacr.2021.02.008

29. Rainey, C., Bond, R., McConnell, J. et al. (2024) Reporting Radiographers' Interaction with Artificial Intelligence—How do different forms of AI Feedback Impact Trust and Decision Switching? PLoS Digital Health. https://doi.org/10.1371/journal.pdig.0000560

30. Corfmat, M., Martineau, J.T., Régis, C. (2025) BMC High-reward, High-Risk Technologies? An Ethical and Legal Account of AI Development in Healthcare. Med Ethics. 26(1):4. https://doi.org/10.1186/s12910-024-01158-1

31. Elgin, C.Y., Elgin, C. (2024) Ethical Implications of AI-Driven Clinical Decision Support Systems on Healthcare Resource Allocation: A Qualitative Study of Healthcare Professionals' Perspectives. BMC Med Ethics. 25(1):148. https://doi.org/10.1186/s12910-024-01151-8

32. Walsh, G., Stogiannos, N., van de Venter, R. et al. (2023). Responsible AI Practice and AI Education are Central to AI Implementation: A Rapid Review for all Medical Imaging Professionals in Europe. BJR|Open. 5(1):0033. https://doi.org/10.1259/bjro.20230033

33. World Health Organisation. (2015) Global Strategy on People-Centred and Integrated Health Services. WHO; Geneva, Switzerland. https://iris.who.int/handle/10665/155002

34. Kotter, E., D'Antonoli, T.A., Cuocolo, R. et al. (2025) Guiding AI in Radiology: ESR's Recommendations for Effective Implementation of the European AI Act. Insights Imaging. 16:33. https://doi.org/10.1186/s13244-025-01905-x [accessed 30 June 2025]

35. International Society of Radiographers and Radiological Technologists (2020) The European Federation of Radiographer Societies. Artificial Intelligence and the Radiographer/Radiological Technologist Profession: A Joint Statement of the International Society of Radiographers and Radiological Technologists and the European Federation of Radiographer Societies. Radiography (Lond). 26(2):93–95. https://doi.org/10.1016/j.radi.2020.03.007

36. Kenny, L.M., Nevin, M. and Fitzpatrick,K. (2021) Ethics and Standards in the Use of Artificial Intelligence in Medicine on Behalf of the Royal Australian and New Zealand College of Radiologists. J Med Imaging Radiat Oncol. 65(5):486–494. https://doi.org/10.1111/1754-9485.13289

37. Van Kolfschooten, H. and van Oirschot, J. (2024) The EU Artificial Intelligence Act (2024): Implications for Healthcare. Health Policy. 149:105152. https://doi.org/10.1016/j.healthpol.2024.105152

38. Van Leeuwen, K.G., Doorn, L. and Gelderblom, E. (2025) The AI Act: Responsibilities and Obligations for Healthcare Professionals and Organizations. Diagn Interv Radiol. https://doi.org/10.4274/dir.2025.252851

39. Digital Health and Care Northern Ireland-HSC Goes Digital (2025) My Care – DHCNI [accessed 30 June 2025]

40. Van Veen, D., Van Uden, C., Blankemeier, L. et al. (2024) Adapted Large Language Models can Outperform Medical Experts in Clinical Text Summarization. Nat Med. 30:1134–1142. https://doi.org/10.1038/s41591-024-02855-5

41. Holstead, R.G. (2024) Utility of Large Language Models to Produce a Patient-Friendly Summary from Oncology Consultations. JCO Oncol Pract. 20(9):1157–1159. https://doi.org/10.1200/OP.24.00057

42. Jeblick, K., Schachtner, B., Dexl, J. et al. (2024) ChatGPT Makes Medicine Easy to Swallow: An Exploratory Case Study on Simplified Radiology Reports. Eur Radiol. 34:2817–2825. https://doi.org/10.1007/s00330-023-10213-1

3 Background to Technology Used in Healthcare

Holly Toner

3.1 THE EVOLUTION OF AI

3.1.1 Historical Background/Introduction

The field of artificial intelligence (AI) has come a long way from its early beginnings, with important developments shaping its role in healthcare and other industries today. AI traces its roots back to the mid-20th century, when the concept was first explored by pioneers like Alan Turing. In 1956, the term 'artificial intelligence' was officially coined at the Dartmouth Conference, an event that laid the foundation for AI as an academic discipline.

The early development of AI was largely theoretical, focusing on problem-solving and decision-making in controlled environments. Researchers created early AI systems known as expert systems in the 1960s and 1970s, which aimed to replicate the decision-making processes of human experts. These systems relied heavily on rule-based algorithms, allowing machines to process specific information and provide conclusions in narrowly defined contexts. However, the complexity of real-world applications often exceeded the capabilities of these early AI systems, limiting their practical use.

AI took a major step forward in the 1980s with the development of machine learning (ML), which enables machines to learn from data rather than relying on fixed rules. The 1990s saw further progress with neural networks, allowing machines to process information in a way similar to the human brain. These advances made AI more adaptable and capable of handling complex tasks.

In the 21st century, deep learning (DL), a form of ML using layered neural networks, revolutionised AI in healthcare. With increased computing power and vast datasets, DL is now used in medical imaging, natural language processing, and predictive analytics. AI is enhancing decision-making, improving diagnostics, and forecasting disease outbreaks.

3.2 TYPES OF AI MODELS

AI is a vast and rapidly evolving field, encompassing a wide array of models and techniques. From ML to DL, the terminology used to describe these systems can be overwhelming. This section will break down these complexities by defining AI clearly and exploring the different types of AI models used today. By understanding how these models are grouped and applied, particularly in healthcare, we can gain a clearer picture of their capabilities and limitations.

3.2.1 Definitions

AI refers to the design of machines or systems capable of performing tasks that previously required human intelligence. These tasks include reasoning, decision-making, problem-solving, and adapting to new information. Broadly speaking, AI can be divided into narrow AI and general AI.

Narrow AI, the most common form today, is designed for specific tasks, such as diagnosing diseases or interpreting medical images. These systems excel in their focused domains but lack the flexibility to generalise beyond them. In contrast, general AI—which remains largely theoretical—aims to perform any intellectual task a human can.

ML and DL represent two critical branches within AI (Figures 3.1 and 3.2). Unlike earlier AI methods, such as expert systems, which relied on explicitly programmed rules and logic, ML allows systems to learn from data patterns without predefined rules. This makes ML much more adaptable and scalable, especially for tasks involving large datasets.

DL, a more advanced form of ML, mimics the structure of the human brain by utilising neural networks with multiple interconnected layers. These layers enable DL models to process vast amounts of complex data, identifying intricate patterns that may not be visible to humans.

For further background and legal context of AI please see Martinez [1]. For a general introduction to AI, Boden [2] is a useful resource. Additional reading in the context of the background to AI development and current use and regulation includes [3–5].

3.2.2 Training Methods

A key component of understanding ML is recognising the various training methods used to develop models. By examining the three primary training approaches—**supervised learning**, **unsupervised learning**, and **reinforcement learning**—we gain insight into how AI systems can be tailored

DOI: 10.1201/9781032709956-3

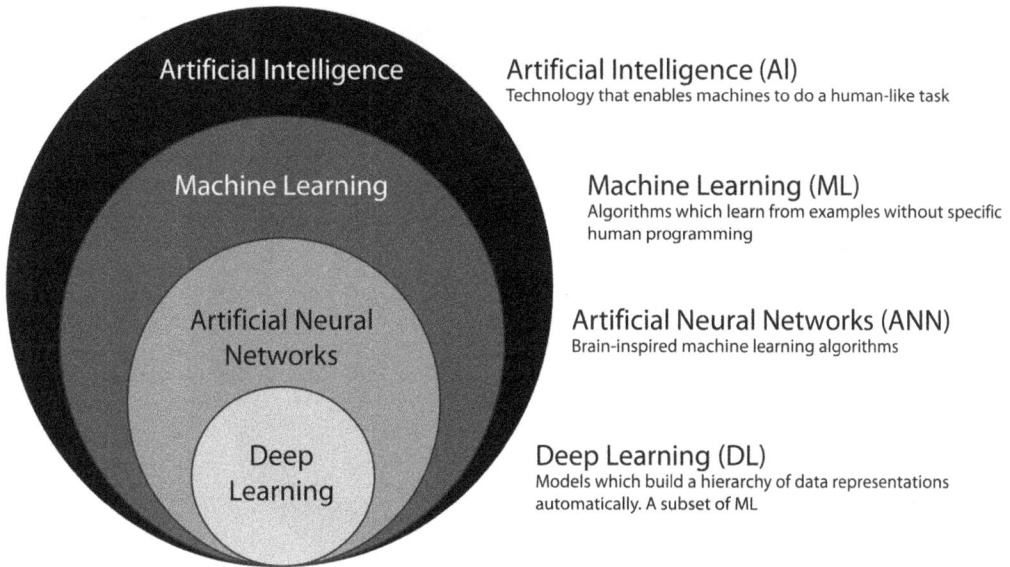

Artificial Intelligence (AI)
Technology that enables machines to do a human-like task

Machine Learning (ML)
Algorithms which learn from examples without specific human programming

Artificial Neural Networks (ANN)
Brain-inspired machine learning algorithms

Deep Learning (DL)
Models which build a hierarchy of data representations automatically. A subset of ML

Figure 3.1 Hierarchy of AI.

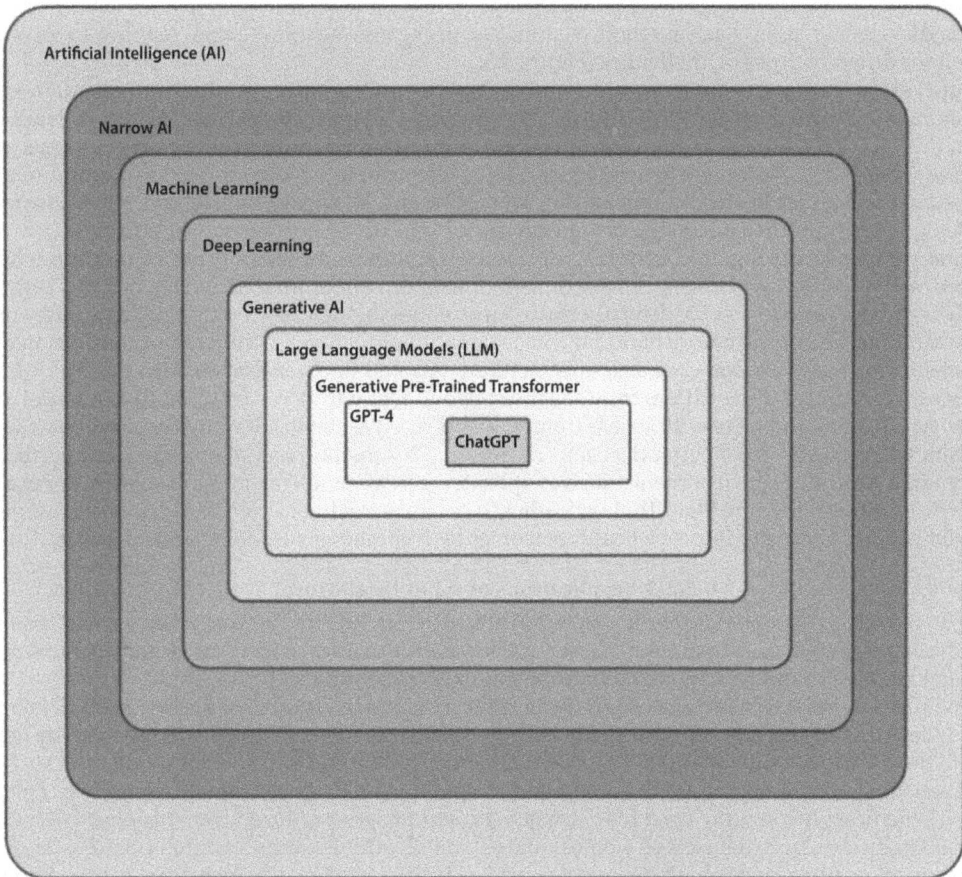

Figure 3.2 Taxonomy of AI.

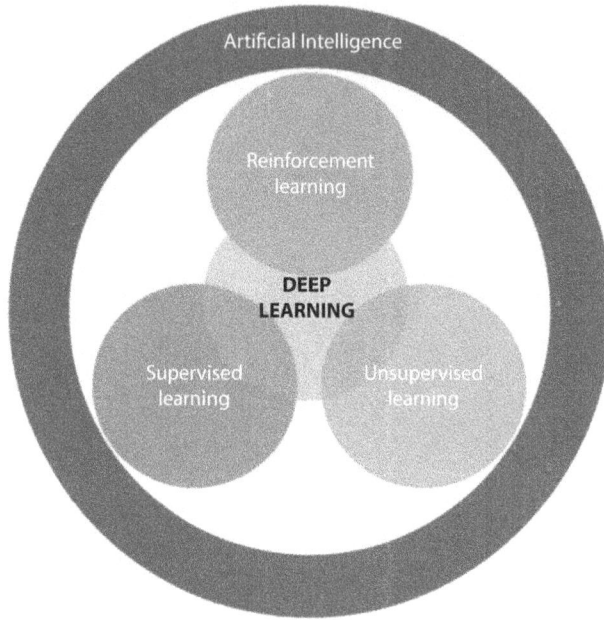

Figure 3.3 Deep learning training approaches.

to handle specific tasks. Each method has unique strengths and limitations, making them well-suited for different types of challenges (Figure 3.3).

Supervised learning is the most widely used approach in healthcare AI. In this method, models are trained on labelled datasets, where both the input and the correct output are known. By learning from this labelled data, supervised learning algorithms can map inputs to the correct outputs and then generalise this knowledge to new, unseen data. For example, a model trained to detect tumours in medical images learns from thousands of labelled scans, allowing it to recognise malignancies with high accuracy when analysing new images.

Unsupervised learning, in contrast, is used when data lacks labelled outputs. Here, the model is tasked with identifying patterns or structures in the data without guidance. This method is especially useful for uncovering hidden patterns in large datasets, such as grouping patients with similar symptoms. Clustering algorithms and dimensionality-reduction techniques are common in this approach, helping to process complex, unstructured data and find hidden relationships.

Reinforcement learning differs from the other two in that it involves learning through trial and error. An AI agent interacts with its environment and receives feedback in the form of rewards or penalties, learning to make better decisions over time. This method has shown significant promise in dynamic healthcare environments, such as optimising treatment strategies in real time. For example, reinforcement learning algorithms can adjust a patient's treatment plan based on their response to medications, aiming to improve health outcomes by continuously learning and adapting.

3.2.3 Applications of AI in Healthcare

AI has numerous potential applications in healthcare, from improving diagnostics to optimising patient management and treatment planning. However, the most widely used and impactful AI technologies are computer vision and natural language processing (NLP).

Computer vision involves the use of AI to interpret and analyse visual data, such as medical images and videos. In healthcare, computer vision plays a crucial role in assisting with diagnostics by helping to detect diseases and anomalies in medical images produced from various modalities, such as magnetic resonance imaging (MRI), computed tomography (CT), projectional radiography ('plain' X-rays), medical photography used for dermatology, and images produced from histology slides. AI models trained on large datasets of medical images can identify patterns and abnormalities, such as tumours or fractures, with a high degree of accuracy. This technology is widely used to speed up the diagnostic process, providing clinicians with valuable support in identifying conditions that may be difficult to detect through human observation alone.

Natural language processing focuses on enabling machines to process and interpret human language, both written and spoken. In healthcare, NLP models are employed to analyse unstructured text data, such as clinical notes, electronic health records, and medical literature. These models extract key information, helping clinicians make data-driven decisions. Common applications include identifying drug interactions, summarising patient histories, and automating administrative tasks like medical coding and insurance claims.

3.2.4 Interpretability: White-Box vs. Black-Box Models

A major challenge in AI, especially in healthcare, is interpretability—the ability to understand how a model makes its decisions. AI models are often categorised as white-box or black-box based on how transparent they are.

White-box models are highly interpretable, allowing users to trace the steps taken to arrive at a decision. Models like decision trees and linear regression are examples, providing clear pathways that explain how inputs lead to outputs. This transparency is crucial in healthcare, where clinicians need to understand and trust the reasoning behind diagnoses or treatment recommendations.

On the other hand, black-box models, such as those used in DL, are far more complex and less interpretable. While these models often deliver superior accuracy, particularly in areas like medical imaging, their internal workings are not easily understood. This lack of transparency can be concerning in healthcare, where explainability is important for ensuring trust and accountability.

Balancing accuracy and interpretability is an ongoing challenge in AI. Black-box models can excel in performance but may raise concerns when used in critical areas like patient care. Conversely, white-box models provide clearer insights into their decision-making processes but might not always match the accuracy of more complex systems. Researchers are working to bridge this gap by developing models that are both highly accurate and interpretable or incorporate some form of reliable explainability to present to the user.

3.3 GENERATIVE AI

Generative AI (GenAI) refers to a subset of narrow AI that focuses on creating new content, such as text, or images, based on patterns learned from existing data. This contrasts with other AI models—such as those used for classification or prediction—which primarily analyse existing data to make decisions or identify patterns. GenAI models, on the other hand, create entirely new outputs, making them especially valuable in fields like healthcare where innovation and the ability to simulate real-world scenarios are crucial.

GenAI fits within the broader spectrum of ML and DL models, which were described in earlier sections. GenAI models build on the foundational principles of DL by utilising neural networks, particularly transformer architectures, to generate new content (Figures 3.2 and 3.3). Transformers, a type of neural network, are crucial in enabling generative models to process and generate sequences of data, such as text or images, by understanding the relationships amongst data points across long contexts. This is a key advancement over earlier AI models, allowing GenAI to handle more complex and varied tasks.

GenAI training often begins with unsupervised learning, where models learn patterns from unlabelled data. They also incorporate reinforcement learning to refine their outputs, particularly in specialised tasks like healthcare. A notable method used is reinforcement learning from human feedback (RLHF), where human reviewers guide the model to improve accuracy and reliability, ensuring that AI-generated content meets high standards for quality and ethical compliance.

A well-known example of GenAI is the generative pre-trained transformer (GPT), a language model that generates human-like text by predicting the next word or sentence based on prior context. In healthcare, these models can be fine-tuned for specific tasks such as generating clinical reports, summarising medical literature, or assisting with patient communication. By adapting to healthcare-specific datasets, GPT models offer a significant advancement in narrow AI, moving beyond standard predictive tasks to create personalised, contextually relevant outputs.

GenAI is not limited to text; it can be applied across various data types, including medical imaging. In healthcare, this technology can be used to simulate new medical images, helping train medical professionals or allowing researchers to create synthetic datasets for analysis without compromising patient privacy.

3.3.1 Training Processes and Applications of GenAI

GenAI models rely on specific training processes to achieve their advanced capabilities. The two primary phases in training are pre-training and fine-tuning, which work together to make these models both powerful and adaptable across various applications, particularly in healthcare.

In the pre-training phase, the model is exposed to vast, diverse datasets to learn general patterns, structures, and relationships within the data. This phase gives the model a foundational understanding of language, concepts, or image patterns. In healthcare, for example, a GenAI model might be pre-trained on large-scale datasets that include medical literature, research studies, or anonymised patient data. This training allows the model—often referred to as a foundation model—to understand the core language and concepts that are common across the field, making it versatile for future tasks.

After pre-training, the model undergoes fine-tuning to specialise its knowledge for more specific tasks. During this phase, the model is further trained on targeted, domain-relevant datasets to adapt its outputs to the precise needs of a particular area. In healthcare, fine-tuning might involve training the model on clinical records or disease-specific data, enabling the AI to perform highly specialised tasks. For example, fine-tuning could allow the model to generate precise diagnostic reports or provide treatment recommendations based on current medical practices.

A particularly powerful method when applying GenAI is retrieval-augmented generation (RAG). RAG enhances the model's ability by not only generating responses from its pre-trained knowledge but also retrieving real-time information from trusted, up-to-date sources. This combination makes RAG highly effective in healthcare (or any specialised context), where the latest clinical guidelines or research findings are critical. For instance, when generating treatment suggestions, RAG can pull in the most current studies or clinical data, allowing it to offer recommendations that reflect the latest advancements in medicine. This real-time augmentation makes the generated output more accurate and relevant, helping clinicians make more informed decisions.

GenAI's potential applications in healthcare are broad. One notable use is the generation of synthetic medical data for research purposes. This allows researchers to create artificial datasets that mimic real patient data without exposing sensitive information, thus maintaining privacy while ensuring the data remains useful for analysis. Another important application is the ability to simulate clinical scenarios. These simulations offer a risk-free environment for healthcare professionals to practice procedures or analyse potential outcomes, greatly improving medical training. Additionally, GenAI plays a growing role in drug discovery and development, where it can propose new molecular structures or simulate drug interactions. This significantly speeds up the research process, helping scientists identify promising drug candidates more efficiently.

GenAI, especially when paired with tools like RAG, represents a major advancement in healthcare. Its ability to generate dynamic, accurate, and creative solutions to complex medical challenges offers promising avenues for improving diagnostics, treatment planning, and research innovation.

3.3.2 AI Access and Public Perceptions

GenAI has significantly broadened access to advanced AI tools, allowing individuals, small businesses, and creators to leverage AI without needing extensive technical knowledge. Intuitive platforms have made AI-driven innovation more accessible across sectors like marketing, content creation, education, and research, reshaping industries by democratising creativity and streamlining workflows.

As AI becomes more integrated into everyday operations, concerns about reliability and quality control have grown. Non-experts may face challenges with biased or inaccurate outputs, affecting decision-making. Ensuring these systems are accurate, unbiased, and secure is crucial as reliance on AI for critical tasks increases.

Awareness of AI has rapidly grown among both clinicians and patients, leading to a mix of optimism and concern. Clinicians are increasingly recognising the potential of AI to improve diagnostics, treatment planning, and patient outcomes. Patients, too, are becoming more familiar with AI-powered tools like chatbots and predictive analytics in healthcare. However, alongside this optimism comes fear—concerns about accuracy, data privacy, and the potential for AI to replace human judgement in critical decisions. The opportunities for significant advances in medicine are substantial, but they come with risks. It is crucial that we educate both healthcare providers and patients on AI's capabilities and limitations and implement safeguards to mitigate risks. Only through responsible use and clear communication can we fully harness AI's potential while minimising its challenges.

3.4 RESPONSIBLE IMPLEMENTATION OF AI IN HEALTHCARE

The implementation of AI in healthcare offers significant opportunities to enhance diagnostics, streamline workflows, and improve patient outcomes. However, realising these benefits requires careful attention to ethical design, risk management, and regulatory compliance. As AI becomes more deeply integrated into clinical decision-making and patient care, ensuring that these systems are reliable, transparent, and accountable is critical. Balancing the promise of AI with the need for safety, fairness, and trust will be essential for its long-term success in healthcare.

3.4.1 Ethical Design and Risk Management

Ethical design is critical for AI implementation in healthcare. AI models must be built with a robust ethical framework that prioritises fairness, transparency, and accountability. One of the most significant risks in healthcare AI is the potential for biased outputs, which could disproportionately affect underrepresented or vulnerable populations. To address this, it is crucial to train AI systems on diverse datasets that reflect a broad range of demographics, medical conditions, and care environments. This ensures that AI models are not only accurate but also equitable, avoiding the perpetuation of existing healthcare disparities.

Risk management should be woven into every stage of AI development and deployment. This begins with thorough impact assessments to identify and mitigate potential risks, including concerns around data privacy, the accuracy of diagnoses, and the over-reliance on AI in clinical decision-making. Ensuring that AI supports rather than replaces human judgement is essential to maintaining trust and safety in medical environments.

Furthermore, healthcare providers must be actively involved in understanding and addressing these risks. Education and training for clinicians on the capabilities and limitations of AI are crucial for reducing unintended consequences. By emphasising a balanced approach that combines human expertise with AI-driven insights, healthcare systems can foster a safer and more ethical integration of AI into clinical practice.

3.4.2 Regulatory Compliance and Governance

The implementation of AI in healthcare within the UK and EU must adhere to strict data privacy and AI-specific regulations to ensure patient safety, transparency, and accountability. Both the UK General Data Protection Regulation (UK GDPR) and the EU General Data Protection Regulation (GDPR) set stringent requirements for the processing of personal data in AI systems. These regulations mandate that healthcare AI systems handle sensitive patient data responsibly, ensuring consent, security, and transparency in all applications.

In addition to data privacy laws, the EU's Artificial Intelligence Act (AI Act), which came into force in August 2024, introduces a comprehensive legal framework for AI systems across all member states. The AI Act classifies AI systems based on their potential risk to health, safety, and fundamental rights. Healthcare AI models, often considered high-risk, must meet strict requirements related to data quality, transparency, human oversight, and robustness. The Act also establishes specific transparency obligations for AI systems that interact directly with individuals or generate synthetic content, ensuring users are aware they are engaging with AI.

In the UK, AI technologies must comply with safety standards regulated by the Medicines and Healthcare Products Regulatory Agency (MHRA), ensuring that AI-based medical devices meet high standards for efficacy, safety, and performance. As the UK develops its own approach to AI regulation, frameworks such as the UK AI Strategy aim to support the responsible development of AI while fostering innovation.

Effective governance is essential to oversee the development and deployment of AI in healthcare. Organisations must establish clear guidelines for the testing, validation, and continuous monitoring of AI models. Regular audits are critical for assessing both the performance and ethical implications of AI systems. This ensures that AI systems are held accountable to both regulatory bodies and healthcare professionals.

REFERENCES

1. Martinez, R. (2019) Artificial Intelligence: Distinguishing Between Types & Definitions. 19 Nev. L.J. 1015. Available at: https://scholars.law.unlv.edu/nlj/vol19/iss3/9
2. Boden, M.A. (2018) What Is Artificial Intelligence? In: Artificial Intelligence: A Very Short Introduction, Very Short Introductions. Oxford Academic, Oxford. https://doi.org/10.1093/actrade/9780199602919.003.0001
3. Sheikh, H., Prins, C., Schrijvers, E. (2023) Artificial Intelligence: Definition and Background. In: Mission AI. Research for Policy. Springer, Cham. https://doi.org/10.1007/978-3-031-21448-6_2
4. European Commission. (December 2018) High-Level Expert Group on Artificial Intelligence. A Definition of AI Main Capabilities and Scientific Disciplines. Available at: https://ec.europa.eu/futurium/en/system/files/ged/ai_hleg_definition_of_ai_18_december1.pdf [accessed September 2024]
5. The European High Performance Computing Joint Undertaking (EuroHPC JU). (2023) AI and HPC: Enhancing Research Possibilities. Available at: https://eurohpc-ju.europa.eu/ai-and-hpc-enhancing-research-possibilities-2023-09-12_en [accessed September 2024]

4 Statistical Analyses and Reporting of Performance of AI Models
An Introduction to AI Statistics

Vanessa Otti and Siegfried Wagner

4.1 DESCRIPTIVE STATISTICS

While detailed knowledge of medical statistics is not required for this chapter, you should be familiar with some concepts. We will briefly review these at the beginning of the chapter.

- Types of data
- Sampling and the concept of inference
- Basic summary statistics (mean, median, mode)
- Confidence intervals
- Bias

4.1.1 Categorical and Numerical Data

Data can be of many different types, but in general we can divide most data into categorical and numerical. Categorical, or qualitative, data describes characteristics. They can be divided into binary, ordinal and nominal, depending on the number of categories available and their natural ordering (Figure 4.1).

Numerical data are also termed quantitative data. This type of data can be counted and are described as either discrete or continuous (Figure 4.2).

4.1.2 Sampling, Inference and Bias

It is almost impossible to collect data on a whole population, so we generally take a sample and make inferences about the population based on that sample (Table 4.1).

One analogy for this is when you're making soup. During the process, you might take a spoonful (sample) of soup to give you an idea of how the whole soup tastes (population). This concept is inference.

Another important epidemiological concept in sampling is bias. Bias can be defined as a systematic error in methodology that leads to incorrect estimates and is therefore a very important factor to consider and attempt to mitigate against.

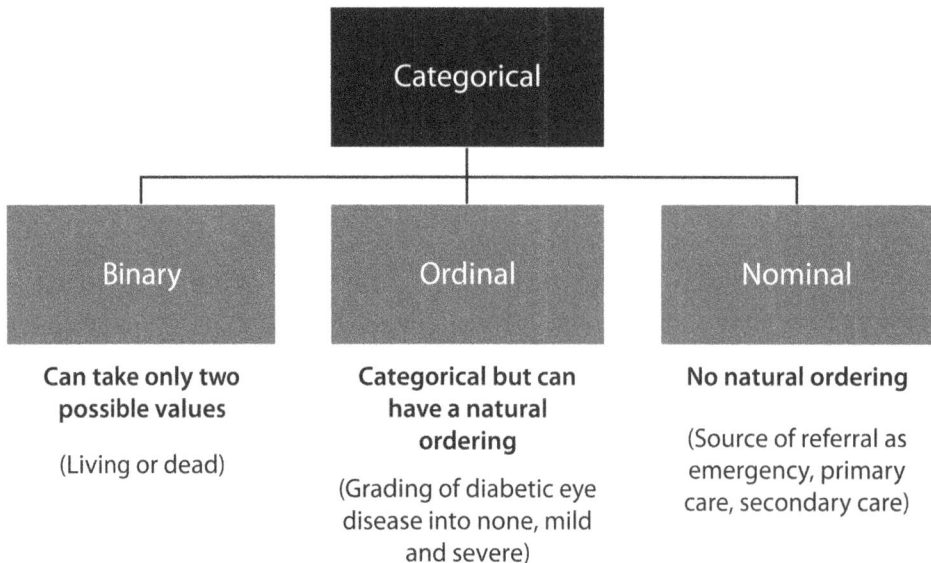

Categorical

Binary

Ordinal

Nominal

Can take only two possible values

(Living or dead)

Categorical but can have a natural ordering

(Grading of diabetic eye disease into none, mild and severe)

No natural ordering

(Source of referral as emergency, primary care, secondary care)

Figure 4.1 Subdivisions of categorical data types.

DOI: 10.1201/9781032709956-4

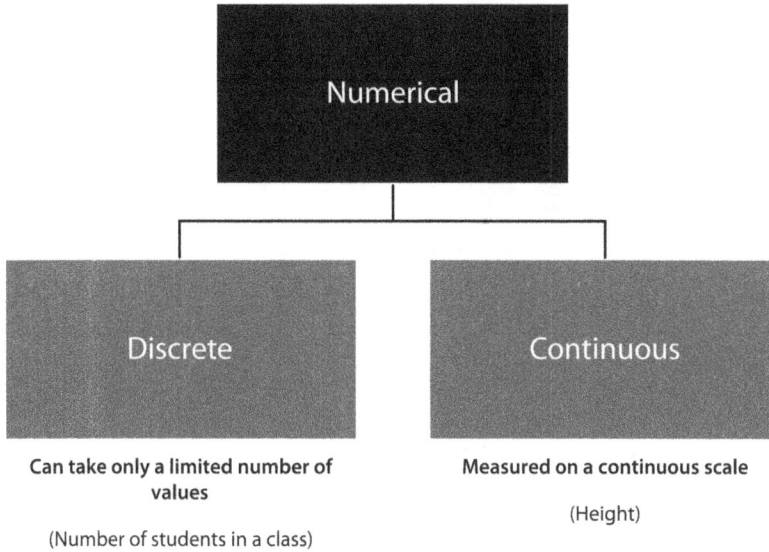

Figure 4.2 Subdivisions of numerical data types.

Table 4.1 Sampling and Inference

Sample	Inference
Set of observations collected from a population using some method	Using analysis of data to deduce information about the underlying probability distribution

Bias can take many forms. One of the major forms is selection bias, in which the methods used to select data are flawed in such a way that the findings are not representative of the population a researcher intends to analyse. Another important consideration and form of bias is information bias. One common type of this is misclassification bias. In machine learning, this could be where there are systematic differences in the labelling of data leading to errors in the model's output. Examples of this will be presented later in this chapter.

4.1.3 Averages, Standard Deviation and Confidence Intervals

We can summarise the data from our sample in different ways (Table 4.2) to produce values of central dispersion. The terms *mean, median, mode* and *standard deviation* are frequently used to describe where the centre of data values may be and as such help us understand what the data is describing.

Table 4.2 Methods of Data Summary (Mean, Median, Mode and Standard Deviation)

Statistic	Definition
Mean (or arithmetic mean)	The average of the observations. This is calculated by summing the observations (must be numerical) and dividing by the total number of observations.
Median	The middle observation if you were to line observations in ascending order. If there is an even number of observations (e.g. four), then take the mean of the middle two observations, e.g. 2, 4, 6, 13, 17, 19, 36, 87, 88, 94 The 'middle' two values are 17 and 19. The sum of 17 and 19 is 36. 36/2 = 18. The median is therefore 18.
Mode	The most common observation seen: 11, 15, 18, 3, 7, 27, 34, 3, 18, 3, 34, 76 In this case the mode would be 3 as this value has been observed most frequently. This would be best represented on a frequency table.
Standard Deviation (SD)	A measure of the spread or variation in the data, i.e. the distance of each observation from the mean.

A final important concept is the confidence interval. We can calculate summary measures on our sample but how confident can we be that this relates to that of the population? Confidence intervals provide a range of values within which we can be confident that the population summary value lies. Confidence intervals are typically presented as the upper and lower 95% confidence limits. They are calculated using the summary parameter (e.g. mean) and the standard error (the standard deviation divided by the square root of the sample size).

4.2 PREDICTIVE STATISTICS

4.2.1 Prediction Models

Artificial intelligence (AI) is generally used for prediction rather than description. In prediction statistics, we use our understanding of the observed data to make predictions on future data.

Prediction modelling has been around for some time. You may be familiar with traditional approaches, such as logistic regression and random forests. In many ways, modern AI-based approaches, such as deep learning, are similar; however, the interpretation of some results may be more nuanced. The principles we will cover here are generally the same across all clinical prediction models.

4.2.2 A Word About Data

Earlier, you reviewed the different types of data (e.g. continuous numerical, ordinal categorical). One advantage of modern deep learning methods is the ability to use more complex data types, such as images/video or audio, e.g. voice recordings (Figure 4.3). These complex data types usually act as inputs* (termed input variable/independent variable/predictor variables).

*There are some deep learning methods where you might generate data, but they are outside the scope of this chapter. An introduction to these concepts can be found in Chapter 3 of this book.

The input data are usually treated as (or converted to) either numerical or categorical data. The type of output most suitable for the task determines the type of model. There are two main types of prediction models: regression or classification (Figure 4.4).

Regression models output a numerical value. Classification models output a categorical variable.

For example, Menzies et al. [1] trained a mobile phone–based deep learning model with skin lesion images as input. The output was pigmented skin cancer diagnosis (categorical) and therefore a classification model. In radiology, classification models are also used to provide predictions from images, many of which are now in use clinically.

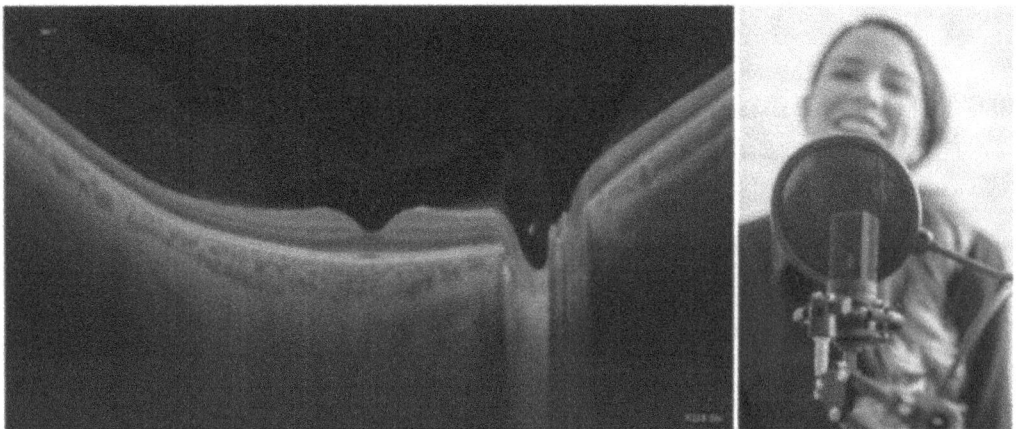

Images   Voice Recordings

Figure 4.3 Examples of types of data input.

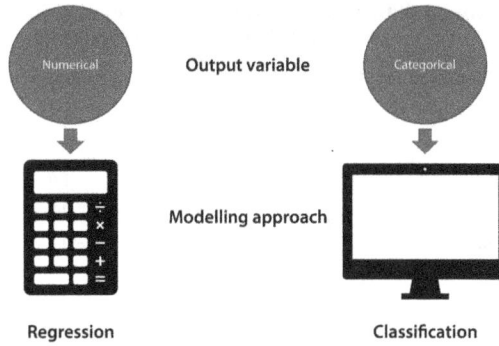

Figure 4.4 Model choice in relation to format of desired output.

4.3 MEASURES OF PERFORMANCE

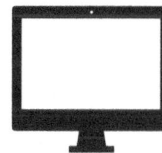

Performance measures generally ascertain how much the model outputs compare to the real values. We can do this numerically and graphically. The methods of measuring performance may differ between regression and classification AI models.

We can measure model performance numerically and graphically, outlined in Figure 4.5. We will now go through each of these methods in the next sections.

4.3.1 Regression Models

As described previously, regression models output a numerical prediction. A common method of measuring performance is to see how the predicted value differs from the actual observed value. This difference is known as a residual. The most common methods are the root mean squared error (RMSE), mean absolute error (MAE) and the coefficient of determination (R^2) (Table 4.3).

The value for both RMSE and MAE can be anything between 0 and infinity. For both, the lower the value, the better the performance of a model.

For example, imagine that you've developed a model that predicts haemoglobin level from a picture of the retina.

Table 4.4 presents the results of your model.

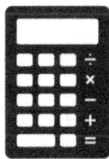

Regression		Classification	
Numerical	**Graphical**	**Numerical**	**Graphical**
Mean absolute error		Sensitivity / Area under the curve	
Root mean squared error	Bland-Altman Plots	Specificity / Precision	ROC Curve
R2		Positive predictive value / Recall	
		Negative predictive value / Kappa	

Figure 4.5 Differentiation of performance measures of regression and classification models.

Table 4.3 Root Mean Squared Error and Mean Absolute Error

Root Mean Squared Error	Mean Absolute Error
We calculate the difference between the predicted and observed value (residual). The residuals for all observations are squared, summed and then divided by the number of compared values. The square root of this is then calculated.	We again calculate the residuals but we then sum the absolute values (so the figures are always positive).

**Table 4.4 Haemoglobin Levels in the Retina
– Example Experimental Findings**

Predicted (mg/dL)	Observed (mg/dL)	Residual
8.1	6.8	−1.3
9.5	9.0	−0.5
6.5	11.1	4.6
10.0	10.4	0.4
9.2	8.4	−0.8

- Each row represents a single image.
- The first column details the predicted haemoglobin level from your model.
- The second column shows the actual value.
- The third column is the residual, i.e. the difference between the actual value and predicted value.

Using the values in the Table 4.4, calculate both the root mean squared error and the mean absolute error. The worked example is below:

Root mean squared error can be calculated as follows:

Square each residual and add them together

$(−1.3)^2 + (−0.5)^2 + (4.6)^2 + (0.4)^2 + (−0.8)^2 = 23.9$

Divide by the number of compared values: $23.9/5 = 4.78$

Take the square root of the value: $\sqrt{4.78}$

RMSE = 2.19

Mean absolute error is also calculated from the data collected:

Take the absolute values of the residuals

And add them together: $1.3 + 0.5 + 4.6 + 0.4 + 0.8 = 7.6$

Divide by the number of compared values: $7.6/5$

MAE = 1.52

The coefficient of determination (R^2) is another common metric used in regression model performance. It measures how the difference in one variable is explained by the difference in another variable. It is similar to a correlation coefficient (R). R^2 is a number between 0 and 1. The closer the value is to 1, the more the variation in the output can be explained by the input, i.e. the stronger the relationship.

Now that we've covered calculating measures of regression model performance, let's look at an example of how to apply these to assess the performance of a particular model. Please type the following URL into your browser search bar: https://youtu.be/g4iZF4gQxCg

An image as below should appear:

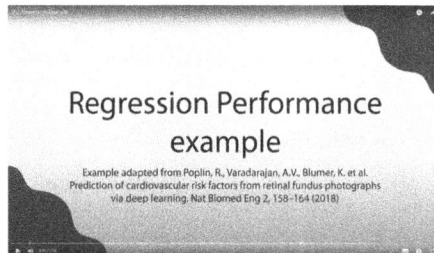

Regression Performance example

Example adapted from Poplin, R., Varadarajan, A.V., Blumer, K. et al.
Prediction of cardiovascular risk factors from retinal fundus photographs
via deep learning. Nat Biomed Eng 2, 158–164 (2018)

The data used in this example is based on the study by Poplin et al. [2].

4.3.2 Limits of Agreement

We can also measure the performance of regression models using graphical methods such as Bland–Altman plots. Please see an explanation in this video: https://youtu.be/o7nhLbZcKQk – the below image should appear.

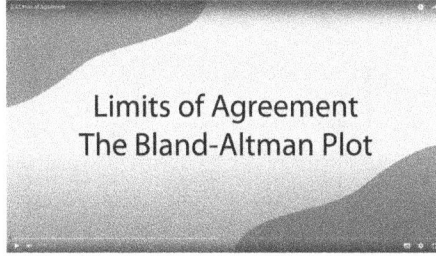

The data used in this example is adapted from Jin et al. [3] where the authors use the Bland–Altman method to assess agreement between an AI virtual ruler to measure the diameter of oesophageal varices compared to visual observation carries out by endoscopists.

A further example is provided by Ludbrook [4] with particular focus on how to quantify elements of bias with some worked examples.

4.3.3 Classification Models

The output in classification models is known as a *category* (also known as a *class* in machine learning) (Figure 4.6).

We cannot numerically compare this output to the actual output, so we need different methods to assess performance. Other measures of classification model performance are needed, such as sensitivity, specificity, positive predictive value and negative predictive value.

Classification models can be of different types, but we will focus on the main types (Table 4.5).

Medical AI research often uses performance measures of binary classification for many multiclassification tasks, using a "one vs. all" approach. We will discuss this later in this chapter.

4.3.3.1 Let's Focus on Binary Classification First

Imagine you've just developed a new prediction model that classifies an image as a dog or cat. Now, you want to assess its performance. You test your model on 10 new unseen photographs of dogs and cats. The results are shown in Figure 4.7.

How can we assess the performance of our model?

- One simple way is to see how many it got right; in other words, how many AI outputs were the same as the 'ground truth'?

- This model classified seven correctly and three incorrectly.

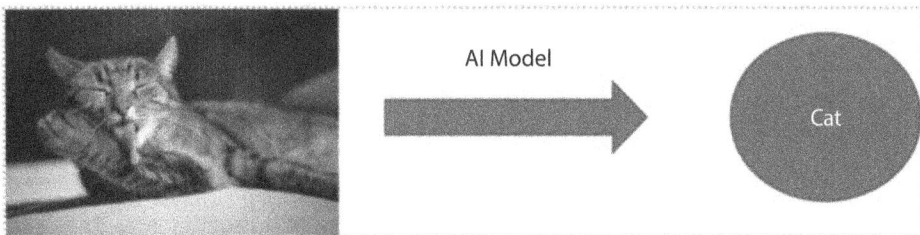

Figure 4.6 Input to output flow.

Table 4.5 Types of Classification Model

Binary	Multiclassification
Output can take one of two possible classes.	Output can take multiple classes.
Example: Dog or cat	Example: Dog, cat, pig, horse

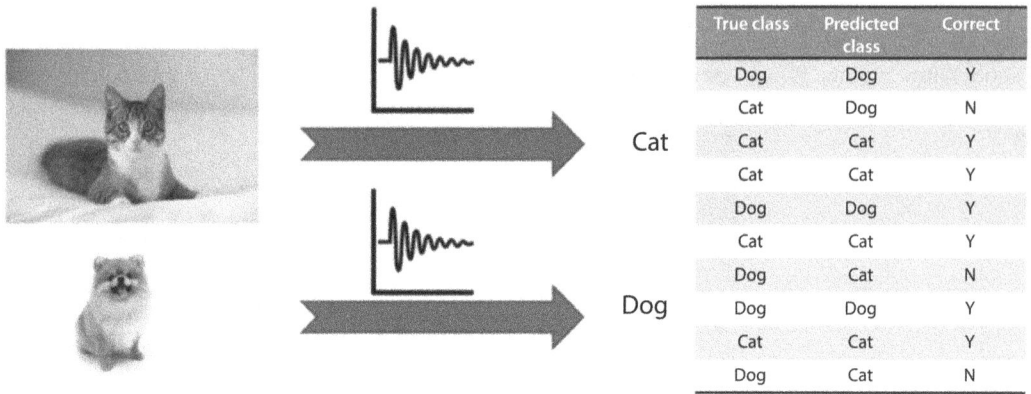

True class	Predicted class	Correct
Dog	Dog	Y
Cat	Dog	N
Cat	Cat	Y
Cat	Cat	Y
Dog	Dog	Y
Cat	Cat	Y
Dog	Cat	N
Dog	Dog	Y
Cat	Cat	Y
Dog	Cat	N

Figure 4.7 Example outputs from binary classification model.

- We could therefore say it was correct seven out of ten times, i.e. 70% of the time.

- This is accuracy.

Accuracy is simple to measure but not ideal in datasets where the number in each class differs significantly (class imbalance). This may be the case with medical data, where the pathology class may represent the minority class, particularly in rare diseases.

Imagine now that you use another dataset, which consists of eight cats and two dogs. The model you test (developed by someone else of course) just outputs cat every single time. The accuracy would be 80%!

One of the best ways to assess performance is through a *confusion matrix*, also termed a *contingency table* (Figure 4.8).

We can use confusion matrices to calculate the following:

- True positives

- True negatives

- False positives

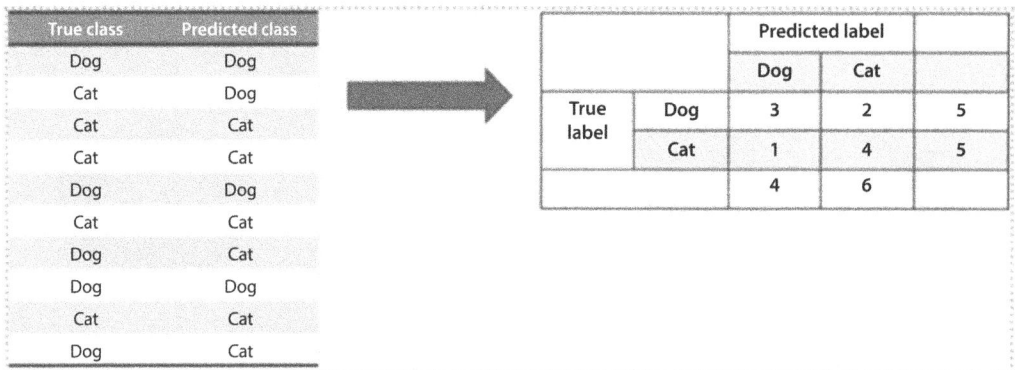

Figure 4.8 Example outputs from binary classification model and associated confusion matrix. An example of a confusion matrix is shown on the right of the figure.

- False negatives
- Sensitivity
- Specificity
- Positive predictive value
- Negative predictive value
- Accuracy

When using a confusion matrix, one class is nominated as the positive class. This is often obvious as it usually refers to a disease being present.

In this example, we will use *Dog* as our positive class.

Once you have correctly identified the true positives, true negatives, false positives and false negatives, it is very easy to calculate the other metrics.

Two key measures of performance are sensitivity and specificity.

Sensitivity

- Sensitivity is a proportion of positive cases that are correctly identified as positive.
- It is sometimes also referred to as the *true positive rate.*
- So, it is the number of true positives divided by all the actual positive cases (true positives and false negatives).
- Sensitivity = true positives/(true positives + false negatives)

4.3.3.2 *Positive Predictive Value and Negative Predictive Value*

Another key metric is positive predictive value (PPV) and negative predictive value (NPV). Respectively, upon a positive and negative predicted label, what are the chances of being truly positive or negative?

Importantly, these measures take into account how common the condition is in the dataset (the prevalence). A commonly used example of this is the diagnosis of human immunodeficiency virus (HIV). In a community where the prevalence of HIV is 0.04%, the PPV of a typical HIV assay test is only 44%. The paper has been linked below for further reading [5].

PPV = true positives/(true positives + false positives)

NPV = true negatives/(true negatives + false negatives)

Refer to the confusion matrix earlier – can you calculate the PPV and NPV of our dog/cat classifier?

Whilst some of these reporting metrics are familiar to clinicians, some are not. One challenge with engaging with the literature in the field of machine learning and statistics is that there can be different terms for the same thing. Machine learning work often refers to precision and recall, where precision is the same as the positive predictive value, and recall is the same as sensitivity or the true positive rate. We often see precision and recall used in machine learning research while medical papers report specificity and sensitivity. Since precision (positive predictive value) takes into account the prevalence of a condition, it may be more informative in imbalanced datasets.

Occasionally, machine learning literature will report the F score of a model. *The F score is a performance metric composed of the harmonic mean of recall and precision.*

$$F\,score = 2 * (precision * recall) / (precision + recall)$$

Sometimes it is adapted as the adjusted F score when more weighting is given to either precision or recall. (As always, it depends on the purpose of your test!) When the importance of both precision and recall are equal, F_1-score is calculated. Where recall is deemed more important than precision, a heavier weight is assigned to it, and F_2-score should be calculated; conversely, when greater weight should be assigned to precision, $F_{0.5}$- score is appropriate. It is therefore very important to consider which is more important to answer the research question – sensitivity/specificity, precision/recall?

The answer is, as you might imagine, that it depends. What is the purpose of your test? Back to our dog/cat example:

If you are trying to find photos of dogs but don't want to go through the manual process of checking the predictions, you'd want a highly specific model (i.e. most of the predicted dogs will be dogs).

On the other hand, if you wanted as many dog images as possible and didn't mind checking them, you would want a highly sensitive (high recall) model.

Screening and diagnostic tools have different purposes, and different sensitivities may be of value. A screening tool requires a high sensitivity to detect most potential cases. A moderate specificity is acceptable as further diagnostic procedures can clarify results. A diagnostic tool requires both a high specificity to confirm the diagnosis and high sensitivity to ensure no cases are missed. By tailoring the sensitivity and specificity threshold to the tool's purpose, healthcare providers can balance the risks of false positives and false negatives.

BUT…You can't have it all!

- Sensitivity and specificity are intimately related.

- As we increase the model sensitivity, the specificity will decline and vice versa. This concept is known as the sensitivity–specificity trade-off. It is essential to interpret the value of one in the context of the other.

Imagine you use the C-reactive protein (CRP) to investigate active vasculitis. Setting a CRP cut-off of 4 mg/L (within the normal range) will recognise virtually all cases of active vasculitis (high sensitivity), but many of the predicted cases will be normal (low specificity). In contrast, setting the CRP cut-off at 50 will mean many more cases will correctly be active vasculitis (high specificity), but at the cost of many missed cases (low sensitivity). In practice, low-specificity screening tools can significantly burden healthcare systems by increasing investigation and follow-up workload, potentially misallocating resources and contributing to patient stress. Greig [5] offers an example of this in practice and highlights how the low prevalence of HIV affects the positive predictive value of a typical HIV assay. In another example, Devaraj et al. [6] report several iterations of a model to screen for cataracts to find an acceptable sensitivity and specificity.

4.3.4 The ROC Curve

One of the most common graphical representations of classification model performance is the receiver operating characteristics (ROC) curve. The video at https://youtu.be/iW0y8ZN973w will explain the importance of the ROC curve and area under the curve for assessing classification model performance. De Fauw et al. [7] report on their deep learning model for the multiclassification of retinal scans into four categories – urgent, semi-urgent, routine and normal. They assessed area under the receiver operating characteristic curve, confusion matrices and accuracy to evaluate models. Additionally, Al-Timemy et al. [8] report on their deep learning model for detecting keratoconus; images were classified as normal, suspect and keratoconus. They assessed area under the receiver operating characteristic curve (AUC), confusion matrices, accuracy, and F1 score to evaluate models.

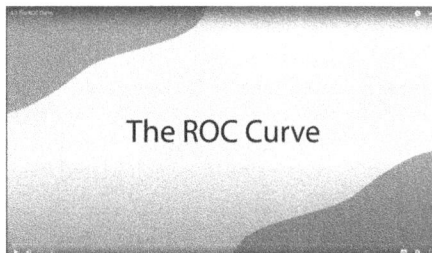

The ROC Curve

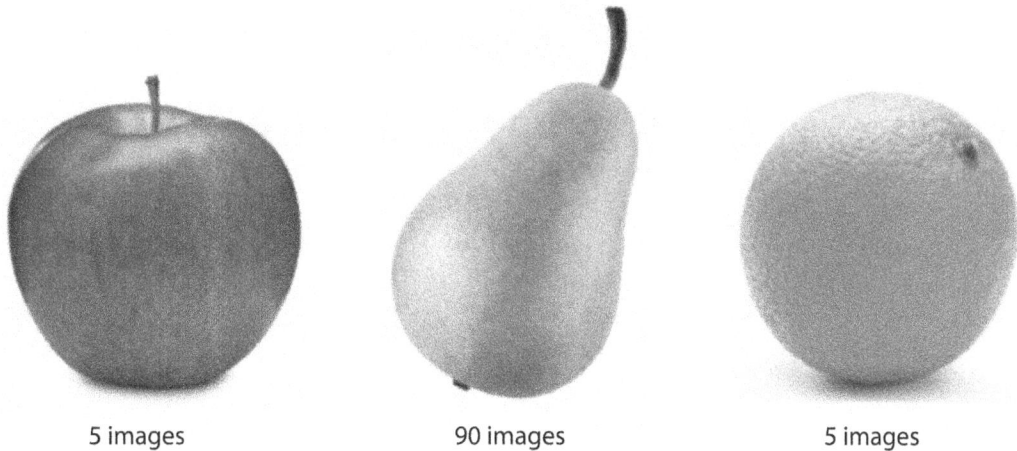

| 5 images | 90 images | 5 images |

Figure 4.9 Image input examples – apple, pear and orange.

4.3.5 Multiclassification Performance

As mentioned in the ROC curve video, with the one-vs-all approach, you can evaluate the performance of a multiclassification model using measures for binary classifiers.

However, there are specific performance measures for multiclassification.

Cohen's kappa statistic is one such measure. Cohen's kappa statistic takes into account the prevalence of different classes, by comparing the model performance to a random multiclassification based on the class distribution.

As an example, imagine you have a dataset of pictures (e.g. Figure 4.9) and want to develop an image classifier:

There are three classes, but the majority of images are of one particular class (pears). As mentioned earlier, a classifier that outputs pears every time will have a high accuracy but obviously isn't very helpful. Cohen's kappa takes this class imbalance into account by incorporating that probability.

$$\mathbf{Kappa} = 1 - \big((1 - \rho 0) / (1 - \rho e) \big)$$

$\rho 0$ is the observed agreement (your classifier).

ρe is what you would expect based on randomly guessing according to the prevalence of the class.

4.4 METHODS OF MODEL VALIDATION

We've covered the different ways of measuring the performance of a model but what data do you use to test its performance?

■ Random parts of the same data?

■ Unseen data from the dataset?

■ An entirely different dataset?

The process of evaluating model performance is called *validation*.

Validation can take different forms. For evaluating how a model generalises, external validation is of the greatest value (ideally even performed by another set of investigators).

In internal validation, the measures of performance are generally restricted to the same overall dataset from which the model was developed (Figure 4.10).

In machine learning research, this is usually through a split-sample approach where a pre-specified subset of the full dataset (usually 10–20%, termed the *test set*, but can also be called the *validation set*) is set aside for testing the performance. This is therefore a completely unseen dataset but sourced from the same original full dataset.

An alternative approach for internal validation is to use resampling methods. These methods involve resampling data multiple times. There are two main types:

1. Bootstrapping – lots of small subsets are made from a dataset with replacement. Each subset is the same size as the original dataset.

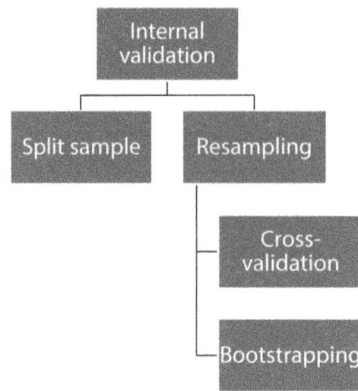

Figure 4.10 Internal validation options flowchart.

2. Cross validation – the dataset is divided into many groups and each group can be used as a potential test set. The number of divisions can be stipulated but is often either five or ten (you may see in papers, for example, that a 'ten-fold cross validation' was performed).

One of the benefits of these methods is that they can produce multiple estimates of the population parameter. Remember our soup analogy? It's like taking multiple spoonsful of soup to get an idea of the variability of the taste.

4.4.1 Validation and Model Fit

Here's a video example of external validation and model fit. As before, please type this URL into your search engine: https://youtu.be/oyeBdf7ryTU

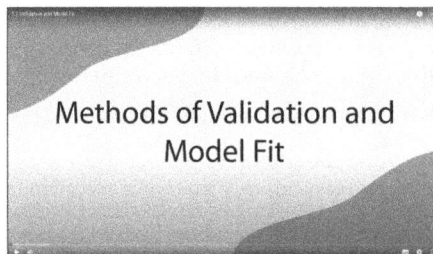

In the examples offered in the video, Ting and Wong [9] report the external validation of the model by Poplin et al. [2]. The external validation was carried out by an independent group. Additionally, Attia et al. [10] demonstrate that an AI-enabled ECG acquired during normal sinus rhythm permits point-of-care identification of individuals with a high likelihood of atrial fibrillation, with the external validation of the model reported by Gruwez et al. [11].

4.5 SUMMARY

This chapter covered descriptive statistical concepts, prediction models and the most commonly used performance metrics for evaluating them. Other performance metrics exist, such as Dice coefficients and Frechet inception distance, but these are beyond the scope of this chapter.

Some of the key takeaways are as follows:

- Measure of performance depends on whether the task is classification or regression.

- Performance of regression models is through MAE, RMSE, R2 and visually through Bland–Altman plot.

- Performance of classification models is through sensitivity, specificity, positive/negative predictive value and visually through the ROC curve.

- Sensitivity should be interpreted only in the context of the associated specificity for machine learning models.

- Validation can be internal or external. External validation provides a way of assessing generalisability of a model.

The receiver operating characteristics curve and confusion matrices are the most common displays of model performance that you will see in the literature. If you want to delve further into the subject, take a look at the further readings at the end of this chapter.

Reporting guidelines – Transparent Reporting of a multivariable prediction model for Individual Prognosis Or Diagnosis (TRIPOD) – were published in 2015 to provide the minimum reporting recommendations for studies developing or evaluating the performance of a prediction model. TRIPOD was updated with an AI extension in 2024. You will find this in the further reading section below. The Standards for Reporting of Diagnostic Accuracy Study (STARD) guidelines, published in 2015, were developed to improve the completeness and transparency of reporting in studies investigating diagnostic test accuracy. An AI extension should be published soon.

4.6 EDITORS' COMMENTS

This chapter introduced the reader to many of the performance metrics used in the reporting of AI studies. Understanding these metrics is particularly important for clinicians assessing model performance prior to clinical implementation. Some of the reporting metrics used in AI studies may not be immediately familiar to clinicians, including precision, recall and F-score; however, measures such as these and other 'prevalence agnostic' measures are vitally important when considering imbalanced classes, as is frequently the case in medicine, where the pathology class is usually the minority class. Class balancing may be included in the methodology in some studies, but this will not always be the case. The implications of missed pathology may have unfavourable outcomes for the patient; however, overdiagnosis can also have service provision implications through wasted resources as well as impacting the patient through unnecessary additional investigations. Knowledge of the most important reporting metrics is therefore essential when evaluating the performance of a model relative to the clinical task. This is further addressed in the context of computer vision in radiology by Rainey et al. [12]. There is no requirement for all clinicians to be statisticians, however, and adequate knowledge is required for critical engagement with the literature.

REFERENCES

1. Menzies, S.W., Sinz, C., Menzies, M. et al. (2023) Comparison of Humans Versus Mobile Phone-Powered Artificial Intelligence for the Diagnosis and Management of Pigmented Skin Cancer in Secondary Care: A Multicentre, Prospective, Diagnostic, Clinical Trial. Lancet Digit. Health. 5:e679–e691. https://doi.org/10.1016/S2589-7500(23)00130-9
2. Poplin, R., Varadarajan, A.V., Blumer, K. et al. (2018) Prediction of Cardiovascular Risk Factors from Retinal fundus Photographs via Deep Learning. Nat Biomed Eng. 2:158–164. https://doi.org/10.1038/s41551-018-0195-0
3. Jin, J., Dong, B., Ye, C. et al. (2023) A Noninvasive Technology Using Artificial Intelligence to Measure the Diameter of Esophageal Varices Under Endoscopy. Surg Laparosc Endosc Percutan Tech. 33:282. https://doi.org/10.1097/SLE.0000000000001168
4. Ludbrook, J. (2010) Confidence in Altman–Bland Plots: A Critical Review of the Method Ofdifferences. Clin Exp Pharmacol Physiol. 37:143–149. https://doi.org/10.1111/j.1440-1681.2009.05288.x
5. Greig, J.R., Batchelor, D., Wallis, M. (2013) Positive Predictive Value Is Poor in Low-Riskpopulations Seen in Universal Screening for HIV Infection. BMJ. 346:f3575. https://doi.org/10.1136/bmj.f3575
6. Devaraj, M., Namasivayam, V., Srichandan, S.S. et al. (2024) Development and Testing of Artificial Intelligence-Based Mobile Application to Achieve Cataract Backlog-Free Status in Uttar Pradesh, India. Asia Pac J Ophthalmol. 13:100094. https://doi.org/10.1016/j.apjo.2024.100094
7. De Fauw, J., Ledsam, J.R., Romera-Paredes, B. et al. (2018) Clinically Applicable Deep Learning for Diagnosis and Referral in Retinal Disease. Nat Med. 24:1342–1350. https://doi.org/10.1038/s41591-018-0107-6
8. Al-Timemy, A.H., Mosa, Z.M., Alyasseri, Z. et al. (2021) A Hybrid Deep Learning Construct for Detecting Keratoconus from Corneal Maps. Transl Vis Sci Technol. 10:16. https://doi.org/10.1167/tvst.10.14.16
9. Ting, D.S.W., Wong, T.Y. (2018) Eyeing Cardiovascular Risk Factors. Nat Biomed Eng. 2(3):140–141. https://doi.org/10.1038/s41551-018-0210-5
10. Attia, Z.I., Noseworthy, P.A., Lopez-Jimenez, F. et al. (2019) An Artificial Intelligence-Enabled ECG Algorithm for the Identification of Patients With Atrial Fibrillation During Sinus Rhythm: A Retrospective Analysis of Outcome Prediction. Lancet. 394:861–867. https://doi.org/10.1016/S0140-6736(19)31721-0
11. Gruwez, H., Barthel, sM., Haemers, P. et al. (2023) Detecting Paroxysmal Atrial Fibrillation From an Electrocardiogram in Sinus Rhythm: External Validation of the AI Approach. JACC Clin Electrophysiol. 9:1771–1782. https://doi.org/10.1016/j.jacep.2023.04.008
12. Rainey, C., McConnell, J., Hughes, C. et al. (2021) Artificial Intelligence for Diagnosis of Fractures on Plain Radiographs: A Scoping Review of Current Literature. Intell Based Med. 5:100033. https://doi.org/10.1016/j.ibmed.2021.100033

CHAPTER 4 FURTHER READING

TRIPOD-AI Guidance

Collins, G.S., Moons, K.G.M., Dhiman, P., Riley, R.D., Beam, A.L., Calster, B.V. (2024) TRIPOD+AI Statement: Updated Guidance for Reporting Clinical Prediction Models That Use Regression or Machine Learning Methods. BMJ. 385:e078378. https://doi.org/10.1136/bmj-2023-078378

A Clinician's Guide to Artificial Intelligence: How to Critically Appraise Machine Learning Studies (2020)

Faes, L., Liu, X., Wagner, S.K. et al. (2020) A Clinician's Guide to Artificial Intelligence: How to Critically Appraise Machine Learning Studies. Transl Vis Sci Technol. 9(7). https://doi.org/10.1167/tvst.9.2.7

On Evaluation Metrics for Medical Applications of Artificial Intelligence

Hicks, S.A., Strümke, I., Thambawita, V., Hammou, M., Riegler, M.A., Halvorsen, P., Parasa, S. (2022) On Evaluation Metrics for Medical Applications of Artificial Intelligence. Sci Rep. 12:5979. https://doi.org/10.1038/s41598-022-09954-8

Receiver Operating Characteristic Curve: Overview and Practical Use for Clinicians

Nahm, F.S. (2022) Receiver Operating Characteristic Curve: Overview and Practical Use for Clinicians. Korean J Anesthesiol. 75:25–36. https://doi.org/10.4097/kja.21209

STARD-AI Protocol (guidance should be published soon)

Sounderajah, V., Ashrafian, H., Golub, R.M. et al (2021) Developing a Reporting Guideline for Artificial Intelligence-Centred Diagnostic Test Accuracy Studies: The STARD-AI Protocol. BMJ Open. 11:e047709. https://doi.org/10.1136/bmjopen-2020-047709

5 Human–Computer Interaction and Biases Associated with Technology Use in the Context of Healthcare

Avneet Gill and Clare Rainey

5.1 HUMAN–COMPUTER INTERACTION

Human–computer interaction (HCI) concerns the usability and experience of technology from a human perspective. The study of HCI focuses on the improvement of experience with technology. This field of study is increasingly important as our everyday lives become more intertwined with computers. Subsequently, the promotion of a user-friendly experience becomes critical [1].

The study of HCI combines both psychology and the social sciences with technology. Due to its multidisciplinary and pluralistic nature of encompassing many different disciplines, there has been continuous debate around the defined disciplinary nature of HCI [2, 3]. Dix [4] outlined the importance of focusing on the methodological components of HCI research, conducting this in an organised and robust way, in maintaining the disciplinary nature of HCI. The unique nature of HCI is the connection between theory, i.e., ideas and concepts, with practice. Many studies have outlined the complicated and overlapping relationships HCI has with components such as user experience, interaction design, behavioural sciences and engineering [5]. It also continues to have a wide societal impact through the investigation of HCI in the context of education, healthcare and environmental sciences.

One of the key factors studied by HCI researchers is human cognitive bias [6]. Cognitive biases go hand in hand with human decision-making and affect the way an individual perceives the world. This may not be logical or rational as it is not based on objective facts. Tversky and Kahneman [7] pioneered the work on cognitive bias and heuristics, identifying that heuristics, or mental shortcuts, could be misconceived or inferred incorrectly leading to non-logical and simplistic cognitive biases in humans. There are many different types of cognitive biases, such as confirmation, anchoring, automation and availability bias [8]. Some examples of known human biases in the healthcare context are presented in Table 5.1 [9].

This also relates heavily to the deployment of artificial intelligence (AI) in everyday life, as this has increased rapidly over the past decade, specifically in assisting human experts in settings such as healthcare, finance and the criminal justice system [8]. Humans faced with basic and more cognitive tasks want to optimise the benefits of their surroundings, using the most important information available and disregarding extraneous data. Modern forms of AI attempt to mimic this rationality; however, when humans use their own 'mental shortcuts', they organically establish their own 'subjective social reality'. This means that, as humans, we tend to make decisions based on myriad subjective factors which are, at times, inexplicable, even to ourselves. This could imply that AI systems

Table 5.1 Human Biases in the Context of Radiological Image Interpretation

Bias	Definition
Attribution bias	Diagnosis of a clinical condition based on known attributes of the presenting patient (i.e., stereotyping)
Alliterative bias	Bias caused by the findings from previous examinations impacting the findings of the current examination.
Availability bias	Diagnostic decisions based on other, unrelated recent cases which may have come to the attention of the reader
Regret bias	Overdiagnosis of a condition resulting from a previous miss or underdiagnosis
Framing bias	Error resulting from the reader viewing the examination through the lens of the clinical question ('framing') and therefore potentially missing other information from the examination
Premature closure/ Satisfaction of search	Initial findings accepted as final diagnosis without further scrutiny or verification of findings
Anchoring bias	Related to the above, where the reader becomes fixated on their first opinion/ diagnosis and discounts other information which disputes initial diagnosis
Confirmation bias	The reader seeks out supporting information to support initial finding, related to anchoring bias

DOI: 10.1201/9781032709956-5

are also susceptible, and potentially magnify, human cognitive biases as many of them are trained on human-generated datasets [8, 10]. When considering the impact of cognitive biases within the human–computer interaction element of AI, there subsequently exists a complicated relationship affected by many factors. An understanding of these cognitive biases is a step towards human acceptance, responsible engagement with and integration of the technology, where appropriate.

5.2 HUMAN–COMPUTER INTERACTION RELATING TO ARTIFICIAL INTELLIGENCE

The field of HCI is involved in the development, design and evaluation of user studies in relation to computing systems. This also involves engagement with user-experience (UX) research to improve the usability of technology [11]. In the past few decades, HCI has made significant milestones from the introduction of the graphical user interface (GUI) from the previous text-based interface and is now used commonly for all technology, such as computers and mobile phones [12, 13]. Human–computer interaction devices include, for example, the keyboard, mouse, pressure pen and joystick, whereas 'computer–human interactive' devices include printers, monitors and speakers [12]. Previously, there has been confusion around the scientific core of HCI and queries around the methodological thinking in HCI as the technological and social context of the field has rapidly expanded [4]. More recently, the combination of voice, vision and text multimodal information has been used to influence the upgrade of HCI technology, with gesture interaction technology becoming an increasingly important part of the field [12]. With the introduction of machine learning (ML) and deep learning (DL), there has been an acceleration around research in HCI. ML and DL are now commonly referred to as 'AI' [14]. DL is essentially based on the building of models that emulate neural connections in the human brain and the learning techniques relating to deep neural networks (DNNs). (See Chapter 2 for more detail [12, 14, 15]). Research has suggested that the adoption of DL in the field of HCI could improve the accuracy of speech/image recognition and, importantly, make interactions more realistic [12]. Interestingly, the concept of human-centred machine learning (HCML) is an emerging research field which gained popularity in the mid-2010s, alongside the beginning of the DL era. This is a research field exploring the methods of aligning ML systems with human goals and ways of working. It has been proposed to bridge the divide between model performance and end-user integration [14]. HCML forms a subset of the field of human-centred AI (HCAI), which has a primary focus on optimisation of intelligent systems' interaction and design [16]. It has been suggested that HCAI requires a better understanding of the societal impact of AI to enhance user experience [17]. Though research gaps and existing challenges have been identified considering HCML and HCAI [14, 16], there exist similarities with the field of HCI and the field of AI. This has importance due to the fast-growing field of AI and the need for the field of HCI involvement to create mutually beneficial outcomes for humans.

5.3 HUMAN BIASES: DIFFERENT TYPES OF COGNITIVE BIASES

Human bias, as a general term, has been defined as a systematic tendency to repeat the same error in different settings or as time progresses [18]. Interestingly, people are usually unaware of their own biases and there may be an inclination to rationalise our own biased tendencies. In the field of statistics, bias refers to 'systematic distortion of a statistic' [19]. AI algorithms are subject to algorithmic bias through the ingestion of unchecked and biased information or samples, leading to biased predictions. There are many different biases that can be introduced during AI development. One example is 'iterative algorithmic bias' which can occur during the human labelling process for the construction of training sets for ML models. As the human is used to provide a 'label' for the data, the biases or inaccuracies originating in the human are retained in the dataset. This data are then used to update the machine learning algorithm prediction model and consequently affect the learned model with bias in following iterations, particularly if the same data are used repeatedly in training [19]. Although this type of algorithmic bias occurs as a result of human input, the nuances of human biases are, in general, difficult to study due to the complexities of the human condition, for instance, cultural background, education, work and contextual programming environment [18].

5.3.1 The Impact of Human Biases on Cognition

There is an existing body of literature that demonstrates how cognitive bias affects human deliberations [20]. Why cognitive biases occur has been explained with dual-processing theories – automatic (System 1/'bottom-up') and controlled (System 2/'top down') processes [21]. The brain's preferred cognitive state is 'System 1', i.e., fast or automatic thinking, that relies on heuristics and works outside of conscious awareness. Human or cognitive biases result when System 1 is used in situations of uncertainty, i.e., in algorithmic development, when System 2 should be used instead. System 2

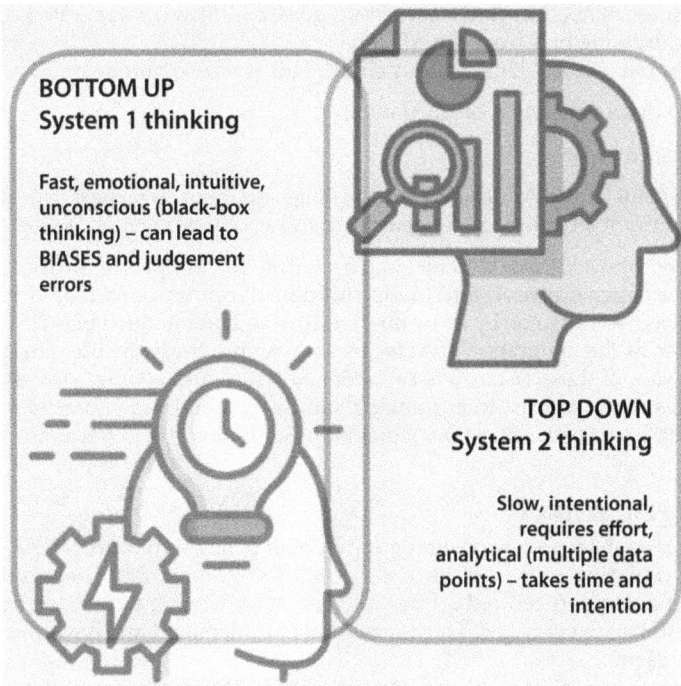

Figure 5.1 Differentiation between bottom-up (System 1) and top-down (System 2) thinking (see also [21]) has direct impact on the patients and can lead to fatality, misdiagnoses and an inability to generalise findings of the technology [23].

employs a slower analytical and cognitive process, though this mode is not easily attained and requires conscious effort (Figure 5.1). Cognitive bias ultimately reduces the amount of information that requires processing and is therefore efficient [6, 18, 21]. Cognitive bias results when processing information in AI development that is too complex or the volume of the information is too high. It can also occur for humans having to make a judgement in a short amount of time or not having enough information to make a full judgement [18].

There are several groups of the human population that have a long history of misrepresentation and absence from existing biomedical datasets, which introduced gender, sexual orientation and socio-economic standing biases. Data-driven bias exists commonly in most fields of human research, with a bias towards participants that fit the Western, educated, industrialised, rich, democratic (WEIRD) profile [22]. With many AI datasets used to train AI algorithms being collected in this context, algorithmic bias is introduced, as described in the previous paragraph [23]. Unfortunately, it is objectively impossible to quantify the number of different biases within a dataset. For example, socioeconomic standing or sexual orientation is unable to be identified within a biomedical dataset unless collected as additional metadata within AI development. This may carry significant weight in healthcare, causing the detriment of AI reinforcing these biases.

Furthermore, the transfer of bias is not strictly unidirectional. It has also been found that humans can inherit bias from AI. Humans can do this through the reproduction of AI models' bias in their own decisions, despite moving to a scenario without AI [24]. Conformity bias is the tendency to listen to others' opinions, hence confirm and conform to them, and essentially consider others more expert than they factually are [25, 26]. This conformity bias in the context of human–computer interaction in AI development can lead to conformity in two contexts: trust in a human second opinion or trust in the AI technology decision (also known as automation bias, as described by, e.g., Bond et al. [27] and Rainey et al. [28]). Research on a study investigating ECG and humans' conformity bias to AI for ECG abnormality detection suggested that opinions should not be displayed to doctors involved in second opinion services before their own interpretation has been made, as conformity and prejudice result from either the AI or second human opinion [25]. Novel research on generative AI, specifically large language models (LLMs), commonly used AI technology in information-seeking or decision-making for productivity improvement, found similar biases noted with other forms of AI. Techniques such as devil's advocate questioning were suggested to be appropriate interventions at addressing bias from the AI [26].

There is the question of a resultant 'vicious circle'. This is due to humans

1. contributing to the construction of an AI dataset,

2. labelling the data and/or

3. having involvement in the AI design process alongside their own cognitive biases, i.e., conformity, gender, authority, cultural, socio-economic and sexual orientation biases.

These in turn feed into a biased AI model and are ultimately trained on further biased data from humans, in the case of generative AI and LLMs, through algorithmic and data-driven biases. These AI findings are then over-relied on by some humans, through automation bias [25, 28], and the cycle continues. However, as the integration of AI technology within everyday life is in its infancy, we are becoming more aware of these issues. We can identify issues and attempt, as best as humans can, to design the biases out or at least to minimise them. For example, members of underrepresented groups can contribute to the identification of bias alongside solutions, in the matter of AI design and deployment [23].

5.4 ETHICAL IMPLICATIONS

Traditional AI research had a focus on emulating human behaviour; however, AI engineering currently focuses on replacing human tasks, e.g., speech recognition, facial recognition and natural language processing. Human-centred AI has a focus on enhancing human performance to make systems reliable and trustworthy [29]. This is essential to understand and have awareness of human cognitive biases present.

It is vitally important to ensure that adherence to ethical standards is central to the implementation and deployment of AI in healthcare. This is, in part, due to the impact that AI can have on both the patient directly and other health economics-based factors such as resource allocation [30]. The ethical considerations of AI include both functional and quality requirements [31]. Research exploring ethical AI has begun to grow significantly since 2018 and this will continue as AI modifies to meet the needs of the users [32].

Shneiderman [29] offers a three-layer structured framework to govern HCAI systems to maintain reliability, safety and trustworthiness. It is suggested that concepts such as privacy, environmental protection, human rights, security and social justice are also concerns that need to be addressed during technology development. Other recommendations such as Ethically Aligned Design (EAD) from the Institute of Electrical and Electronic Engineers (IEEE), focus on ethical principles such as human well-being and reduction of bias in the development of autonomous and intelligent systems [33]. Six 'grand challenges' have also been identified by researchers, with a recommendation to produce HCAI that is centred in

1. improving human well-being,

2. utilisation of responsible design principles,

3. adherence to privacy standards,

4. appropriate co-design and evaluation of models with humans whilst respecting their cognitive capacities,

5. adherence to HCAI standards through all stages of the AI life cycle, including inception of the idea to implementation and

6. strict governance and external oversight (for further information: Garibay et al. [34], Figure 5.2).

5.4.1 Sensitive Data

In the context of healthcare, a major ethical concern in AI and ML development, implementation and ongoing clinical use is the use of sensitive medical data. This includes the use of patient data for the training dataset used to train the ML algorithm, monitoring the post-deployment dataset in practice and ethical use of the data thereafter [29, 30, 35].

Furthermore, to mitigate the risks associated with human and data-driven biases, there is a need for in-depth testing of training datasets to ensure the data is up to date and is representative of the target population [29]. Another ethical dilemma that needs more investigation is the use of AI

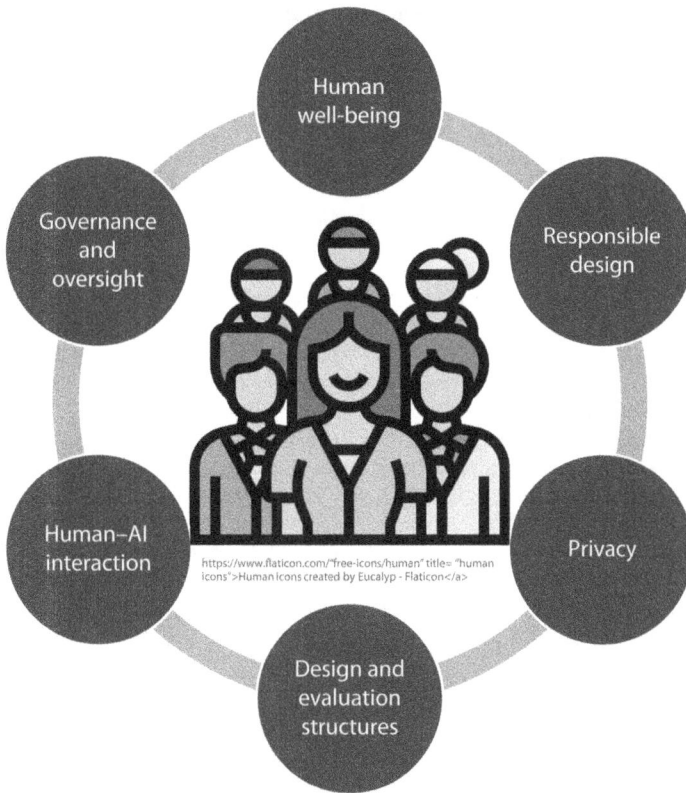

Figure 5.2 'Six grand challenges' for human-centred AI. (See also [34].)

technology in improving the lives of people with disabilities through the removal of obstacles. Any security breaches, data anonymisation issues and data storage strategies need to be focused on the mitigation of risks linked to AI applications. This is in line with international data use regulations, such as the General Data Protection Regulations (GDPR) in the European Union and the Health Insurance Portability and Accountability (HIPAA) in the United States [30].

5.4.2 Transparency and Explainability

Opacity, scale and harm are three important components of AI and ML algorithms when there are consequential applications of the technology, such as granting parole or processing mortgage applications [29]. This opacity could relate to the transparency of AI technology, which is the *openness and accessibility of information about the decision-making processes of AI* [30]. Shneiderman's three-layer governing ethical framework for AI development includes trustworthiness as an integral component, which is aligned closely with transparency [29]. Additionally, the use of transparent and explainable AI and interpretable ML could allow identification of bias evident in the dataset, thus enabling stakeholders to develop strategies to address these [30].

Explainability differs to transparency as this refers to stakeholders' ability to understand AI outputs in a meaningful way. Both concepts are integral to trust [30]. Research has found a close relationship amongst explainability, transparency and trustworthiness of AI technology [31]. There is a requirement for user trust to support the integration of the technology into practice. Currently explainability in AI is a growing research field; however, much of the literature is concerned with the design/technical challenges, rather than the human-related facets of implementation [32]. Interestingly, it has been suggested that the explainable AI (XAI) field, though it adds explainability to models, does not take a human-centred approach. An approach, therefore, is needed in design that combines both human-centred AI and XAI [14].

Further research is subsequently needed in the field; however, it is evident that explainability and transparency are part of the ethical grounding needed to guide the design of ethically robust explainable AI systems [32, 36].

5.4.3 Governing Frameworks

Due to the differences AI and ML algorithms have in comparison to other interventions in the medical field, no clinical trials are permitted before regulatory approval to ensure the safety of the products. There is, therefore, a subsequent need for standardised frameworks to validate the technology, including rigorous testing, standardisation of performance metrics, model development and validation of study design [30]. Research has suggested the use of sound technical and software engineering practices to produce reliable HCAI systems [29]. Recommendations also suggest that AI developers need to employ 'algorithmic fairness techniques' to identify and address biases in ML models, e.g., fairness-aware training algorithms which aim to optimise AI models for metrics such as demographics [30]. Additionally, there should be adoption of findable, accessible, interoperable and reusable (FAIR) principles when building AI datasets, training AI models and testing (Figure 5.3). Transparency of the training and testing of AI, and the resultant possibility for reproducibility and independent testing, may increase acceptance. Cerejo and Carvalhais [37] suggest the use of anticipatory design principles in the field of AI and ML, i.e., for AI designers to involve human-centred design principles and understand the user's future desires and needs whilst developing the technology. This could prove useful in future governing frameworks encompassing the ethical considerations of AI for users.

As detailed in the previous section, data or human biases can have detrimental effect on the industry that deploys AI technology. There is a subsequent need for all stakeholders involved in technology deployment to take this responsibility and be involved. For example, in the medical field, this would include healthcare providers, patient advocate groups and others, not solely those involved in technology design [30]. Especially in environments such as healthcare, ethical principles are integral to responsible AI integration, with a wider scope than AI affecting solely patients. AI in healthcare may have a wide potential societal impact concerning health inequalities and disparities. Further to this, there is a need for the different HCAI techniques to be applied to the different domains of AI development, including education, healthcare and environmental protection. There is not a 'one size fits all' approach that can be taken, as each avenue requires an adapted approach to HCAI [29, 38].

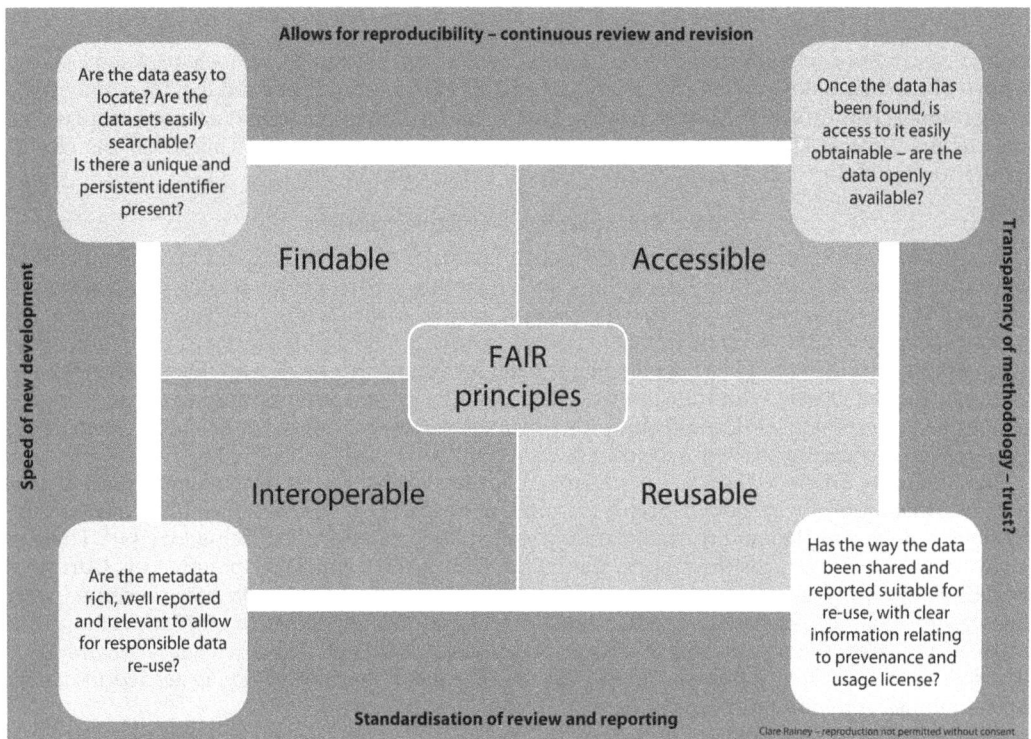

Figure 5.3 FAIR principles in relation to the AI development cycle.

5.5 USER DESIGN AND USER EXPERIENCE WITHIN HCI AND AI

The importance of incorporating the components of HCI into the design and use of AI has been high-lighted as integral to ensure as little harm to humans as possible [16, 38]. Non-automated AI-based systems may have some autonomous features and, therefore, the ability to perform specific tasks independently. This evolution into human-like features, and results that can be non-deterministic and autonomous, can be used to understand the technology's level of intelligence. This has brought a paradigmatic shift within the human–machine relationship and there is a fear that, if humans are not involved in the design process of the technology, there could be issues with safety. Despite its wide number of uses in applications across all industries, there are threats posed to human health and well-being via political, economic, social and more determinants of health using AI [39]. Fortunately, the field of HCI is becoming an inherent part of the creation of ethical and trustworthy AI technology. Interestingly, it has been suggested that human-like features on AI-powered chat-bots are a positive predictor of social presence and psychological ownership. These factors indicate a continuation intention of the technology [40], indicating that AI technology with human features and likeness will encourage use.

There is a pressing need to focus designs on user needs and overall usability, which should be tested continually [41]. This aligned with Norman and Draper's [42] concept of User-Centred Design. User-centred design (UCD) is the methodology or discipline that encompasses the inclusion of end users throughout the development process, to ensure the design accurately meets user needs and goals. UCD practices underline the importance of an iterative process when concerned with design alongside gaining valuable insights from users [43]. Currently, UCD is used in many dif-ferent industry applications, including e-learning modules for education and mobile phone appli-cations encompassing user-centred principles. These are used to form evaluation metrics such as questionnaires [44, 45]. UCD also incorporates life-cycle-stage design, including identification of the problem, testing and maintenance. The design is essentially formed with continuous feedback to be better [45]. UCD has also been suggested as a type of design principle to be used in the cre-ation of AI to address user concerns and issues, particularly in healthcare AI [46, 47]. User-centred designs address unmet needs and break barriers, especially in the case of assistive technologies [46]. Helpfully, Gulliksen et al. [48] identified 12 principles that should be incorporated within UCD:

- User focus
- Active user involvement
- Evolutionary system development
- Simple design representations
- Prototyping
- Evaluation of use in context
- Explicit and conscious design activities
- A professional attitude
- Usability champion
- Holistic design principles
- Processes customisation
- User-centred attitude to be established throughout

An understanding of how AI can be used for user experience has significant implications for research and practice. Research bringing the two together has grown over the past few years [49]. The use of datasets containing user data essentially enables AI to facilitate the creation of adaptive user interfaces that evolve based on the changing requirements of end users. This is especially important as inferior UX can lead to non-use by users and is associated with technological stress, fatigue and misuse. Contrarily, there has also been argument that use of AI in UX design pro-cesses could be a risk factor for lack of autonomy, misalignment and potential job displacement [49]. Despite concern over setbacks from junior designers affected by creativity exhaustion or skill degra-dation, there is a way forward encompassing responsible human-AI collaboration in UX design [50].

AI development with a focus on empathy, creativity and iterative design processes can result from a human-centred approach [50, 51]. Similarly, design thinking (DT) has understanding and empathy with end users at the forefront of the practice through centring the design process around needs of people. Integrating AI with design thinking maintains a human-centred view by fusing insights that are driven by data with sympathetic comprehension. For example, successful ventures using both design thinking and AI include the PillPack, a medication-dispensing process, or Spotify, a music streaming service. Spotify uses AI to make song recommendations and uses design thinking to create playlists customised to each user's preference. Spotify's UX design is simple and promotes ease of use to relieve cognitive burden and enhance user engagement [51]. The same principles could be suggested in AI development, incorporating UCD and DT as contributors.

As the complexity of the contributions of AI technology increase, the effective communication between users becomes imperative [12]. The level of complication of the user interface affects engagement directly [52]. User interface is the way the user engages with a device. A few of the different user interfaces in the field of AI include intelligent or adaptive user interfaces (IUIs, AUIs) and explanation user interfaces (EUIs) [53, 54]. Some of the important usability factors in intelligent user interfaces include accuracy, predictability, task complexity and interaction frequency. These may differ to a non-AI user interface [53]. There are many differences that need to be considered with AI interfaces in comparison to the conventional methods, particularly including design methodologies [55]. This is largely because AI interfaces invest more into the longer-term interactions compared to conventional interfaces; i.e., training a model takes time before the benefit of the learning is demonstrated. However, with AI interfaces, a system–user collaboration is cultivated [55].

Interestingly, older perceptions about AI user interfaces suggested concern that the heuristic nature of AI would lead to an unreliable interface or that AI's focus on mimicking human decision-making would override the users' decisions [55]. More recent research suggests that there are two ways that can be taken to design a user interface: either intelligently adaptive or separately tailor-made to the user [52]. These fears surrounding human decision-making being overridden by the AI remain; however, the design of user interfaces of AI has developed to be agile following user feedback. This outlines the importance of the amount of adaptation required to ensure an interface is usable for users from cross-cultural backgrounds and the essentiality of considering the accessibility of a user interface for people with a disability, non-technical professional people and older adults [52].

Cognitive workload is a concept to consider when concerned with UX research within the field of HCI. It is seen as a factor that should be kept to a minimum or engaging level to enhance the user experience [11]. Acknowledgement of cognitive load has been found useful in the design of user interfaces, through a constructive approach where cognitive workload is measured to improve designs, or a summative approach using existing systems to evaluate the cognitive workload with different visualisations [11, 56]. Despite acknowledgement of cognitive workload within the HCI field, there are no universal definitions or measures currently. The NASA-Task Load Index questionnaire, which has commonly been used to assess cognitive load, is a multidimensional subjective tool encompassing subjects such as mental load and frustration [11]. The understanding of cognitive load for tasks is a topic of primary concern in healthcare AI, due to short staffing amongst many different healthcare professions and the sentiment that a higher cognitive load is associated with clinician burnout [56]. AI technology relating to electronic health records that is designed effectively and efficiently could reduce this cognitive load on clinicians. Designed poorly, this could have a negative effect on clinicians, and this solidifies the need for AI to be designed with end-user input to reduce and improve existing biases [56].

User interfaces in AI have also been suggested to have a focus on transparency and explanations, due to the existing complexities of machine learning algorithms [53]. (See also Chapter 3.) Additionally, the usefulness of AI user interfaces has been suggested to be dependent on factors including bias, motivation of users, the learning curve needed, the cultural background of users, the technology used to service the interface and the mode of interaction [52]. Plasticity is a more recent development used by designers to ensure user interfaces mould to the past experiences and present needs of the user. These dynamic techniques can enhance user experience [52], which in turn encourages usability. This is especially important to reduce the amount of human bias introduced during user interface development. Chromik [54] also recommended four principles to be incorporated in EUIs: responsiveness, sensitivity, naturalness and flexibility. This is in addition to transparency components such as progressive disclosure. Progressive disclosure is where an interaction with a user is kept track of and resultant data organised hierarchically to consequently disclose information progressively, e.g., a user clicks another button to allow a multi-dimensional visual explanation [54, 57]. Despite the iterative, transparent and explainable recommendations for AI user interfaces, there is still a lack of standardisation of testing tools and evaluation protocols [53]. Due to the nature of AI and personalised interfaces and difficulty in making comparisons between users, the evaluation of these must differ to the conventional processes [55]. There exists an opportunity for the joint evaluation of UX- and AI-related user interfaces [53]. The sphere of AI user interfaces requires further research to establish a standardised evaluation measures and further work on the inclusion of all users.

5.6 CONCLUSION

In this chapter we explored human–computer interaction and the different aspects of artificial intelligence that merge with the field. Human cognitive biases are one of the key factors studied by HCI researchers and common amongst everyone [6]. This could imply that AI systems are also susceptible to human cognitive biases, as many of them are trained on human-generated datasets [8, 10]. There was an establishment of the need to approach the integration of AI and ML to uphold high ethical standards, due to impact the technology has, e.g., streamlining patient pathways in the healthcare setting [30]. The ethical considerations of AI importantly were noted to have both functional and quality requirements [31]. Continuous evaluation and security around AI datasets for humans and the subsequent requirement for a governing framework are key in supporting high ethical standards. This should include considerations in relation to explainability, transparency and trustworthiness of AI technology and refers to the human trust of the technology to allow integration into a variety of industries [31]. Principles such as explainability in AI are emerging and require more of a human-related implementation strategy, instead of the focus that is maintained on the design and technical challenges [32]. This in turn could allow for a clearer vision when addressing human cognitive biases in the development of AI and ML algorithms. Discussion around user experience and user-centred design allow for insight into the different human cognitive biases that can result from a user perspective when using AI. The importance of integrating AI with design thinking maintains a human-centred view, by fusing insights that are driven by data with sympathetic comprehension of the human perspective [51]. Finally, the most important part of AI technology to humans, the user interface, allows identification of nuances that are needed to support the interface, such as datasets covering wide populations and cultures alongside the different features necessary for success, e.g. responsiveness, sensitivity, naturalness and flexibility [52, 54]. It is evident that more focussed research in this field will help developers and users in their ongoing struggle to develop AI that incorporates HCI principles and limits human bias. Although human bias cannot be avoided in the development of AI, it should be considered and recognised as a necessary component of the process.

5.7 EDITORS' COMMENTS

It is clear, from this chapter, that an understanding of the human–AI relationship is key. This is not only for a consideration of the use of AI tools, which is an obvious area of focus, but also for the design of the technology. Design of AI tools that assist humans, whilst allowing them to maintain their 'humanness,' will support responsible AI use and deployment. Human oversight of the ongoing requirements of the AI tools will be an iterative process, requiring review and revision at regular intervals during the life cycle of the system. This chapter also reminds us that inherent human biases can present substantial problems when using data generated by humans to train AI. With a limited volume of data available, this human-generated data can be used repeatedly to exacerbate any bias introduced in the AI model. Ongoing vigilance will be required with user-centric design to ensure that clinicians can rely on systems developed for clinical use.

REFERENCES

1. Lawrence, D. and Ashleigh, M. (2019) Impact of Human-Computer Interaction (HCI) On Users in Higher Educational System: Southampton University as a Case Study. International Journal of Management Technology. 6(3):1–12. Available at: https://eprints.soton.ac.uk/436645/1/Impact_of_Human_Computer_Interaction_HCI_On_Users_in_Higher_Educational_System.pdf.
2. Carroll, J.M. (1997) Human Computer Interaction: Psychology as a Science of Design. Annual Review of Psychology. 48(1):61–83. https://doi.org/10.1146/annurev.psych.48.1.61
3. Diaper, D. (1989) The Discipline of HCI. Interacting With Computers. 1(1):3–5. https://doi.org/10.1016/0953-5438(89)90002-7
4. Dix, A. (2010) Human–computer Interaction: A Stable Discipline, a Nascent Science, and the Growth of the Long Tail. Interacting With Computers. 22(1):13–27. https://doi.org/10.1016/j.intcom.2009.11.007.
5. Reeves, S. (2015) Human-Computer Interaction as Science. Aarhus Series on Human Centered Computing. 1(1):12. https://doi.org/10.7146/aahcc.v1i1.21296
6. Saygi, I. and Saygi, B. (2021) The Impact of Cognitive Biases on User 21 Making in Human-Computer Interaction: A Review of the Literature. EURAS Journal of Engineering and Applied Sciences. 3(2):69–83. https://doi.org/10.17932/ejeas.2021.024/ejeas_v03i2001

7. Tversky, A. and Kahneman, D. (1974) Judgment Under Uncertainty: Heuristics and Biases. Science, New Series. 185(4157):1124–1131. https://doi.org/10.1126/science.185.4157.1124
8. Rastogi, C., Zhang, Y., Wei, D. et al. (2022) Deciding Fast and Slow: The Role of Cognitive Biases in AI-Assisted Decision-Making. Proceedings of the ACM on Human-Computer Interaction. 6(CSCW1):1–22. https://doi.org/10.1145/3512930.
9. Rainey, C. (2023) Artificial Intelligence in Radiographic Image Interpretation: An Investigation of the Impact of an AI Model on Diagnostic Accuracy, Trust and Decision Switching in Radiographers [PhD thesis]. Ulster University. Available from: https://pure.ulster.ac.uk/en/studentTheses/artificial-intelligence-in-radiographic-image-interpretation
10. Brem, A. and Rivieccio, G. (2024) Artificial Intelligence and Cognitive Biases: A Viewpoint. Journal of Innovation Economics & Management. 44(2):223–231. https://doi.org/10.3917/jie.044.0223
11. Kosch, T., Karolus, J., Zagermann, J. et al. (2023) A Survey on Measuring Cognitive Workload in Human-Computer Interaction. ACM Computing Surveys. 55(13s). https://doi.org/10.1145/3582272
12. Lv, Z., Poiesi, F., Dong, Q. et al. (2022) Deep Learning for Intelligent Human–Computer Interaction. Applied Sciences. 12(22):11457. https://doi.org/10.3390/app122211457.
13. Wersényi, G. (2010) Auditory Representations of a Graphical User Interface for a Better Human-Computer Interaction. In: Ystad S., Aramaki M., Kronland-Martinet R., Jensen K. (eds) Auditory Display. CMMR ICAD 2009 2009. Lecture Notes in Computer Science, vol 5954. Springer, Berlin, Heidelberg. https://doi.org/10.1007/978-3-642-12439-6_5
14. Kaluarachchi, T., Reis, A. and Nanayakkara, S. (2021) A Review of Recent Deep Learning Approaches in Human-Centered Machine Learning. Sensors. 21(7):2514. https://doi.org/10.3390/s21072514
15. Sarker, I.H. (2021) Deep Learning: A Comprehensive Overview on Techniques, Taxonomy, Applications and Research Directions. SN Computer Science. 2(240). https://doi.org/10.1007/s42979-021-00815-1
16. Xu, W., Dainoff, M.J., Ge, L. et al. (2022) Transitioning to Human Interaction With AI Systems: New Challenges and Opportunities for HCI Professionals to Enable Human-Centered AI. International Journal of Human–Computer Interaction. 39(3):494–518. https://doi.org/10.1080/10447318.2022.2041900
17. Bingley, W.J., Curtis, C., Lockey, S. et al. (2023) Where is the Human in Human-Centered AI? Insights from Developer Priorities and User Experiences. Computers in Human Behavior. 141:107617. https://doi.org/10.1016/j.chb.2022.107617
18. Johansen, J., Pedersen, T. and Johansen, C. (2023) Studying Human-to-Computer Bias Transference. AI & Society. 38:1659–1683. https://doi.org/10.1007/s00146-021-01328-4
19. Sun, W., Nasraoui, O. and Shafto, P. (2020) Evolution and Impact of Bias in Human and Machine Learning Algorithm Interaction. PLoS One. 15(8):e0235502. https://doi.org/10.1371/journal.pone.0235502
20. Korteling, J.E., Paradies, G.L. and Sassen-van Meer, J.P. (2023) Cognitive Bias and How to Improve Sustainable Decision Making. Frontiers in Psychology. 14(1129835). https://doi.org/10.3389/fpsyg.2023.1129835
21. Kahneman, D. (2011) Thinking, Fast and Slow. New York. Farrar, Straus and Giroux.
22. Henrich, J., Heine, S.J. and Norenzayan, A. (2010) The Weirdest People in the World? Behavioral and Brain Sciences. 33:61–83. https://doi.org/10.1017/S0140525X0999152X
23. Norori, N., Hu, Q., Aellen, F.M. et al. (2021) Addressing Bias in Big Data and AI for Health Care: A Call for Open Science. Patterns. 2(10):100347. https://doi.org/10.1016/j.patter.2021.100347
24. Vicente, L. and Matute, H. (2023) Humans Inherit Artificial Intelligence Biases. Scientific Reports. 13:15737. https://doi.org/10.1038/s41598-023-42384-8
25. Cabitza, F. (2019) Biases Affecting Human Decision Making in AI-Supported Second Opinion Settings. Modeling Decisions for Artificial Intelligence. 283–294. https://doi.org/10.1007/978-3-030-26773-5_25
26. Zhu, X., Zhang, C., Stafford, T. et al. (2024) Conformity in Large Language Models. arXiv (Cornell University). https://doi.org/10.48550/arxiv.2410.12428
27. Bond, R.R., Novotny, T., Andrsova, I. et al. (2018) Automation Bias in Medicine: The Influence of Automated Diagnoses on Interpreter Accuracy and Uncertainty When Reading Electrocardiograms. Journal of Electrocardiology. 51(6):S6–S11. https://doi.org/10.1016/j.jelectrocard.2018.08.007
28. Rainey, C., Bond, R., McConnell, J. et al. (2025) The Impact of AI Feedback on the Accuracy of Diagnosis, Decision Switching and Trust in Radiography. PLoS One. 20(5):e0322051. https://doi.org/10.1371/journal.pone.0322051
29. Shneiderman, B. (2020) Bridging the Gap Between Ethics and Practice. ACM Transactions on Interactive Intelligent Systems. 10(4):1–31. Available at: https://dl.acm.org/doi/abs/10.1145/3419764
30. Tilala, M.H., Chenchala, P.K., Choppadandi, A. et al. (2024) Ethical Considerations in the Use of Artificial Intelligence and Machine Learning in Health Care: A Comprehensive Review. Cureus. 16(6):e62443. https://doi.org/10.7759/cureus.62443
31. Balasubramaniam, N., Kauppinen, M., Rannisto, A. et al. (2023) Transparency and Explainability of AI Systems: From Ethical Guidelines to Requirements. Information and Software Technology. 159(159):107197. https://doi.org/10.1016/j.infsof.2023.107197
32. Vainio-Pekka, H., Ori-Otse Agbese,M., Jantunen, M. et al. (2023) The Role of Explainable AI in the Research Field of AI Ethics. ACM Transactions on Interactive Intelligent Systems. 13(4). https://doi.org/10.1145/3599974
33. Shahriari, K. and Shahriari, M. (2017) IEEE Standard Review—Ethically Aligned Design: A Vision for Prioritizing Human Wellbeing with Artificial Intelligence and Autonomous Systems. 2017 IEEE Canada International Humanitarian Technology Conference (IHTC), Toronto, ON, Canada, pp. 197–201. https://doi.org10.1109/IHTC.2017.8058187
34. Garibay, O., Winslow, B., Andolina, S. et al. (2023) Six Human-Centered Artificial Intelligence Grand Challenges. International Journal of Human–Computer Interaction. [online] 39(3):391–437. https://doi.org/10.1080/10447318.2022.2153320
35. Rhem, A.J. (2023) Ethical Use of Data in AI Applications. IntechOpen eBooks. https://doi.org/10.5772/intechopen.1001597
36. Nannini,L., Marchiori Manerba, M. and Beretta, I. (2024) Mapping the Landscape of Ethical Considerations in Explainable AI Research. Ethics and Information Technology. 26(3). https://doi.org/10.1007/s10676-024-09773-7
37. Cerejo, J. and Carvalhais, M. (2023) Anticipation as a Tool for Designing the Future. In: Martins, N., Brandão, D. (eds) Advances in Design and Digital Communication IV. DIGICOM 2023. Springer Series in Design and Innovation, vol 35. Springer, Cham. https://doi.org/10.1007/978-3-031-47281-7_4
38. Antona, M., Margetis, G., Ntoa, S. et al. (2023) Special Issue on AI in HCI. International Journal of Human–Computer Interaction. 1–4. https://doi.org/10.1080/10447318.2023.2177421.

39. Federspiel, F., Mitchell, R., Asokan, A. et al. (2023) Threats by Artificial Intelligence to Human Health and Human Existence. BMJ Global Health. [online] 8(5):e010435. https://doi.org/10.1136/bmjgh-2022-010435

40. Jin, S.V. and Youn, S. (2022) Social Presence and Imagery Processing as Predictors of Chatbot Continuance Intention in Human-AI-Interaction. International Journal of Human–Computer Interaction. 1–13. https://doi.org/10.1080/10447318.2022.2129277

41. Gould, J.D. and Lewis, C. (1985) Designing for Usability: Key Principles and What Designers Think. Communications of the ACM. 28(3):300–311. https://doi.org/10.1145/3166.3170

42. Norman, D.A. and Draper, S.W. (1986) User Centered System Design: New Perspectives on Human-Computer Interaction. Hillsdale, NJ: Lawrence Erlbaum.

43. Chammas, A., Quaresma, M. and Mont'Alvão, C. (2015) A Closer Look on the User Centred Design. Procedia Manufacturing. [online] 3(3):5397–5404. https://doi.org/10.1016/j.promfg.2015.07.656

44. Hasani L.M., Sensuse D.I., Kautsarina. et al. (2020) User-Centered Design of e-Learning User Interfaces: A Survey of the Practices. 2020 3rd International Conference on Computer and Informatics Engineering. (IC2IE). https://doi.org/10.1109/ic2ie50715.2020.9274623

45. Wardhana, S., Sabariah, M.K., Effendy, V. et al. (2017) User Interface Design Model for Parental Control Application on Mobile Smartphone Using User Centered Design Method. 2017 5th International Conference on Information and Communication Technology (ICoIC7). https://doi.org/10.1109/icoict.2017.8074715

46. Goerss, D., Köhler, S., Rong, E. et al. (2024) Smartwatch-Based Interventions for People with Dementia: User-Centered Design Approach. JMIR Aging. 7(1):e50107. https://doi.org/10.2196/50107

47. Fan, X., Chao, D., Zhang, Z. et al. (2021) Utilization of Self-Diagnosis Health Chatbots in Real-World Settings: Case Study. Journal of Medical Internet Research. 23(1):e19928. https://doi.org/10.2196/19928

48. Gulliksen, J., Göransson, B., Boivie, I. et al. (2003) Key Principles for User-Centred Systems Design. Behaviour & Information Technology. 22(6):397–409. https://doi.org/10.1080/01449290310001624329

49. Stige, Å, Zamani, E.D., Mikalef, P. et al. (2024) Artificial Intelligence (AI) for User Experience (UX) Design: A Systematic Literature Review and Future Research Agenda. Information Technology & People. 37(6):2324–2352. https://doi.org/10.1108/ITP-07-2022-0519

50. Li, J., Cao, H., Lin, L. et al. (2024) User Experience Design Professionals' Perceptions of Generative Artificial Intelligence. https://doi.org/10.1145/3613904.3642114

51. Sreenivasan, A. and Suresh, M. (2024) Design Thinking and Artificial Intelligence: a Systematic Literature Review Exploring Synergies. International Journal of Innovation Studies. 8(3). https://doi.org/10.1016/j.ijis.2024.05.001

52. Miraz, M.H., Ali, M. and Excell, P.S. (2021) Adaptive User Interfaces and Universal Usability Through Plasticity of User Interface Design. Computer Science Review. 40:100363. https://doi.org/10.1016/j.cosrev.2021.100363

53. Brdnik, S., Heričko, T. and Šumak, B. (2022) Intelligent User Interfaces and Their Evaluation: A Systematic Mapping Study. Sensors. 22(15):5830. https://doi.org/10.3390/s22155830

54. Chromik, M and, Butz, A. (2021) Human-XAI Interaction: A Review and Design Principles for Explanation User Interfaces. In: Ardito, C., et al. Human-Computer Interaction – INTERACT 2021. Lecture Notes in Computer Science. vol 12933. Springer, Cham. https://doi.org/10.1007/978-3-030-85616-8_36

55. Lieberman, H. (2009) User Interface Goals, AI Opportunities. AI Magazine. 30(4):16. https://doi.org/10.1609/aimag.v30i4.2266

56. Gandhi, T.K., Classen, D.C., Sinsky, C.A. et al. (2023) How can Artificial Intelligence Decrease Cognitive and Work Burden for Front Line Practitioners? JAMIA Open. 6(3). https://doi.org/10.1093/jamiaopen/ooad079

57. Springer, A. and Whittaker, S. (2018) Progressive Disclosure: Designing for Effective Transparency. arXiv.org. https://doi.org/10.48550/arXiv.1811.02164

6 Educating Clinicians of the Future in AI

Jordan Perchik

6.1 BRIEF HISTORY OF AI IN HEALTHCARE

The concept of artificial intelligence (AI) has grown to encompass a wide and diverse range of algorithms and tasks that would have been unimaginable less than a century ago. AI can be defined as a computer system that has the capability to perform human-level reasoning or perform tasks that would traditionally require human intelligence. The origins of AI can be traced back to the 1950s, with the first applications of AI in healthcare occurring in the 1970s [1]. These early AI tools included INTERNIST-1, a diagnostic assistance algorithm that could receive patient symptoms as inputs and generate a differential diagnosis [2], and MYCIN, an algorithm that used a system of input criteria to analyse patient clinical data to suggest antibiotic therapy and suggest diagnoses for infectious disease [3]. With additional advancements in machine learning techniques, convolutional neural networks, the digitisation of the health record and medical images, and the work of the Human Genome Project, AI evolved in leaps and bounds over the following decades [4, 5]. Healthcare AI now boasts applications in every specialty of medicine and promises to be the generation-defining breakthrough of medical practice in the 21st century.

Some of the most highly targeted areas for AI integration in the medical field have been in the areas of radiology, cardiology, and pathology [6], but radiology has been the dominant force in the healthcare AI marketplace [7]. This is not to say that AI research and development is not occurring in the other medical specialties. In fact, AI research and publication experienced a steady annual increase in every medical subspecialty from 2000 and 2020 [8]. However, in the early 2000s, one fundamental change set radiology and AI on a collision course, and this was the rise of picture archiving and communication systems (PACS) and the transition to a digitised radiology department [8–10].

There are several other reasons that radiology may be considered a natural fit for AI integration. Radiology is a technology-driven specialty with a number of informatics steps in the electronic health record (EHR) and non-interpretive processes that occur between exam ordering, patient scheduling, and exam acquisition. AI integration can increase efficiency between these multiple systems and multiples steps in the radiology exam life cycle. Additionally, modalities like computed tomography (CT) and magnetic resonance imaging (MRI) require extensive image processing which can be optimised by AI techniques. Even the radiologist's interpretive role mirrors how AI applications can learn patterns from images and make diagnoses. AI can provide a "second-read" of some radiology exams and assist the radiologist in making their diagnosis. Computer-aided detection algorithms (CAD) existed even before the age of digital radiology. An AI application that detected and highlighted suspicious breast lesions on mammograms first acquired Food and Drug Administration (FDA) clearance in 1998 and was the first AI application to gain FDA clearance in radiology. The modern history of AI has been inexorably linked to radiology, and as such, the field of medicine can look to the mutual evolution of AI and radiology as a roadmap to how other specialties can embrace, integrate, and evolve with AI.

6.2 INNOVATION AND THE AI HYPE CYCLE

Three breakthroughs in the field of AI and radiology occurred in the mid-2010s which precipitated an AI research and development boom that has continued into the 2020s. First, advancements in machine learning techniques, the rise of convolutional neural networks, and deep learning allowed computer systems to perform more advanced tasks than ever before. One area where these algorithms excelled was pattern recognition and image processing [5]. Second, the publication of large, publicly available, anonymised data sets made AI development and testing more feasible for AI researchers [11, 12]. Aggregating and anonymising sufficient training and testing data for AI was, and continues to be in many disciplines, a substantial barrier to AI development. These large, anonymised data sets, particularly for chest radiographs and head CT, provided AI developers the opportunity to train their algorithms on diverse and publicly available data rather than having to aggregate and anonymise data from individual hospital systems. In fact, cardiothoracic and neuro imaging are two of the most highly represented subspecialties of radiology in the AI marketplace, and it is likely that the availability of these large data sets contributed to their position in the marketplace today [13]. Finally, the first deep learning enabled AI application, Arterys, gained FDA clearance in 2016 and a Conformité Européenne (CE) mark in 2017 [8].

DOI: 10.1201/9781032709956-6

While this was not the first AI-enabled device to gain clearance for medical use, the approval of the Arterys tool, which performs automated segmentation of ventricle volumes on cardiac MRI, served as a precedent for medical AI approval through a "software as a medical device (SaMD)" pathway. This opened the door for dozens of AI applications which would be cleared in the following year, and the number of FDA-cleared AI tools per year has increased ever since.

These rapid advancements generated anxiety in the field of medicine, with publications purporting applications that performed "as well or better than radiologists" at detecting pneumonia, intracranial haemorrhage, breast cancer, and so on. The prospect of an "AI future" prompted some in radiology to wonder if there would be a day where radiologists would be replaced by AI [14]. This anxiety was only heightened by individuals outside of the field who proclaimed that the days of the human radiologist would soon be over. They often suggested that human radiologists would and *should* be replaced by an AI algorithm that never sleeps, never takes breaks, and never asks for a higher salary [14, 15]. All the while, leaders in the field of radiology and AI experts made more modest predictions of a future with radiologists working in tandem with AI to make their practice better, safer, and more efficient [16, 17]. Certainly, the field of radiology would change, but as Curtis Langlotz, a radiologist at Stanford University, would say, "AI will not replace radiologists, but radiologists who use AI will replace radiologists who don't" [18]. However, the fears of replacement caused ripple effects through the field of radiology, with fewer applicants applying to the field and a majority of medical students in 2017 reporting that the uncertainty of AI in radiology negatively affected their choice of radiology [19].

The discordance between the hype and reality of radiology AI provided an opportunity for radiologists to establish a more collaborative relationship with AI developers and rethink how AI could be integrated into radiology. As radiologists entered the AI research and development space in greater numbers, the conversation on the future of AI in radiology shifted from "Will AI replace radiologists?" to "How can AI make radiologists better?" AI became more accepted and viewed as a tool that would augment and assist the radiologist and allow the radiologist to provide better patient care rather than replacing their services. Pathologies which require urgent diagnosis and intervention like stroke, intracranial haemorrhage, pulmonary embolus, and pneumothorax have been highly targeted by AI developers; if these AI tools can demonstrate even a small improvement in accuracy, interpretation time, and/or time to treatment, then vendors can report that their tool increases patient safety and improves patient outcomes [20, 21].

Radiology, despite the initial fears, has largely embraced the role that AI will play in the future of their field. Research and publication of AI exponentially increased in the radiology literature since 2000, and this was followed by a boom of AI entrepreneurship and increasing AI integration into daily radiology workflow. Radiology experienced the breath of the AI hype cycle, and this cycle is beginning to repeat itself in other medical specialties, including internal medicine, primary care, ophthalmology, dermatology, pathology, and more [22–25]. As AI advances in these medical specialties and other medical specialties begin preparing for the future of AI in healthcare, how can these specialties learn from the experience of radiology? Figure 6.1 below highlights the increase in publications in AI in many medical domains, with pathology and radiology reaching in excess of 2000 in 2020.

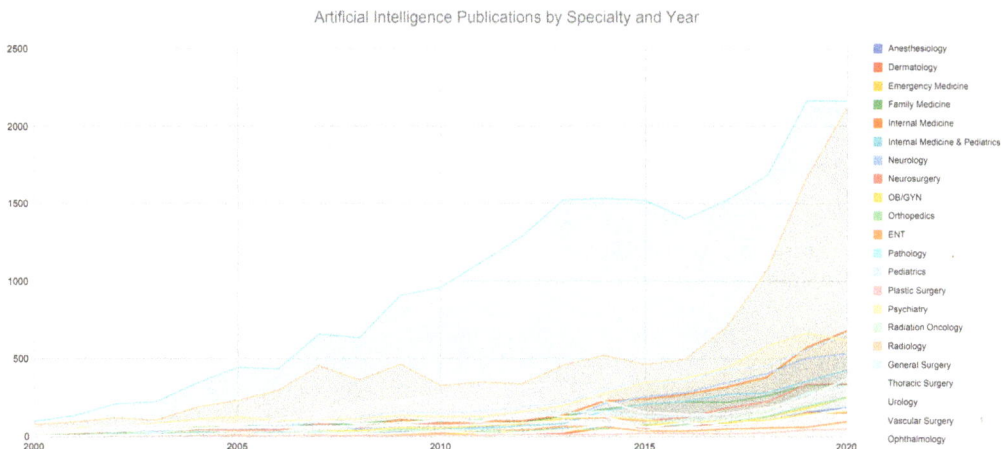

Figure 6.1 AI publications by speciality and year.

6.3 CRITICAL ROLE OF EDUCATION

One of the most significant lessons from radiology's relationship with AI is that education and hands-on experience with AI are crucial to successful integration. It has been demonstrated that fear of replacement by AI decreases with increasing experience with AI, so it was no coincidence that the anxiety of replacement decreased as radiologists became increasingly involved in AI research and became more engaged with AI developers [26, 27]. Despite the importance of early exposure and a guided AI education curriculum, there continues to be an unmet need for AI education at all stages in medical training. Surveys of pre-medical undergraduate students, medical students, and residents all report that AI education is important to the careers of these doctors-in-training but is infrequently available at their training institutions [28–32]. There are a number of reasons that fundamental topics of AI are not more widely integrated into medical education. Some of the frequently cited reasons include a lack of faculty with expertise in AI, a lack of guidance from governing organisations on how to teach AI topics, and limited space to integrate a new topic, like fundamentals of healthcare AI, into an already-packed medical education curriculum. Progress is being made, with AI education resources becoming more widely available through online courses, and some institutions have already begun to integrate AI into their medical education and residency curricula [33]. It should be noted, however, that these resources for AI education can be cost prohibitive or exclusive to the students at the universities that host the course. A new health disparity may be on the horizon, as AI education resources are disproportionately limited to institutions with higher resources, more AI expertise, and more opportunity for research and hands-on experience, and opportunities for AI education are not as available for learners from lower-resource programs.

Turning back to radiology, hundreds of AI algorithms have already entered the marketplace, but a relatively small proportion of practising radiologists have had dedicated AI training. Radiology is in an unusual position where AI availability has vastly outpaced AI education. In 2020, a survey of American radiologists demonstrated that approximately one-third of radiologists in practice use AI in some capacity in their daily practice [34]. The same year, a survey of US radiology residencies showed that only 3% of residency programs had AI integrated into their education curricula [35]. AI users without a baseline knowledge of AI are more prone to automation bias (accepting results they know to be false because they trust the AI result over their own knowledge). Fundamental AI education enables users to recognise errors when they occur, override the AI when there is a false positive or false negative, and understand the monitoring and quality control steps that are needed to ensure an AI application continues to perform as intended. AI education for healthcare providers should focus on fundamental methods and terminology, practical applications, recognising and troubleshooting errors when they occur, and understanding the primary pitfalls of clinical AI; importantly, AI education resources must be made open, accessible, and relevant to users in different settings around the world.

6.4 AI IN RADIOLOGY EDUCATION AND THE AI LITERACY COURSE

As an example, to address the AI education gap in radiology, Artificial Intelligence in Radiology Education (AIRE) was founded in 2020 to produce accessible and sustainable AI programming for radiology trainees [36, 37]. AIRE hosted the first AI Literacy Course in November 2020, and the AI Literacy Course progressively grew from a single-institution program at the University of Alabama at Birmingham to become a regional, then national, and now international course. The AI Literacy Course is a free, one-week course on the fundamentals of AI in radiology, and the course now serves as the largest free program for AI education in radiology, worldwide. For the majority of participants, the AI Literacy Course is their first experience with AI, so this course plays an important part in advancing AI competency in the field of radiology. This model has a proven record of increasing learners' subjective comfort with and objective knowledge of fundamental AI terms, methods, and applications in radiology.

6.4.1 Course Goals

One of the primary objectives of the AI Literacy Course is to provide a more realistic expectation of what the clinical integration of AI will look like in radiology. Participants should realise that AI is not an "all-purpose solution," and that the initial hype of the AI future (and fears of replacement by AI) substantially outpaced the reality of AI. The course directors emphasise that it is as important for learners to gain exposure to the different AI applications and techniques in their subspecialty as it is for learners to grasp the pitfalls of AI. AI applications, especially in the late 2010s and early 2020s, were often narrow, brittle, and biased – three of the major pitfalls to the clinical implementation of AI. These pitfalls are illustrated with case scenarios during the AI Literacy Course, with an example of one such case scenario below:

6.4.2 Curriculum

The AI course is a one-week series of lectures focused on AI in radiology; two 30-minute lectures are given per day for a total of 10 lectures during each course (Figure 6.2). Each year, the course begins with a review session on fundamental terms and methods of AI. Topics covered in this session include key terms and definitions, a brief review of important statistical methods, concepts in data preparation and algorithm training, as well as expectations for the course. The course discusses the applications of AI in seven radiology subspecialties (neuroradiology, breast imaging, chest imaging, abdominal imaging, musculoskeletal imaging, paediatric imaging, and molecular imaging/therapeutics). These subspecialties are rotated on a biennial basis, to allow sufficient time for new applications or topics to develop and mature in the interim. For example, if one year covered AI applications in neuroradiology, breast imaging, chest imaging, and abdominal imaging, the following year would cover musculoskeletal imaging, paediatric imaging, and molecular imaging/therapeutics; this cycle would repeat, meaning that two years would pass before any subspecialty topic was repeated. The remainder of the course lectures would be dedicated to special topics such as "The AI Marketplace", "Quality Assurance and AI", and "Ethics of AI in Radiology". On the final day of the course, AIRE would work with an industry partner to provide a hands-on event, so that participants could experience what an AI algorithm would look like in their daily workflow.

The fundamental concepts discussed on the first day of the course are revisited and expanded during the different subspecialty and special topics lecturers throughout the week. Learners are expected to understand the different categories of AI applications and the different types of tasks

Day 1 (October 3, 2022)

Course introduction (10 minutes) – 12:00pm CST

1. Introduction to Terms and Methods of AI (30 minutes) – 12:10pm CST – Dr. Houman Sotoudeh

   (5-minute break)

2. Introduction to Terms and Methods of AI 30 minutes) – 12:45pm CST – Dr. Houman Sotoudeh

Day 2 (October 4, 2022)

1. AI in Nuclear Medicine (25 minutes) – 12:00pm CST – Dr. Jordan Perchik

   (5-minute break)

2. The Future of AI in Radiology (25 minutes) – 12:30pm CST – Dr. Andrew Smith

Day 3 (October 5, 2022)

1. Special Topic: Federated Learning in AI (20 minutes) – 12:00pm CST – Vishwa Parekh

   (5-minute break)

2. Pitfalls in MSK Imaging (20 minutes) – 12:25pm CST – Dr. Paul Yi

   (5-minute break)

3. Feedback (10 minutes), 12:50pm CST

Day 4 (October 6, 2022)

1. AI in Pediatric Imaging (25 minutes) – 12:00pm CST – Dr. Marcelo Straus Takashi

   (5-minute break)

2. Special Topic: Economics of AI (25 minutes) – 12:30pm CST – Dr. Hari Trivedi

Day 5 (October 7, 2022)

1. Course review (10 minutes) – 12:00pm CST – Dr. Jordan Perchik

   (5-minute break)

2. Hands-On Event (45 minutes) – 12:15pm CST – AI Metrics

Figure 6.2 The AI course schedule and curriculum.

they can perform. To revisit the example of the intracranial haemorrhage algorithm, this tool, a computer aided detection (CAD or CADe) application, could detect a haemorrhage, allowing the radiologist to provide a quicker interpretation. This could lead to a shorter time to treatment, and in theory, better patient outcomes. This tool could be further optimised to provide worklist integration and "flag" studies that the AI screened as positive for intracranial haemorrhage; this would be an example of a subcategory called computer-aided triage, or CADt. This alert would prompt the radiologist to interpret these positive studies more rapidly, and again, reduce time to treatment for patients with these acute findings. Another subtype of CAD is computer-aided diagnosis (CADx), which would assist the radiologist in making their diagnosis, such as in cases of prostate cancer on prostate MRI or breast cancer on mammography. Additional examples of algorithms discussed during the course include medical image management and processing systems (MIMPS), which could be applications ranging from image reconstruction applications to AI-guided 3D reconstructions, to automated reports and other workflow optimisations.

6.4.3 Building Partnerships

The AI Literacy Course was poised to grow rapidly in the early 2020s. The course began in a remote format, so adding additional partner programs could be accomplished at no cost to the host institution. Radiology training programs throughout the country had a need for AI education, but most programs did not have expertise in every subject area and therefore could not provide a complete curriculum for their residents. The AI Literacy Course served as a hub for institutions to be able to share expertise and aggregate resources, and for programs without AI expertise or infrastructure in their institutions, the course provided fundamental knowledge for them to broach the world of AI with a baseline level of understanding.

As a remote, free resource, AI Literacy Course was particularly well suited to international deployment. This is of particular importance, as the existing disparities in AI education and exposure between high and low resource programs becomes even more pronounced between high-income countries and low- and middle-income countries (LMICs). There is a great need for AI education in LMICs because AI can produce some of its most significant impacts in areas with fewer doctors, lower resources, and limited subspecialist support. To increase accessibility of the AI Literacy Course to the international community, AIRE partnered with two radiology non-governmental organisations (NGOs), RadAID and Health4theWorld to distribute the course to radiology education programs internationally [38]. As of 2024, learners from over 25 countries have participated in the AI Literacy Course (Figure 6.3).

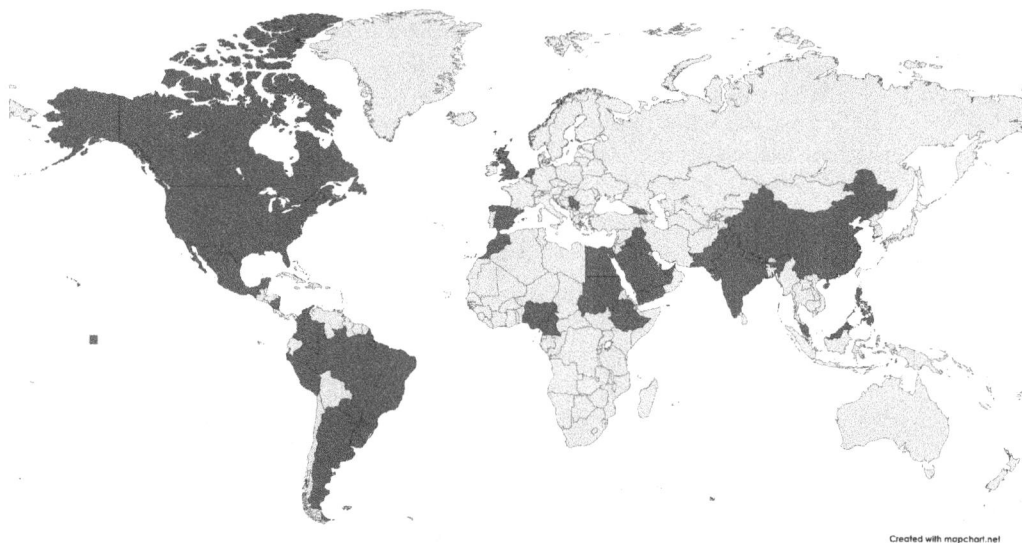

Figure 6.3 Map of participants and home countries (dark shaded countries). Participants represented a total of 28 countries from Asia, Africa, Europe, and North America.

6.4.4 Learner Evaluation

A survey and evaluation are distributed to course participants before and after completion of the course each year. The survey captures demographic information as well as information on prior AI experience and learner opinions on AI in radiology. Participants' general knowledge of AI terms and methods is assessed in the pre- and post-course evaluation, which contains 15 questions on key terms, definitions, and applications of AI in radiology discussed in the course. The survey and evaluation provide subjective and objective data on the effectiveness of the course, and each year, participants have demonstrated increased subjective and objective knowledge of AI after completion of the course. Notably, the participants who have completed the course previously score significantly higher than new participants, suggesting that the lessons learnt in the course endure from year to year. The course is consistently well received, with over 90% of participants reporting that they would be interested in continuing the course the following year [38].

6.4.5 Challenges and Future Directions

As the course has grown to an international community, several gaps in the course curriculum and organisation have become apparent. First, the course was previously delivered only in a live format which proved challenging for observers in different time zones to participate. To address these limitations, the course lectures are now recorded and available free online, and the course can be completed asynchronously. The course was previously available only in English, which served as a limitation for non-English speaking countries and learners without a high level of English proficiency. The hosting website for the lectures provides accessibility features such as closed captioning and live translation; however, these services have been noted to be imperfect and are suboptimal as an enduring solution [39–41]. To build a network of parallel programs, AIRE has published its curriculum on the course to enable leaders in non-English speaking regions to create and adapt their own course using a proven, successful curriculum. AIRE has since led a Spanish-language AI Literacy Course in February 2024, with additional courses, in Portuguese, French and Arabic, planned in the future.

Finally, as one of the primary resources for AI education for radiologists and radiology trainees in LMICs, AIRE recognises its responsibility to provide practical and relevant resources for radiologists in these countries. In lower-resource healthcare settings with limited subspecialist support, AI can provide a vital service supporting healthcare providers to provide a higher level of care [42]. Paradoxically, these areas where AI could make the most impact are also the areas that are least represented in algorithm training and therefore would require a higher level of oversight by its users. So, while AI could be a breakthrough for healthcare in LMICs, it also has the potential to perpetuate the vicious cycle of health disparities and bias that exists today. Because AI promises to make an even more substantial impact on healthcare in lower-resource settings, it is crucial that users in these countries have adequate training and a baseline understanding of radiology AI [43, 44].

6.5 OPPORTUNITIES AND PITFALLS

The integration of AI into healthcare has shown great promise to augment the abilities of practising physicians and alleviate the stress of an already overburdened healthcare system. Physician education, and especially early exposure in medical and pre-medical education, is key to successful deployment. Not all AI tasks have to be as sophisticated or far-reaching as a "doctor in a box" that can diagnose and treat every known disease. Even small-scale algorithms that automate repetitive or low-cognitive-load tasks can make significant impacts on workflow and increase physicians' quality of life. AI is particularly efficient at aggregating and condensing data, so AI could assist physicians in analysing years' worth of clinical data when determining a treatment plan, and AI could integrate with clinical trial databases to assist with treatment regimens for cancer or other diseases. AI's capability to analyse medical images has already yielded many applications in radiology, but other types of medical images are also being targeted for AI integration. In ophthalmology, AI algorithms can analyse digital images from an ophthalmological exam to detect diabetic retinopathy [45]. While this is not necessarily a tool that is needed by an ophthalmologist, a primary care physician could use this tool to increase their diagnostic confidence and prevent the need for a secondary referral and a delayed diagnosis. This ability to provide a higher level of care is especially important in lower-resource settings, in rural areas that are far from major academic centres, and in LMICs where there may not be any subspecialist care available [45]. Continued advancements in wearable technology, precision medicine and remote healthcare will provide fodder for a sustained AI boom that will expand well beyond radiology into all medical specialties in the near future.

As the AI future becomes the AI present, healthcare providers must understand the inherent risks of AI integration. Again, education is the key to unlocking the promise of AI while mitigating the risks of harm. Algorithmic bias, algorithm drift, automation bias, and brittle algorithms all provide pitfalls that could serve as stumbling blocks to realising the promise of AI in healthcare [46, 47]. Gone unchecked, these pitfalls could not only degrade confidence in clinical AI in the long term but also cause harm to patients in the short term. It is crucial for healthcare providers to be able to see through the hype of these new technologies and make more measured and informed decisions on how AI can be used to improve patient care. Access to AI education is becoming more widely available, but additional steps are needed to ensure that resources for practical and relevant AI education are accessible for healthcare providers across the world. The medical community can look to radiology and to the AI Literacy Course for a proven framework for embracing AI, increasing accessibility to AI education, and demonstrating that the fears of AI replacement can yield opportunities for AI integration.

6.6 EDITORS' COMMENTS

The importance of AI education is clear and multifaceted. AI education will equip clinicians to be able to harness the potential of the tools currently available and promote those at an earlier stage of development. Furthermore, AI education may reduce the concerns of radiologists' jobs being taken and quell any fears of doctors considering radiology as a specialism.

All too often there is a discrepancy in education provision internationally, so a more connected curriculum, with input from world-leading experts, will help iron out global education disparities, but only if education provision can be accessed equitably. However, budgets are finite especially in low- to middle-income countries, so disparities will remain. The course described here has quality and accessibility at its core; with careful consideration of curriculum content delivered by international experts in languages other than English (and with additional languages planned), the free access to learning will enable the widest outcomes to be achieved for the benefit of all.

REFERENCES

1. Hirani, R., Noruzi, K., Khuram, H. et al. (2024) Artificial Intelligence and Healthcare: A Journey Through History, Present Innovations, and Future Possibilities. Life. https://doi.org/10.3390/life14050557
2. Miller, R.A., Pople, H.E., Myers, J.D. (1982) Internist-1, an Experimental Computer-Based Diagnostic Consultant for General Internal Medicine. N Engl J Med. 307:468–476. https://doi.org/10.1056/nejm198208193070803
3. Shortliffe, E.H. (1977) A Knowledge-Based Computer Program Applied to Infectious Diseases. Proc Annu Symp Comput Appl Med Care., 3–5:66–69.
4. Hamamoto, R. (2021) Application of Artificial Intelligence for Medical Research. Biomol. 11(1):90. https://doi.org/10.3390/biom11010090
5. Rajpurkar, P., Chen, E., Banerjee, O. et al. (2022) AI in Health and Medicine. Nat Med. 28:31–38. https://doi.org/10.1038/s41591-021-01614-0
6. US Food and Drug Administration (FDA). (2025) Artificial Intelligence and Machine Learning (AI/ML)-Enabled Medical Devices. https://www.fda.gov/medical-devices/software-medical-device-samd/artificial-intelligence-and-machine-learning-aiml-enabled-medical-devices. Accessed 18 June 2024.
7. Perera, N., Perchik, J.D., Perchik, M.C. et al. (2022) Trends in Medical Artificial Intelligence Publications from 2000–2020: Where Does Radiology Stand? Open J Clin Med Images. 2(2):1052.
8. Driver, C.N., Bowles, B.S., Bartholmia, B.J. et al. (2019) Artificial Intelligence in Radiology: A Call for Thoughtful Application. Clin Transl Sci. https://doi.org/10.1111/cts.12704
9. Thrall, J.H. (2005) Reinventing Radiology in the Digital Age Part 1. The All-Digital Department. Radiol. 236(2):382–385. https://doi.org/10.1148/radiol.2362050257
10. Kohll, M., Dreyer, K.J., Geis, J.R. (2015) Rethinking Radiology Informatics. Am J Roentgenol. 204(4):716–720. https://doi.org/10.2214/AJR.14.13840
11. Willemink, M.J., Koszek, W.A., Hardell, C. et al. (2020) Preparing Medical Imaging Data for Machine Learning. Radiol. https://doi.org/10.1148/radiol.2020192224
12. Tang, A., Ram, R., Cadrin-Chênevert, A. et al. (2018) Canadian Association of Radiologists White Paper on Artificial Intelligence in Radiology. Can Assoc Radiol J. 69(2):120–135. https://doi.org/10.1016/j.carj.2018.02.002
13. Dreyer, K.J., Wald, C., Allen, B. Jr. et al. (2021) Evaluation and Real-World Performance Monitoring of Artificial Intelligence Models in Clinical Practice: Try It, Buy It, Check It. JACR, 18(11):1489–1496. https://doi.org/10.1016/j.jacr.2021.08.022
14. Chockley, K., Emanuel, E. (2016) The End of Radiology? Three Threats to the Future Practice of Radiology. J Am Coll Radiol. 13(12 Pt A):1415–1420. https://doi.org/10.1016/j.jacr.2016.07.010
15. Mukherjee, S. (2017) A.I. versus M.D. What Happens When the Diagnosis is Automated? The New Yorker.
16. Siegel, E. (2017) Rest Assured, João, You are Safe from Artificial Intelligence. Appl Radiol. https://appliedradiology.com/articles/rest-assured-jo-o-you-are-safe-from-artificial-intelligence. Accessed 5 June 2024.
17. Gichoya, J.W., Nuthakki, S., Maity, P.G. et al. (2024) Phronesis of AI in radiology: Superhuman meets natural stupidity. arXiv. https://doi.org/10.48550/arXiv.1803.11244. Accessed 17 June 2024.
18. Langlotz, C.P. (2019) Will Artificial Intelligence Replace Radiologists? Radiol Artif Intell. 1(3) https://doi.org/10.1148/RYAI.2019190058
19. Gong, B., Nugent, J.P., Guest, W. et al. (2019) Influence of Artificial Intelligence on Canadian Medical students' Preference for Radiology Specialty: A National Survey Study. Acad Radiol. 26(4):566–577. https://doi.org/10.1016/j.acra.2018.10.007

20. Mouridsen, K., Thurner, P., Zaharchuk, G. (2020) Artificial Intelligence Applications in Stroke. Stroke. 51(8):2573–2579. 10.1161/STROKEAHA.119.027479
21. Savage, C.H., Elkassem, A.A., Hamki, O., Sturdivant, A., Benson, D., Grumley, S. et al. (2024) Prospective Evaluation of Artificial Intelligence Triage of Incidental Pulmonary Emboli on Contrast-Enhanced CT Examinations of the Chest or Abdomen. Am J Roentgenol. 223(3):e2431067. https://doi.org/10.2214/AJR.24.31067
22. Mainous, A.G. III (2022) Will Technology and Artificial Intelligence Make the Primary Care Doctor Obsolete? Remember the Luddites. Front Med. 9:878281. https://doi.org/10.3389/FMED.2022.878281
23. Korot, E., Wagner, S.K., Faes, L. et al. (2020) Will AI Replace Ophthalmologists? Transl Vis Sci Technol. 9(2). https://doi.org/10.1167/TVST.9.2.2
24. Elkhader, J., Elemento, O. (2022) Artificial Intelligence in Oncology: From Bench to Clinic. Sem Canc Biol. 84:113–128. https://doi.org/10.1016/j.semcancer.2021.04.013
25. Li, Z., Koban, K.C., Schenck, T.L. et al. (2022) Artificial Intelligence in Dermatology Image Analysis: Current Developments and Future Trends. J Clin Med. 11(22):6826. https://doi.org/10.3390/jcm11226826
26. Sit, C., Srinivasan, R., Amlani, A. et al. (2020) Attitudes and Perceptions of UK Medical Students Towards Artificial Intelligence and Radiology: A Multicenter Survey. Insights Imaging. 11(14). https://doi.org/10.1186/S13244-019-0830-7
27. Reeder, K., Lee, H. (2022) Impact of Artificial Intelligence on US Medical students' Choice of Radiology. Clin Imaging. 81:67–71. https://doi.org/10.1016/j.clinimag.2021.09.018
28. Paranjape, K., Schinkel, M., Panday, R.N. et al. (2019) Introducing Artificial Intelligence Training in Medical Education. JMIR Med Educ. 5(2):e16048. https://doi.org/10.2196/16048
29. Ejaz, H., McGrath, H., Wong, B.L. (2022) Artificial Intelligence and Medical Education: A Global Mixed-Methods Study of Medical Students' Perspectives. Digital Health. 2(8). https://doi.org/10.1177/20552076221089099
30. Masters, K. (2019) Artificial Intelligence in Medical Education. Medical Teacher. 41(9):976–980. https://doi.org/10.1080/0142159X.2019.1595557
31. Civaner, M.M., Uncu, Y., Bulut, F. et al. (2022) Artificial Intelligence in Medical Education: A Cross-Sectional Needs Assessment. BMC Med Educ. 22:772. https://doi.org/10.1186/s12909-022-03852-3
32. Hu, R., Fan, K.Y., Pandey, P. et al. (2022) Insights from Teaching Artificial Intelligence to Medical Students in Canada. Commun Med. Published online: June 3, 2022. https://doi.org10.1038/s43856-022-00125-4
33. Charow, R., Jeyakumar, T., Younus, S. et al. (2021) Artificial Intelligence Education Programs for Health Care Professionals: Scoping Review. JMIR Med Educ. Published online: 13 December 2021. https://doi.org/10.2196/31043
34. Allen, B., Agarwal, S., Coombs, L., Wald, C., Dreyer, K. (2021) 2020 ACR Data Science Institute Artificial Intelligence Survey. J Am Coll Radiol. 18(8):1153–1159. https://doi.org/10.1016/j.jacr.2021.04.002
35. Li, D., Morkos, J., Gage, D., Yi, P.H. (2022) Artificial Intelligence Educational and Research Initiatives and Leadership Positions in Academic Radiology Departments. Curr Probl Diagn Radiol. 51(4):552–555. https://doi.org/10.1067/j.cpradiol.2022.01.004
36. Perchik, J.D., Smith, A.D., Elkassem, A.A. et al. (2023) Artificial Intelligence Literacy: Developing a Multi-Institutional Infrastructure for AI Education. Acad Radiol. 30(7):1472–1480. https://doi.org/10.1016/j.acra.2022.10.002
37. Perchik, J.D., Sotoudeh, H., Rothenberg, S.A. et al. (2024) Going Global: Scaling the Artificial Intelligence Literacy Course to an International Audience. J Glob Radiol. Published online: 24 May 2024. https://doi.org/10.7191/jgr.783
38. Lanier, M.H., Wheeler, C.A., Ballard, D.H. (2021) A New Normal in Radiology Resident Education: Lessons Learned from the COVID -19 Pandemic. Radiographics. 41(3). Published online: May 3, 2021. https://doi.org/10.1148/rg.2021210030
39. Saxena, A., Khamis, S. (2020) "I'll See you on Zoom!" International Educators' Perceptions of Online Teaching Amid, and Beyond, Covid-19. Arab Media Soc. 30:1–21. https://doi.org/10.70090/ASSK20ZI
40. Parton, B.S. (2016) Video Captions for Online Courses: Do YouTube's Auto-Generated Captions Meet Deaf Students' Needs. J Open Flexible Distance Learn. 20(1):8–18. https://doi.org/10.61468/jofdl.v20i1.255
41. Ciecierski-Holmes, T., Singh, R., Axt, M. et al. (2022) Artificial Intelligence for Strengthening Healthcare Systems in Low- and Middle-Income Countries: A Systematic Scoping Review. NPJ Digit Med. 5(162). Published online October 28, 2022. https://doi.org/10.1038/s41746-022-00700-y
42. Mollura, D.J., Culp, M.P., Pollack, E. et al (2020) Artificial Intelligence in Low and Middle-Income Countries: Innovating Global Health Radiology. Radiology. 297:513–520. https://doi.org/10.1148/radiol.2020201434
43. Abuzaid, M.M., Elshami, W., McConnell, J. et al. (2021) An Extensive Survey of Radiographers from the Middle East and India on Artificial Intelligence Integration in Radiology Practice. Health Technol. 11:1045–1050. https://doi.org/10.1007/s12553-021-00583-1
44. Rajiv, R., Dasgupta, D., Ramasamy, K. et al. (2021) Using Artificial Intelligence for Diabetic Retinopathy Screening: Policy Implications. Indian J Ophthalmol. 69(11):2993–2998. https://doi.org/10.4103/ijo.IJO_1420_21
45. Celi, L.A., Cellini, J., Charignon, M.L. et al. (2022) Sources of Bias in Artificial Intelligence That Perpetuate Healthcare Disparities – A Global Review. PLoS Digit Health. Published online 31 March 2022. https://doi.org/10.1371/journal.pdig.0000022
46. Goirand, M., Austin, E., Clay-Williams, R. (2021) Implementing Ethics in Healthcare AI-Based Applications: A Scoping Review. Sci Eng Ethics. Published online: 3 September 2021. https://doi.org/10.1007/s11948-021-00336-3
47. Li, F., Ruijs, N., Lu, Y. (2022) Ethics & AI: A Systematic Review on Ethical Concerns and Related Strategies for Designing With AI in Healthcare. AI. 4(1):28–53. https://doi.org/10.3390/ai4010003

7 Opportunities and Equity in Imaging AI

Implications for Indigenous and Underrepresented Populations

Ziba Gandomkar and Patrick Brennan

7.1 INTRODUCTION

Healthcare disparities remain a widespread challenge in medicine, disproportionately affecting minorities and underrepresented and Indigenous populations [1, 2]. These disparities manifest across a wide range of outcomes, from preventable hospitalizations and chronic disease burdens [3–6] to inequities in cancer outcomes [7]. For Indigenous peoples—such as Aboriginal and Torres Strait Islander populations in Australia, Māori in Aotearoa New Zealand, and Native Americans in North America—diagnostic inequities are especially pronounced. Many of these communities face higher incidence and earlier onset of complex diseases, yet they experience significantly lower rates of diagnostic imaging, slower referral processes, and more limited access to specialized services [8–12].

Artificial intelligence (AI) has emerged as a promising tool to advance equity in healthcare [13–24]. It offers potential to close the gaps by enabling faster, more scalable imaging diagnostics, particularly in areas lacking specialists. AI systems can be embedded in mobile units, telehealth platforms, or community-based screening programs, offering flexibility that conventional models of care cannot.

However, if fairness is not prioritized, AI may worsen disparities [25]. Biased training data, narrow evaluation metrics, or culturally insensitive deployment can reinforce existing inequities. This is especially true in the context of Indigenous health, where histories of colonization, systemic racism, and data misuse have left many communities justifiably cautious about new health technologies. As such, ethical AI development must prioritize inclusivity, transparency, and community governance.

7.2 CONCEPTUALIZING FAIRNESS IN AI FOR UNDERREPRESENTED AND INDIGENOUS POPULATIONS

Fairness in AI must address both process and outcomes [26, 27]. For Indigenous and underrepresented communities, this involves

1. *Procedural fairness*: Ensuring that underrepresented and Indigenous communities are involved in decisions about how AI is designed, data are collected, and consent is obtained. Considering ethical frameworks like OCAP® [28, 29] and CARE [30, 31] is critical.

2. *Distributive fairness*: Guaranteeing that the benefits and harms of AI are equitably distributed. If tools underperform or are unavailable for underrepresented and Indigenous communities, fairness is violated.

3. *Individual fairness*: Making sure that individuals with similar clinical profiles receive similar predictions, regardless of ethnicity or background.

4. *Group fairness*: Striving for equal performance across demographic groups. Disparities in diagnostic accuracy or false positive rates reflect group-level bias.

These categories are interrelated and often overlap in real-world scenarios. A single AI tool can fail across multiple dimensions, compounding inequities. Table 7.1 presents these fairness types with definitions, their implications in Indigenous healthcare contexts, and examples drawn from low-dose computed tomography (CT) lung cancer screening.

For instance, an AI model for lung cancer screening may perform worse for Indigenous patients due to underrepresentation (violating group and distributive fairness), be developed without Indigenous input (a failure of procedural fairness), and generate inconsistent predictions for similar patients based on background (a breach of individual fairness).

7.3 CONTEXTUALIZING HEALTH DISPARITIES IN MEDICAL IMAGING

Disparities in access to diagnostic imaging services are a critical component of broader health inequities for Indigenous communities.

Australia (Aboriginal and Torres Strait Islanders) and New Zealand (Māori and Pacific Peoples): Indigenous Australians have lower uptake of vital imaging-based screening programs.

DOI: 10.1201/9781032709956-7

Table 7.1 Fairness Dimensions in AI and Examples from Lung Cancer Screening

Fairness Type	Definition	In Context of Aboriginal Populations and AI	Example
Procedural	Who is involved in development and decision-making?	Were Indigenous communities consulted? Were principles like OCAP® or CARE followed?	Model developed without Indigenous input or data governance consultation.
Distributive	Are benefits and harms shared equitably?	Does the AI system yield accurate results for Indigenous patients?	AI performs worse for Indigenous patients due to underrepresentation in training data.
Individual	Are similar individuals treated similarly?	Do Indigenous and non-Indigenous patients with similar findings receive consistent predictions?	Patients with similar nodules get different risk scores due to bias in training.
Group	Are outcomes comparable across groups?	Are diagnostic performance metrics consistent across Indigenous and non-Indigenous populations?	Indigenous patients have systematically lower model accuracy.

Participation in screening mammography (BreastScreen) is far lower for Aboriginal and Torres Strait Islander people than for non-Indigenous Australians. Usage of follow-up diagnostic tests is also lower in Indigenous groups, with timely access often limited, especially in remote areas [32]. Geography plays a major role—people in rural/remote Indigenous communities must often travel great distances for advanced imaging, and historically many communities had only intermittent or basic radiography services [33]. Cultural and socioeconomic barriers compound the problem. A recent pediatric imaging study in an Australian tertiary hospital found non-attendance rates for imaging appointments were *significantly higher* among First Nations children, pointing to unmet needs and the importance of culturally safe, family-centered strategies [34].

Māori health inequities mirror many Australian patterns. Māori and Pacific Islander populations face disproportionate burdens of disease but often fewer diagnostic procedures [35]. Even in urban hospitals, subtle inequities emerge; for instance, an Auckland study [36] showed indigenous Māori patients had a higher incidence of acute aortic syndrome but were less likely to receive the indicated CT aortography scans compared to other ethnic groups. Such examples underscore an imbalance in diagnostic imaging services, where Indigenous patients may be underserved or receive investigations later despite greater need. Other research in New Zealand highlights lower rates of certain interventions and diagnostics for Māori, contributing to worse outcomes. Recognizing this, initiatives by radiology professional bodies (like RANZCR [37]) stress various initiatives required to close the gap.

North America: Indigenous communities in the U.S. and Canada similarly experience limited access to diagnostic radiology due to geographic isolation and under-resourced health systems [38–40]. For example, many remote First Nations in Canada rely on small clinics with basic X-ray or ultrasound and infrequent specialist visits [41]. *Teleradiology* networks have partly bridged this gap by enabling off-site radiologists to read images taken in far-flung Indigenous communities, but challenges remain [42]. In the U.S., American Indian and Alaska Native (AI/AN) women have the lowest mammography screening rates among ethnic groups and often present with more advanced breast cancers at younger ages [43]. Over the past 30 years, breast cancer mortality declined for most groups but remained unchanged for AI/AN women, attributable in part to less-timely screening and treatment [43]. Barriers include the limited scope and chronic underfunding of the Indian Health Service, long travel distances to imaging facilities, and historical mistrust due to past unethical research and care [43]. These factors illustrate how systemic issues translate into diagnostic disparities. A review on cancer care in AI/AN populations emphasizes that improving access to imaging and early detection (i.e., breast, lung, and colorectal imaging) is critical to reducing mortality [44]. In short, across regions, Indigenous peoples face a pattern of *under-utilization* of medical imaging relative to health needs—whether due to logistical barriers, cultural disconnection, or inequitable service distribution.

7.4 OPPORTUNITIES FOR AI TO ADDRESS IMAGING DISPARITIES IN INDIGENOUS AND UNDERSERVED POPULATIONS

AI-driven tools in medical imaging present a transformative opportunity to address long-standing diagnostic inequities for Indigenous and underrepresented populations. This section covers a few use cases that have demonstrated effectiveness in real-world settings or show strong promise in ongoing research.

AI-enhanced screening for chronic conditions: One of the most impactful uses of AI in underserved populations is screening for chronic diseases where early detection can prevent severe complications. Diabetic retinopathy screening is a leading example [13–16]. For instance, in Western Australia's Pilbara region [15], an AI-assisted mobile retinal screening program was co-developed with Indigenous communities. A van equipped with a retinal camera and AI software enabled on-the-spot image grading, delivering immediate results and facilitating telehealth referrals. This approach led to an 11-fold increase in screening uptake, with approximately 10% of patients (over half of whom were Indigenous) identified as needing specialist care. Importantly, the service was culturally accepted, with 96% of participants comfortable with AI involvement. A 2024 Australian study [16] confirmed the cost-effectiveness of AI-driven retinopathy screening in primary care settings, estimating the prevention of over 1,200 cases of blindness and generating nearly 10,000 quality-adjusted life years in Indigenous Australians over four decades. Similar results were seen in a 2021 study by Scheetz et al. [17], which deployed AI in Aboriginal Medical Service clinics. The system achieved over 96% sensitivity and was feasible to implement, highlighting how AI can deliver specialist-level screening in areas with limited ophthalmology services.

Diagnostic decision support in remote settings: AI also holds potential in augmenting telehealth [42] and point-of-care diagnostics, especially where specialists are scarce. In Australia's Northern Territory, researchers developed an AI tool to interpret otoscope images for chronic ear disease—common among Indigenous children [18, 19]. The system achieved diagnostic accuracies of 96–99%, offering a reliable triage method that can integrate with telehealth to ensure timely treatment [20]. Furthering this approach, a recent study in South Australia developed a multimodal machine learning algorithm that combined otoscopic and tympanometry data to diagnose otitis media more accurately in school-aged Indigenous children across 10 remote communities. By integrating both data types, the model's accuracy improved from 78% to 82%, demonstrating how multimodal AI can enhance clinical decision support in remote settings where ENT specialists are unavailable. Similar innovations have been tested for ultrasound imaging. AI-guided handheld echocardiography is being explored for managing cardiovascular diseases [21], which disproportionately affects Indigenous youth. These tools enable even non-experts to capture and interpret scans effectively, potentially expanding access to cardiac care in schools and community clinics.

Teleradiology integration and mobile imaging units: Existing teleradiology infrastructures, especially in Canada's North, already link Indigenous community hospitals to distant radiologists [45]. Embedding AI into these networks can enhance efficiency, for example, by flagging urgent cases like pneumonia or tuberculosis on chest X-rays for prioritized review. Mobile imaging units equipped with AI are also emerging. In New Zealand, proposals to deploy portable low-dose CT scanners with AI nodule detection for Māori populations—who face high lung cancer risk but low screening access—illustrate how AI can bring advanced diagnostics to underserved areas [22]. Though still early stage, such technologies promise to bridge geographic and infrastructure gaps.

Addressing inequities for other minority and underrepresented populations: AI has also shown promise in addressing disparities among other racial and ethnic minority groups. In the U.S., a 2021 study developed an AI model to analyze knee X-rays and better predict osteoarthritis-related pain in African American patients—whose symptoms are often underdiagnosed due to limitations in conventional grading systems [23]. The model explained 43% of the unexplained pain, suggesting it could help close diagnostic gaps in musculoskeletal care.

Similarly, the U.S. Centers for Disease Control (CDC) implemented an AI-assisted TB screening protocol for immigrants and refugees, using chest X-rays from visa applicants [24]. The AI reliably detected abnormalities and acted as a second reader, enhancing accuracy and throughput for a program serving culturally and linguistically diverse populations.

7.5 UNDERSTANDING BIAS IN AI FOR MEDICAL IMAGING AND ITS SOURCES

Bias in medical imaging AI refers to systematic errors that produce unequal outcomes for certain groups, often rooted in issues with data, model design, or clinical use. Left unchecked, these biases risk reinforcing existing health disparities, particularly for Indigenous and underrepresented communities.

Bias in AI for medical imaging can be broadly categorized into three stages (Table 7.2):

1. *Data-related bias:* From imbalanced or inconsistent data collection and labelling.

2. *Model-related bias:* Stemming from training choices, optimization goals, or evaluation practices.

3. *Deployment-related bias:* Arising during real-world use due to setting, infrastructure, or clinician interaction.

Table 7.2 Types of Bias in Medical Imaging AI: Key Fairness Questions and Examples. (D = Data related; M = Model related; De = Deployment Related)

Bias Type	Key Fairness Question	Example (Minority/Indigenous Context)
Selection Bias (D)	Who is represented in the training data, and who is left out?	Chest X-ray models trained on mostly urban, non-Indigenous patients perform poorly on rural Indigenous patients.
Measurement Bias (D)	How is the data collected, and does image quality vary between groups?	AI trained on high-res MRI data fails on scans from underfunded clinics serving Indigenous communities.
Label Bias (D)	How are ground truth labels assigned, and are they equally accurate?	Underdiagnosed cancers in Indigenous patients lead to mislabeled training data, causing AI to miss disease.
Optimization Bias (M)	What performance metric is optimized, and who does it overlook?	Skin lesion AI underperforms on darker skin tones due to majority-weighted accuracy goals during training.
Shortcut Learning (M)	Is the model relying on spurious, non-clinical patterns?	COVID-19 X-ray models incorrectly relied on hospital-specific artifacts instead of clinical features, reducing generalizability in Indigenous settings.
Evaluation Bias (M)	Are subgroup differences tested and reported during validation?	AI for detecting lung nodules validated only on non-Indigenous adults misdiagnoses Indigenous patients.
Deployment Bias (De)	Where and how is the AI system implemented?	AI tools not deployed in remote Indigenous clinics due to infrastructure gaps, widening care disparities.
User Bias (De)	How do clinicians trust and use AI across patient groups?	Clinicians may override AI for Indigenous patients due to bias, or over-trust systems known to underperform for them.

7.5.1 Data-Related Biases

The saying "garbage in, garbage out" applies strongly to AI. If the training data for a medical imaging algorithm is not representative of the patient populations it will serve, performance disparities will result.

Selection bias occurs when training data do not reflect the diversity of the real-world population. Datasets often overrepresent majority populations (e.g., urban, non-Indigenous) and underrepresent others, leading to poor model performance in marginalized groups. For example, Larrazabal et al. [46] showed that chest X-ray models trained mostly on male patients underperformed on female patients, revealing how demographic imbalance can skew diagnostic accuracy. Similar risks exist for Indigenous groups underrepresented in public imaging datasets. This has been observed in practice—an AI for diabetic retinopathy that was trained mostly on Asian (Chinese) patients showed *slightly lower accuracy* when used on Indigenous Australian patients' retinal images, likely due to differences in retinal pigmentation and co-existing disease patterns not seen in the training set [17, 47].

Measurement bias arises when image acquisition varies across sites—such as scanner type, image resolution, or protocol differences. In a multi-site study of prostate magnetic resonance imaging (MRI) [48], feature reproducibility varied significantly across hospitals despite preprocessing. This demonstrates how site-level differences in image capture can degrade AI performance in resource-limited Indigenous settings.

Label bias reflects systemic disparities in labeling accuracy. Labels from radiology reports or treatment decisions can be influenced by local expertise and access. In rural areas, generalists rather than subspecialists may label images, reducing label fidelity. Proxy labels based on healthcare utilization—such as surgery or referrals—may embed access-based disparities. For example, a colorectal cancer study found that utilization-based proxy overestimated recurrence in Black and Hispanic patients due to delayed or non-standard care pathways [49]. Elevated false positive rates among racial and ethnic minority groups may result from a combination of higher prevalence of non-malignant lung conditions and delays in initial care, which are often driven by communication barriers and irregular treatment patterns [49].

7.5.2 Model-Related Biases

Optimization bias refers to how training objectives influence model behavior. Most models aim to maximize overall accuracy, which can disproportionately benefit majority groups if data are imbalanced. This creates a bias–variance trade-off that harms underrepresented populations. Dermatology AIs, for instance, often perform worse on darker skin tones due to optimization on predominantly lighter-skinned data [50].

Shortcut learning is a particularly harmful model behavior where the AI relies on spurious, non-clinical features—like text artifacts or image framing—that correlate with disease in the training data but do not reflect actual pathology [51]. A study by DeGrave et al. [52] showed that COVID-19 chest X-ray models often used dataset-specific artifacts instead of pulmonary features, resulting in high internal accuracy but poor generalization. These models can silently fail when applied to images from different scanners or populations, such as Indigenous clinics with different imaging setups. As another example, Zech et al. [53] evaluated convolutional neural networks (CNNs) trained to detect pneumonia on chest X-rays from three hospitals. Although the models performed well internally, their external performance dropped significantly. The reason: CNNs had learned to identify hospital-specific features—such as text labels or scanner artifacts—that correlated with pneumonia prevalence but were irrelevant to the disease itself. In fact, CNNs correctly identified the hospital system in over 99% of cases, and the hospital site alone predicted pneumonia risk with an area under the curve (AUC) of 0.86, revealing a reliance on shortcut signals rather than anatomical markers. When training data were pooled across hospitals with imbalanced disease prevalence, model accuracy improved on internal data but not on external test sets, further exposing the pitfalls of shortcut learning. These findings are particularly relevant for Indigenous and rural health contexts, where models trained in large urban centers may silently fail due to differing image characteristics or population health patterns.

Evaluation bias occurs when models are not properly validated across subgroups. If performance metrics are reported only in aggregate, poor accuracy in specific populations goes unnoticed. For example, a head CT algorithm validated only on adults may fail in pediatric patients. Regulators like the Food and Drug Administration (FDA) now recommend subgroup analyzes during validation [54], but many AI studies still lack this transparency.

7.5.3 Deployment and User Biases

Deployment bias refers to unequal implementation of AI systems. If tools are validated in urban centers but never deployed in rural or Indigenous clinics due to resource limitations, disparities widen. Furthermore, models used in settings they weren't designed for (e.g., different age groups or scanner types) may degrade in performance. Infrastructure gaps—such as lack of internet or digital health records—also affect equitable rollout.

User bias emerges from how clinicians interact with AI systems, particularly in how much they trust or rely on their outputs. *Overtrust* occurs when clinicians accept AI predictions without sufficient scrutiny, assuming the system is universally accurate. *Undertrust*, by contrast, involves clinicians dismissing or second-guessing AI outputs—often due to lack of familiarity, past errors, or perceived irrelevance to specific patient populations [55]. (See also Chapter 5.)

In clinical practice, these trust dynamics can differ markedly based on patient background. For Indigenous and minority patients, clinicians may override AI recommendations more frequently, suspecting that the system underperforms for these groups—a concern often grounded in reality due to underrepresentation in training data. This undertrust can limit AI's potential benefits for marginalized populations. Conversely, if clinicians are unaware of the model's limitations and apply it uniformly, they may overtrust the system even when it is known to be less accurate for minority patients. This risks the propagation of erroneous outputs and deepening disparities. These patterns differ from the AI's use in majority populations, where clinicians may feel more confident in its reliability, having seen it validated on similar patient profiles. Addressing user bias thus requires not just technical fixes but also clinician education, transparent performance metrics, and user interfaces that communicate AI uncertainty clearly.

7.5.4 Additional Examples from Literature

A growing body of research highlights these bias types:

Selection bias: Burlina et al. [56] demonstrated that diabetic retinopathy models trained predominantly on light-skinned patients performed significantly worse on images from darker-skinned individuals—achieving 73.0% accuracy versus only 60.5%. This performance gap was attributed to inadequate representation of diverse skin tones in the training data, leading to biased detection and diagnostic disparities in patients of color.

Label bias: Seyyed-Kalantari et al. [57] highlighted label-related disparities in a chest X-ray model, which systematically underdiagnosed conditions in Black patients. These false negatives stemmed from training labels shaped by uneven care access and subjective diagnostic judgments. Such underdiagnosis poses a serious risk, as affected patients may be incorrectly reassured and denied critical interventions.

Optimization bias: A 2025 review in the *European Journal of Cancer* found that the vast majority of mammography AI studies failed to report race or ethnicity, and most datasets included predominantly Caucasian patients [58]. This lack of diversity undermines fairness in model training and evaluation. When deployed, such models may misclassify cancers in minority women due to skewed optimization metrics that neglect underrepresented groups.

Model bias and shortcut learning: Gichoya et al. (2022) revealed that AI models could infer patient race from medical images—including chest X-rays and CT scans—with alarming accuracy (AUCs of 0.94–0.96), even after image degradation [59]. Although radiologists cannot visually detect race in these scans, models learned race-associated proxies embedded in the images. This raises serious concerns: if AI systems can covertly learn racial identity, they may also incorporate race as a latent variable in diagnostic predictions, thereby reinforcing or amplifying systemic inequities.

Together, these examples underscore the multifaceted and often hidden nature of AI bias. They highlight why comprehensive fairness assessments must be embedded across the full AI development pipeline—from dataset construction to validation reporting. Without such vigilance, imaging AI systems may not only fail to serve underrepresented populations equitably but may actively harm them.

7.6 TOWARD EQUITABLE AND INCLUSIVE AI SYSTEMS

Achieving fairness in medical imaging AI requires more than technical accuracy—it demands inclusive data practices, culturally grounded governance, and sustained community engagement. Historically, Indigenous and underrepresented populations have been largely excluded from the data and processes that shape AI tools. This has raised ethical concerns and led to practical performance failures when such systems are applied to communities they were not designed to serve.

7.6.1 Challenges of Underrepresentation and Data Sovereignty

Indigenous, culturally and linguistically diverse (CALD) [60], and other racial or ethnic minority populations remain underrepresented in imaging datasets [9, 61, 62]. This underrepresentation stems from systemic barriers, such as disparities in healthcare access, limited participation in research initiatives, language and cultural disconnects, and a history of unethical data practices that have eroded trust. Consequently, AI models trained predominantly on data from non-Indigenous, urban, and majority populations often underperform when applied to these underrepresented groups. This performance gap is not only a technical issue but also intersects with ethical and social concerns—particularly the principle of data sovereignty, which asserts that communities should govern how their health data are collected, used, and shared. These issues extend to migrants, refugees, and other minority populations who often remain invisible in mainstream medical datasets [9, 61, 62]. As a result, AI algorithms may fail to capture group-specific disease patterns, clinical manifestations, or social determinants of health. If population-specific characteristics are missing from training datasets, particularly those of minority groups, AI systems risk misdiagnosing or entirely overlooking disease—ultimately reinforcing, rather than reducing, diagnostic disparities.

Frameworks like OCAP® (Ownership, Control, Access, Possession) [28, 29], CARE Principles (Collective Benefit, Authority to Control, Responsibility, Ethics) [30, 31], and regionally grounded initiatives such as Maiam nayri Wingara in Australia [63, 64] and Te Mana Raraunga in New Zealand [65–67] offer important ethical foundations for more equitable AI development.

OCAP®, established by First Nations in Canada, defines four principles: ownership (data belong collectively to Indigenous communities), control (they decide how data are used), access (they have the right to view and manage their own data), and possession (they maintain physical custody of their data or choose stewards). In practice, an OCAP®-compliant AI project must secure explicit community permission for using Indigenous medical images, involve the community in governance, and ideally store data within Indigenous-controlled systems.

CARE principles, developed by the Global Indigenous Data Alliance [30], extend data ethics beyond openness toward equity. "Collective benefit" ensures that data use supports Indigenous communities; "authority to control" reaffirms their governance rights; "responsibility" calls for transparency and accountability in data use; and "ethics" emphasizes alignment with Indigenous worldviews and values. CARE requires free, prior, and informed consent (FPIC) and a commitment to real, tangible benefits. In AI imaging projects, this could mean involving Māori or Indigenous health leaders in design decisions, aligning outcomes with community health priorities, and maintaining cultural safety in data handling.

Maiam nayri Wingara [63, 64, 68, 69], an Aboriginal and Torres Strait Islander data sovereignty collective in Australia, reinforces these principles in the local context. It promotes Indigenous self-determination in data governance, advocating that data projects reflect Indigenous aspirations and cultural narratives. For example, Aboriginal-led ethics committees should guide AI projects using Indigenous health data, ensuring that research is respectful, relevant, and empowering. In New Zealand, **Te Mana Raraunga** [65–67] plays a similar role for Māori data sovereignty, emphasizing Indigenous control, leadership, and the incorporation of Māori perspectives in all data initiatives.

7.6.2 Strategies for Inclusive and Fair AI

Technical solutions include diversifying datasets, auditing models for subgroup performance, rebalancing training objectives, and adapting tools for new clinical environments [70–73]. For example, using transfer learning or domain adaptation [74, 75] can tailor general models to better fit Indigenous populations. Fairness-aware metrics—such as equal opportunity or minimum subgroup accuracy—help ensure equitable outcomes beyond aggregate accuracy.

Governance strategies involve community-led oversight, transparent reporting, and equitable benefit-sharing. Embedding OCAP® or CARE into project agreements ensures that communities retain control and receive meaningful benefits. These principles can also inform engagement with CALD and other minority populations, who may similarly face exclusion and require protections around data governance, consent, and culturally sensitive implementation.

Capacity building and inclusive design are also critical. This includes involving Indigenous and minority researchers, training developers in cultural competence, and ensuring that affected communities co-design the tools intended for them. **Post-deployment monitoring** is equally essential: AI systems must be continuously evaluated in real-world use to detect emerging biases and update models accordingly—particularly in diverse or evolving demographic contexts.

7.7 EDITORS' COMMENTS

This chapter has reinforced the importance of the correctness of fit of any AI model used in any aspect of patient care. Many examples are presented that highlight the danger of using a model which is not optimal for the target population. These issues, and others, will only come to light via thorough monitoring and scrutiny of the model outputs. Careful consideration of the population the AI is intended to help is needed to minimize risk and maximize benefit. This will involve all stakeholders and end users contributing to the inception, design, and implementation of AI tools in healthcare. Care should be taken to ensure the inclusion of minority and indigenous populations, whilst respecting their cultural preferences in relation to personal data management, and to ensure appropriate and acceptable data governance.

REFERENCES

1. Zhang, X., Pérez-Stable, E.J., Bourne, P.E. et al. (2017) Big Data Science: Opportunities and Challenges to Address Minority Health and Health Disparities in the 21st Century. Ethnicity & Disease. 27(2):95.
2. Sklar, D.P. (2018) Disparities, Health Inequities, and Vulnerable Populations: Will Academic Medicine Meet the Challenge? Academic Medicine. 93(1):1–3. https://doi.org/10.1097/ACM.0000000000002010
3. Doshi, R.P., Aseltine, R.H., Sabina, A.B. et al. (2017) Racial and Ethnic Disparities in Preventable Hospitalizations for Chronic Disease: Prevalence and Risk Factors. Journal of Racial and Ethnic Health Disparities. 4:1100–1106. https://doi.org/10.1007/s40615-016-0315-z
4. Powell, E.E., Skoien, R., Rahman, T. et al. (2019) Increasing Hospitalization Rates for Cirrhosis: Overrepresentation of Disadvantaged Australians. EClinicalMedicine. 11:44–53. https://doi.org/10.1016/j.eclinm.2019.05.007
5. Trivedi, A.N., Bailie, R., Bailie, J. et al. (2017) Hospitalizations for Chronic Conditions Among Indigenous Australians after Medication Copayment Reductions: The Closing the Gap Copayment Incentive. Journal of General Internal Medicine. 32:501–507. https://doi.org/10.1007/s11606-016-3912-y
6. Umaefulam, V., Kleissen, T., Barnabe, C. (2022) The Representation of Indigenous Peoples in Chronic Disease Clinical Trials in Australia, Canada, New Zealand, and the United States. Clinical Trials. 19(1):22–32. https://doi.org/10.1177/17407745211069153
7. Whop, L. (2022) Inequities in Cancer Outcomes for Aboriginal and Torres Strait Islander Peoples With Cancer. Power. 10508:016–0728. https://doi.org/10.1111/ajco.13868

8. Miles, R.C., Onega, T., Lee, C.I. (2018) Addressing Potential Health Disparities in the Adoption of Advanced Breast Imaging Technologies. Academic Radiology. 25(5):547–551. https://doi.org/10.1016/j.acra.2017.05.021
9. Dulaney, A., Virostko, J. (2024) Disparities in the Demographic Composition of the Cancer Imaging Archive. Radiology Imaging Cancer. 6(1):e230100. https://doi.org/10.1148/rycan.230100
10. DeBenedectis, C.M., Spalluto, L.B., Americo, L. et al. (2022) Health Care Disparities in Radiology—A Review of the Current Literature. Journal of the American College of Radiology. 19(1):101–111. https://doi.org/10.1016/j.jacr.2021.08.024
11. Perry, H., Eisenberg, R.L., Swedeen, S.T. et al. (2018) Improving Imaging Care for Diverse, Marginalized, and Vulnerable Patient Populations. Radiographics. 38(6):1833–1844. https://doi.org/10.1148/rg.2018180034
12. Waite, S., Scott, J., Colombo, D. (2021) Narrowing the Gap: Imaging Disparities in Radiology. Radiology. 299(1):27–35. https://doi.org/10.1148/radiol.2021203742
13. Chia, M., Hersch, S., Sayres, R. et al. (2022) Validation of a Deep Learning System for the Detection of Diabetic Retinopathy in Indigenous Australians. Investigative Ophthalmology & Visual Science. 108(2):268–273. https://doi.org/10.1136/bjo-2022-322237
14. Chia, M., Hersh, F., Sayres, R. et al. (2024) Validation of a Deep Learning System for the Detection of Diabetic Retinopathy in Indigenous Australians. British Journal of Ophthalmology. 108(2):268–273. https://doi.org/10.1136/bjo-2022-322237
15. Li, Q., Drinkwater, J.J., Woods, K. et al. (2025) Implementation of a New, Mobile Diabetic Retinopathy Screening Model Incorporating Artificial Intelligence in Remote Western Australia. Australian Journal of Rural Health. 33(2):e70031. https://doi.org/10.1111/ajr.70031
16. Hu, W., Joseph, S., Li, R. et al. (2024) Population Impact and Cost-Effectiveness of Artificial Intelligence-Based Diabetic Retinopathy Screening in People Living with Diabetes in Australia: A Cost Effectiveness Analysis. EClinicalMedicine. https://doi.org/10.1016/j.eclinm.2023.102387
17. Scheetz, J., Koca, D., McGuinness, M. et al. (2021) Real-World Artificial Intelligence-Based Opportunistic Screening for Diabetic Retinopathy in Endocrinology and Indigenous Healthcare Settings in Australia. Scientific Reports. 11(1):15808. https://doi.org/10.1038/s41598-021-94178-5
18. Habib, A.R., Crossland, G., Patel, H. et al. (2022) An Artificial Intelligence Computer-Vision Algorithm to Triage Otoscopic Images from Australian Aboriginal and Torres Strait Islander Children. Otology & Neurotology. 43(4):481–488. https://doi.org/10.1097/MAO.0000000000003484
19. Habib, A.R., Crossland, G., Sacks, R. et al. (2024) Tele-Otology for Aboriginal and Torres Strait Islander People Living in Rural and Remote Areas. The Laryngoscope. 134(12):5096–5102. https://doi.org/10.1002/lary.31624
20. Stephens, J.H., Nguyen, P.P., Machell, A. et al. (2025) A Multimodal Machine Learning Algorithm Improved Diagnostic Accuracy for Otitis Media in a School Aged Aboriginal Population. Journal of Biomedical Informatics. 164:104801. https://doi.org/10.1016/j.jbi.2025.104801
21. Soh, C.H., Wright, L., Baumann, A. et al. (2024) Use of Artificial Intelligence-Guided Echocardiography to Detect Cardiac Dysfunction and Heart Valve Disease in Rural and Remote Areas: Rationale and Design of the AGILE-echo Trial. American Heart Journal. 277:11–19. https://doi.org/10.1016/j.ahj.2024.08.004
22. Parker, K., Bartholomew, K., Sandiford, P. et al. (2025) Te Oranga Pūkahukahu Research Programme: Intentional Steps Towards a National Equity-Focused Lung Cancer Screening Programme in Aotearoa New Zealand. Journal of the Royal Society of New Zealand. 1–16. https://doi.org/10.1080/03036758.2025.2458037
23. Pierson, E., Cutler, D.M., Leskovec, J. et al. (2021) An Algorithmic Approach to Reducing Unexplained Pain Disparities in Underserved Populations. Nature Medicine. 27(1):136–140. https://doi.org/10.1038/s41591-020-01192-7
24. Lee, S.H., Fox, S., Smith, R. et al. (2024) Development and Validation of a Deep Learning Model for Detecting Signs of Tuberculosis on Chest Radiographs Among US-Bound Immigrants and Refugees. PLoS Digital Health. 3(9):e0000612. https://doi.org/10.1371/journal.pdig.0000612
25. Ferrara, E. (2023) Fairness and Bias in Artificial Intelligence: A Brief Survey of Sources, Impacts, and Mitigation Strategies. Science. 6(1):3. https://doi.org/10.3390/sci6010003
26. Morse, L., Teodorescu, M.H., Awwad, Y. et al. (2021) Do the Ends Justify the Means? Variation in the Distributive and Procedural Fairness of Machine Learning Algorithms. Journal of Business Ethics. 1–13. https://doi.org/10.1007/s10551-021-04939-5
27. Pfeiffer, J., Gutschow, J., Haas, C. et al. (2023) Algorithmic Fairness in AI: An Interdisciplinary View. Business & Information Systems Engineering. 65(2):209–222. https://doi.org/10.1007/s12599-023-00787-x
28. Konczi, A.E., Bill, L. (2024) Advancing First Nations Principles of OCAP®. In Indigenous and Tribal Peoples and Cancer. Springer. pp. 37–39. https://doi.org/10.1007/978-3-031-56806-0_8
29. Wright, A.L., Butt, M.L., Miller, V. et al. (2023) The Use of Graphic Facilitation to Support Adherence to OCAP® Principles in Research With Indigenous Communities. International Journal of Qualitative Methods. 22. https://doi.org/10.1177/16094069231190557
30. Carroll, S.R., Garba, I., Figueroa-Rodríguez, O.L. et al. (2023) The CARE principles for indigenous data governance. Open Scholarship Press Curated Volumes: Policy.
31. Carroll, S.R., Herczog, E., Hudson, M. et al. (2021) Operationalizing the CARE and FAIR Principles for Indigenous Data Futures. Scientific Data. 8(1):108. https://doi.org/10.1038/s41597-021-00892-0
32. Health, A.I.O. and Welfare. (2021) BreastScreen Australia Monitoring Report 2021. Australian Institute of Health and Welfare.
33. Mander, G., Starkey, D., Dobeli, K. (2024) Imaging Personnel Are Key to Improved Imaging Service Delivery in Rural Areas. Australian Journal of Rural Health. 32(6):1258–1259. https://doi.org/10.1111/ajr.13197
34. Cleary, M., Edwards, C., Mitchell-Watson, J. et al. (2024) Benchmarking Non-Attendance Patterns in Paediatric Medical Imaging: A Retrospective Cohort Study Spotlighting First Nations Children. Radiography (Lond). 30(2):492–499. https://doi.org/10.1016/j.radi.2024.01.002
35. Sullivan, T., McCarty, G., Wyeth, E. et al. (2023) Describing the Health-Related Quality of Life of Māori Adults in Aotearoa Me Te Waipounamu (New Zealand). Quality of Life Research. 32(7):2117–2126. https://doi.org/10.1007/s11136-023-03399-w
36. Bhat, S., Bir, S., Schreve, F. et al. (2022) Ethnic Disparities in CT Aortography Use for Diagnosing Acute Aortic Syndrome. Radiology: Cardiothoracic Imaging. 4(6):e220018. https://doi.org/10.1148/ryct.220018

37. Royal Australian and New Zealand College of Radiologists (RANZCR). (2023) Action Plan for Māori, Aboriginal and Torres Strait Islander Health. Available at: https://www.ranzcr.com/whats-on/news-media/action-plan-maori-aboriginal-torres-strait-islander-health

38. Adams, S.J., Babyn, P., Mendez, I. (2021) Access to Mammography Among Indigenous Peoples in North America. Academic Radiology. 28(7):950–952. https://doi.org/10.1016/j.acra.2021.04.002

39. Adams, S.J., Babyn, P., Burbridge, B. et al. (2021) Access to Ultrasound Imaging: a Qualitative Study in Two Northern, Remote, Indigenous Communities in Canada. International Journal of Circumpolar Health. 80(1):1961392. https://doi.org/10.1080/22423982.2021.1961392

40. Birly, S., Teeple, A., Illes, J. (2024) The Realization of Portable MRI for Indigenous Communities in the USA and Canada. Journal of Law, Medicine & Ethics. 52(4):816–823. https://doi.org/10.1017/jme.2024.159

41. Adams, S.J., (2021) Improving Access to Ultrasound Imaging in Northern, Remote Communities. Thesis, University of Saskatchewan. Improving Access to Ultrasound Imaging in Northern, Remote Communities

42. Moecke, D.P., Holyk, T., Beckett, M. et al. (2024) Scoping Review of Telehealth Use by Indigenous Populations from Australia, Canada, New Zealand, and the United States. Journal of Telemedicine and Telecare. 30(9):1398–1416. https://doi.org/10.1177/1357633X231158835

43. Kurumety, S.K., Howshar, J.T., Loving, V.A. (2023) Breast Cancer Screening and Outcomes Disparities Persist for Native American Women. Journal of Breast Imaging. 5(1):3–10. https://doi.org/10.1093/jbi/wbac080

44. Peña, M.A., Sudarshan, A., Muns, C.M. et al. (2023) Analysis of Geographic Accessibility of Breast, Lung, and Colorectal Cancer Screening Centers Among American Indian and Alaskan Native Tribes. Journal of the American College of Radiology: JACR. 20(7):642–651. https://doi.org/10.1016/j.jacr.2023.04.007

45. Davidson, M., Kielar, A., Tonseth, R.P., Seland, K., Harvie, S., Hanneman, K. (2024) The Landscape of Rural and Remote Radiology in Canada: Opportunities and Challenges. Canadian Association of Radiologists Journal. 75(2):304–312. https://doi.org/10.1177/08465371231197953

46. Larrazabal, A.J., Nieto, N., Peterson, V. et al. (2020) Gender Imbalance in Medical Imaging Datasets Produces Biased Classifiers for Computer-Aided Diagnosis. Proceedings of the National Academy of Sciences. 117(23):12592–12594. https://doi.org/10.1073/pnas.1919012117

47. Li, Z., Keel, S., Liu, C. et al. (2018) An Automated Grading System for Detection of Vision-Threatening Referable Diabetic Retinopathy on the Basis of Color fundus Photographs. Diabetes Care. 41(12):2509–2516. https://doi.org/10.2337/dc18-0147

48. Chirra, P., Leo, P., Yim, M. et al. (2018) Empirical Evaluation of Cross-Site Reproducibility in Radiomic Features for Characterizing Prostate MRI. In Medical imaging 2018: Computer-Aided Diagnosis. SPIE. https://doi.org/10.1117/12.2293992

49. Khor, S., Heagerty, P.J., Basu, A. et al. (2023) Racial Disparities in the Ascertainment of Cancer Recurrence in Electronic Health Records. JCO Clinical Cancer Informatics. 7:e2300004. https://doi.org/10.1200/CCI.23.00004

50. Montoya, L.N., Roberts, J.S., Hidalgo, B.S. (2025) Towards Fairness in AI for Melanoma Detection: Systemic Review and Recommendations. In Future of Information and Communication Conference. Springer. https://doi.org/10.1007/978-3-031-84460-7_21

51. Banerjee, I., Bhattacharjee, K., Burns, J.L. et al. (2023) "Shortcuts" Causing Bias in Radiology Artificial Intelligence: Causes, Evaluation, and Mitigation. Journal of the American College of Radiology. 20(9):842–851. https://doi.org/10.1117/12.3023603

52. DeGrave, A.J., Janizek, J.D., Lee, S.-I. (2021) AI for Radiographic COVID-19 Detection Selects Shortcuts Over Signal. Nature Machine Intelligence. 3(7):610–619. https://doi.org/10.1038/s42256-021-00338-7

53. Zech, J.R., Badgeley, M.A., Liu, M., Oermann, E.K. et al. (2018) Variable Generalization Performance of a Deep Learning Model to Detect Pneumonia in Chest Radiographs: A Cross-Sectional Study. PLoS Medicine. 15(11):e1002683. https://doi.org/10.1371/journal.pmed.1002683

54. U.S. Food and Drug Administration. (2025) Artificial Intelligence-Enabled Device Software Functions: Lifecycle Management and Marketing Submission Recommendations, in Draft Guidance for Industry and Food and Drug Administration Staff. Silver Spring, MD. Available at: https://www.fda.gov/regulatory-information/search-fda-guidance-documents/artificial-intelligence-enabled-device-software-functions-lifecycle-management-and-marketing

55. Rosenbacke, R., Melhus, Å, McKee, M., Stuckler, D. et al. (2024) How Explainable Artificial Intelligence Can Increase or Decrease Clinicians' Trust in AI Applications in Health Care: Systematic Review. JMIR AI. 3:e53207. https://doi.org/10.2196/53207

56. Burlina, P., Joshi, N., Paul, W. et al. (2021) Addressing Artificial Intelligence Bias in Retinal Diagnostics. Translational Vision Science & Technology. 10(2):13. https://doi.org/10.1167/tvst.10.2.13

57. Seyyed-Kalantari, L., Zhang, H., McDermott, M.B. et al. (2021) Underdiagnosis Bias of Artificial Intelligence Algorithms Applied to Chest Radiographs in Under-Served Patient Populations. Nature Medicine. 27(12):2176–2182. https://doi.org/10.1038/s41591-021-01595-0

58. Miyawaki, I.A., Banerjee, I., Batalini, F. et al. (2025) Global Disparities in Artificial Intelligence-Based Mammogram Interpretation for Breast Cancer: A Scientometric Analysis of Representation, Trends, and Equity. European Journal of Cancer. 220:115394. https://doi.org/10.1016/j.ejca.2025.115394

59. Gichoya, J.W., Banerjee, I., Bhimireddy, A.R. et al. (2022) AI Recognition of Patient Race in Medical Imaging: A Modelling Study. The Lancet Digital Health. 4(6):e406–e414. https://doi.org/10.1016/S2589-7500(22)00063-2

60. Pham, T.T., Berecki-Gisolf, J., Clapperton, A. et al. (2021) Definitions of Culturally and Linguistically Diverse (CALD): A Literature Review of Epidemiological Research in Australia. International Journal of Environmental Research and Public Health. 18(2):737. https://doi.org/10.3390/ijerph18020737

61. Paul, H.Y., Kim, T.K., Siegel, E. et al. (2022) Demographic Reporting in Publicly Available Chest Radiograph Data Sets: Opportunities for Mitigating Sex and Racial Disparities in Deep Learning Models. Journal of the American College of Radiology. 19(1):192–200. https://doi.org/10.1016/j.jacr.2021.08.018

62. Tripathi, S., Gabriel, K., Dheer, S. et al. (2023) Understanding Biases and Disparities in Radiology AI Datasets: A Review. Journal of the American College of Radiology. 20(9):836–841. https://doi.org/10.1016/j.jacr.2023.06.015

63. Summit, I.D.S. (2016) Indigenous Data Sovereignty. Available at: https://www.aigi.org.au/wp-content/uploads/2022/01/Communique-Indigenous-Data-Sovereignty-Summit-1.pdf

64. Walter, M., Lovett, R., Maher, B. et al. (2021) Indigenous Data Sovereignty in the Era of Big Data and Open Data. Australian Journal of Social Issues. 56(2):143–156. https://doi.org/10.1002/ajs4.141

65. Whittaker, Dobson, Jin, C.K. et al. (2023) An Example of Governance for AI in Health Services from Aotearoa New Zealand. NPJ Digital Medicine. 6(1):164. https://doi.org/10.1038/s41746-023-00882-z

66. Poor, A. (2022) Data Sovereignty in Action: Designing Building and Implementing a Radically Distributed Health Information System in Aotearoa New Zealand. Auckland University of Technology. Available at: https://openrepository. aut.ac.nz/server/api/core/bitstreams/83f30b76-2248-4692-abe8-53a3f1c6d88b/content

67. Kukutai, T., Cassim, S., Clark, V. et al. (2023) Māori data sovereignty and privacy. https://doi.org/10.15663/j21.35481

68. Bowman, D.N., Bremner, L. (2024) Indigenous Data Sovereignty: Applying It By, With, For, and Through Indigenous Evaluators and Evaluations. Canadian Journal of Program Evaluation. 39(2):265–287. https://doi.org/10.3138/cjpe-2024-0039

69. Kelly, L.M., Wong, D., Timothy, A. (2024) Measuring What Counts in Aboriginal and Torres Strait Islander Care: A Review of General Practice Datasets Available for Assessing Chronic Disease Care. Australian Journal of Primary Health. 30(4). https://doi.org/10.1071/PY24017

70. Ricci, Lara, M.A., Echeveste, R., Ferrante, E. (2022) Addressing Fairness in Artificial Intelligence for Medical Imaging. Nature Communications. 13(1):4581. https://doi.org/10.1038/s41467-022-32186-3

71. Xu, Z., Li, J., Yao, Q. et al. (2024) Addressing Fairness Issues in Deep Learning-Based Medical Image Analysis: A Systematic Review. NPJ Digital Medicine. 7(1):286. https://doi.org/10.1038/s41746-024-01276-5

72. Chen, R.J., Wang, J.J., Williamson, D.F. et al. (2023) Algorithmic Fairness in Artificial Intelligence for Medicine and Healthcare. Nature Biomedical Engineering. 7(6):719–742. https://doi.org/10.1038/s41551-023-01056-8

73. Drukker, K., Chen, W., Gichoya, J. et al. (2023) Toward Fairness in Artificial Intelligence for Medical Image Analysis: Identification and Mitigation of Potential Biases in the Roadmap from Data Collection to Model Deployment. Journal of Medical Imaging. 10(6):061104. https://doi.org/10.1117/1.JMI.10.6.061104

74. Chaddad, A., Lu, Q., Li, J. et al. (2023) Explainable, Domain-Adaptive, and Federated Artificial Intelligence in Medicine. IEEE/CAA Journal of Automatica Sinica. 10(4):859–876. https://doi.org/10.1109/JAS.2023.123123

75. Tian, Y., Wen, C., Shi, M. et al. (2024) FairDomain: Achieving Fairness in Cross-Domain Medical Image Segmentation and Classification. In European Conference on Computer Vision. Springer. https://doi.org/10.1007/978-3-031-73116-7_15

8 AI in Cardiology

Alicja Jasinska-Piadlo and Sonyia McFadden

8.1 INTRODUCTION

Before we discuss how AI is used in daily practice, it is important to discuss the extent of the prevalence of cardiovascular disease (CVD) and its impact on quality of life and life expectancy. According to the latest data collated by the British Heart Foundation, in the UK alone [1],

- there are 7.6 million people living with heart and circulatory disease

- every 3 minutes someone dies of a heart or circulatory disease

- every 5 minutes someone is admitted to hospital due to stroke

- 13 babies a day are diagnosed with a congenital heart defect

CVD is one of the most common causes of mortality and morbidity worldwide. The term CVD is an umbrella term that includes (i) pathological processes affecting heart muscle, (ii) the heart's own arteries presenting with coronary artery disease, (iii) disease of the cardiac conduction system, including various arrhythmias, (iv) disease of heart valves, and (v) disease of the arterial and circulatory system, including stroke and thrombotic events such as pulmonary embolus and peripheral vascular disease.

The application of AI in cardiology ranges from electrocardiogram (ECG) interpretation and imaging interpretation to risk stratification and treatment planning, marking a significant shift towards precision medicine or personalised medicine using an individual tailored approach to disease prevention [2].

8.2 HISTORICAL CONTEXT AND EVOLUTION

The journey of AI in cardiology began with rule-based systems designed to interpret electrocardiograms in the 1970s [3]. These early tools were limited by their dependence on human-coded logic. With the rise of machine learning (ML) in the early 2000s, AI began to analyse real-world clinical data more effectively. Deep learning, particularly convolutional neural networks (CNNs), emerged as a transformative technology around 2010, especially for image-rich data like echocardiography and CT angiography [4]. Today, AI-driven software solutions are Food and Drug Administration (FDA)-cleared for applications ranging from arrhythmia detection to automated cardiac imaging analysis, marking a pivotal moment in the digital transformation of cardiovascular care [5].

8.3 CURRENT CLINICAL APPLICATIONS OF AI IN DAILY PRACTICE

The utility of AI in cardiology spans multiple domains, including diagnosis, screening, and treatment. Diagnostic tests can be divided into **non-invasive tests,** e.g. using detection of electric potentials produced by the heart, such as an ECG; using ultrasound, such as a surface echocardiogram (transthoracic ECHO); using a magnetic field such as cardiac magnetic resonance imaging (MRI); and using ionising radiation, such as in cardiac computed tomography (CT). There is also a breadth of **invasive cardiac tests** and procedures, such as invasive coronary angiography, percutaneous coronary interventions (PCI), electrophysiology studies, and ablation procedures used to treat arrhythmia. Those invasive and non-invasive tests allow decisions to be made on the need for cardiac intervention, e.g. including coronary artery stent implantation, used as a treatment of blocked coronary arteries that can lead to myocardial infarction, commonly known as heart attack. Cardiologists perform procedures transcutaneously (through the skin) or via access in either the radial artery in the wrist or femoral artery in the groin. Those procedures are performed under fluoroscopy, using ionising radiation and ultrasound. Apart from coronary artery interventions, which aim to deliver treatment to coronary arteries, there are also treatments available for valvular disease. Aortic stenosis (the narrowing of the aortic valve) is the most common valvular disease affecting people aged 70 years and over. Due to advancements in interventional cardiology, patients can receive a new valve through the percutaneous access, avoiding the need for cardiac surgery, which requires open-heart surgery.

AI tools have found great application in cardiology and have been successfully implemented into the following areas.

DOI: 10.1201/9781032709956-8

8.3.1 ECG Interpretation and Arrhythmia Detection

AI-powered ECG interpretation tools are now common in both hospital and outpatient settings. Machine learning models can detect arrhythmias (irregular heartbeat), such as atrial fibrillation (AF), ventricular ectopy, and even subtle patterns suggestive of structural heart disease. These tools provide initial flags for clinicians, aiding in faster triage and reducing interpretation variability among providers. Several FDA-approved algorithms are now routinely embedded in ECG machines and software. For example, GE Healthcare's MUSE™ ECG Management System incorporates AI to interpret ECGs for common arrhythmias, myocardial infarction, and conduction abnormalities.

AI-powered ECG interpretation apps such as AliveCor KardiaMobile™ and Eko DUO™ are also FDA-cleared and widely used in outpatient and telemedicine settings [6]. These tools detect irregular heart rhythms, e.g. AF and other arrhythmias from single-lead ECGs, and can integrate with electronic health records for rapid review. In the UK the National Institute for Health and Care Excellence (NICE), which is a national body tasked with regular clinical practice guidance review, recommended the use of AliveCore Kardia Mobile as a screening tool in general practice and in the community for one of the most common arrhythmias, namely AF. Atrial fibrillation is a heart arrhythmia that significantly increases a risk of stroke if it is undetected and untreated with anticoagulation medication (commonly known as blood thinners). A high accuracy of detection of AF, the ease of use and relatively low cost of the device resulted in the Medical Technologies Guidance (MTG 64) published by NICE in 2023. The main clinical evidence used to support the development of the NICE 2023 guidelines comprises 27 studies, including five randomised controlled trials using a head-to-head comparisons of the accuracy of AF detection using standard of care versus a new care using KardiaMobile, with AI-based algorithm detecting AF. Detecting AF in individuals suspected of having paroxysmal AF typically requires continuous ECG monitoring, often through wearing a Holter monitor for one to two days. The KardiaMobile is a portable ECG recorder that can assist in the detection of AF. Clinical evidence indicates that significantly more cases of AF are detected with the KardiaMobile single-lead device compared to a Holter monitor. Additionally, cost modelling reveals that the KardiaMobile is cost-effective, saving an average of £13.22 per patient over a two-year period for those presenting with symptoms such as palpitations. The cost savings associated with KardiaMobile stem from a reduction in diagnostic expenses, including the cost of the device itself.

8.3.2 Echocardiography

AI is transforming echocardiography by automating image acquisition, segmentation, measurement, and disease detection, which in turn enhances accuracy, reproducibility, and efficiency. AI-powered tools guide probe positioning, assess image quality in real time, and automatically delineate cardiac structures to calculate parameters like left ventricular ejection fraction (LVEF) and global longitudinal strain (GLS). LVEF is one of the features that is used to describe the function of the heart. It is a measurement of how much blood the heart pumps out with each beat (i.e. the fraction of blood ejected from the left ventricle in systole compared to the volume of blood remaining at the end of diastole). It is expressed as a percentage and indicates how efficiently the heart's main pumping chamber, the left ventricle, is working.

- A normal LVEF typically falls between 55% and 70%. Based on the value of LVEF, cardiologists distinguish normal LVEF: A healthy heart pumps out about 55% to 70% of the blood in the left ventricle with each contraction.

- Reduced LVEF: An ejection fraction below 40% may indicate heart failure or other heart conditions

- Mildly Reduced: A range of 41% to 49%

- Moderately Reduced: A range of 30% to 40%

- Severely Reduced: An ejection fraction below 30%

Ejection fraction is a key indicator of how well the heart is pumping blood, and it can be used to diagnose and monitor heart conditions. Low ejection fraction is a common feature of heart failure, a condition where the heart cannot pump enough blood to meet the body's needs. Quantifying the ejection fraction can help doctors determine the best course of treatment for heart problems. While ejection fraction is a valuable measure, other factors like the patient's clinical symptoms, other test results, and individual health status are also considered in diagnosis and treatment. Ejection fraction has been used in many clinical trials as a measure of the response to treatment of multiple cardiac conditions. Traditionally, the measurement of the LVEF has been performed manually, by visually measuring the size of the left ventricle at the beginning and end of a heartbeat and estimating the proportion of blood ejected from the left ventricle. The use of AI to replace this manual task reduces operator dependence and inter-observer variability, allowing for more consistent and faster reporting. This all contributes to reproducibility and speed in diagnosis allowing for quicker treatment/intervention. Moreover, AI algorithms can also flag structural heart diseases such as cardiomyopathies and valvular lesions, providing real-time decision support and improving diagnostic confidence. These advances can be particularly valuable for less-experienced operators and in resource-limited settings where expert echocardiographers are scarce. Despite challenges such as data quality, algorithm bias, and regulatory considerations, AI applications in echocardiography hold great promise for expanding access to high-quality cardiac imaging [7–10].

AI-powered systems such as EchoGo (Ultromics) and Caption Health assist in image acquisition and interpretation. These tools provide real-time guidance for optimal probe positioning and automate LVEF estimation to detect and track heart failure.

8.3.3 Cardiac CT: AI in Coronary Calcium Scoring and Plaque Analysis

AI tools are increasingly used in cardiac computed tomography, especially in CT coronary angiography (CTCA). CTCA is now widely accepted as a noninvasive, highly sensitive **test** for ruling out significant coronary artery disease (CAD), especially in patients where the diagnosis is uncertain. CAD is characterised by the presence of atherosclerotic plaques. Atherosclerotic plaque consists of a buildup of a fatty substance, including cholesterol, fat, calcium, and other materials, such as scar tissue and blood cells. The presence of these plaques causes the narrowing of the lumen of the heart arteries, gradually restricting the flow of oxygenated blood through heart arteries. Eventually, the atherosclerotic plaques can completely block the heart arteries, leading to a myocardial infarction (i.e. a heart attack). The presence of calcium in coronary arteries is a sign of the disease. The buildup of calcium in coronary arteries has been linked to the increased risk of future events of heart attack and angina (recurrent episodes of chest pain). A calcium score, known as coronary artery calcium score, is a measurement, a numerical value (Agatston score) of the amount of calcium-containing plaque in the coronary arteries. A higher calcium score indicates a higher risk of the heart attack; hence, it helps cardiologists to assess patients at risk of developing heart disease. Once that risk is known, a patient can be advised on improving their lifestyle or to start taking medication which slows down the progression of the heart disease and prevents events such as heart attack or stroke. CTCA allows non-invasive first-line assessment of the amount of calcium in the coronary arteries, by calculating the coronary artery calcium score (CAC). It also allows visualisation of the coronary arteries and identification of blockages or narrowings caused by atherosclerotic plaque.

The use of CTCA reduces the need for unnecessary invasive percutaneous coronary angiography and helps guide appropriate further testing or treatment. CTCA has evolved over the years and is now a key diagnostic tool recommended in European, UK, and US guidelines [11–13]. It offers a reliable, non-invasive way to assess coronary artery disease with high accuracy. CTCA has demonstrated a high negative predictive value in excluding coronary artery disease, ranging from 98% to 100% [14–17]. It also has a sensitivity of 89% and a specificity of 96% for detecting CAD [17].

Algorithms can now perform automated CAC scoring with high reproducibility, which is essential for risk stratification in asymptomatic patients. Additionally, AI can identify detailed plaque features, evaluate lesion severity (showing the degree of stenosis in vessels), and even simulate fractional flow reserve (FFR) CT to non-invasively determine the maximum blood flow proximal and distal to a stenosis. The fractional flow reserve is a physiological measurement used to assess the severity of a blockage in coronary artery. It is a ratio of the maximum blood flow through a narrowed artery to the maximum flow that would occur if the artery was normal. Traditionally this measurement is performed invasively, during invasive percutaneous coronary angiography, when small catheters are placed inside heart arteries. This functional information offers cardiologists a more comprehensive understanding of CAD, enhancing decision-making and treatment, for example, whether to place a stent in the artery to open the blood flow or to choose from other options like pharmacotherapy or the need for heart surgery (coronary bypass heart surgery) if there are too many diseased arteries. HeartFlow® FFR-CT is an FDA-approved tool that uses AI to create a non-invasive, colour-coded, 3D model of coronary arteries and simulate FFR [18]. HeartFlow® FFR-CT enables cardiologists to assess lesion significance and defer or plan PCI without invasive pressure wires. AI also improves image reconstruction and reduces radiation exposure, addressing the two common limitations of CT imaging.

Another FDA-cleared platform, Cleerly Coronary™, represents the leading edge of AI-enhanced cardiac CT interpretation. Cleerly, uses machine learning algorithms to quantify total plaque volume, lumen diameter, and lesion location on coronary artery disease. It can also monitor atherosclerotic plaque progression and vessel narrowing over time, critical for primary prevention and the assessment of therapeutic efficacy. AI assists in automated vessel delineation, atherosclerotic plaque characterisation and stent sizing. Tools like HeartFlow FFR-CT use AI to simulate blood flow and identify ischaemia-producing lesions from standard CTA data. AI improves calcium scoring, plaque analysis, and coronary artery segmentation. Aidoc and Zebra Medical Vision offer FDA-cleared tools that identify incidental findings and CAD markers in CT scans. For coronary calcium scoring, tools like Philips' IntelliSpace Portal and Siemens Healthineers AI-Rad Companion automatically compute Agatston scores, stratify risk, and integrate with picture archiving and communication system (PACS) for seamless clinical review.

8.3.4 Cardiac MRI: Automated Image Analysis and Tissue Characterisation

Cardiac magnetic resonance imaging (CMRI) is the gold standard for myocardial tissue characterisation. AI applications in CMRI now allow for automatic segmentation of cardiac chambers, wall motion analysis, and quantification of parameters like ejection fraction, myocardial strain, and late gadolinium enhancement. Deep learning models trained on large datasets can detect subtle myocardial fibrosis or oedema patterns associated with cardiomyopathies or myocarditis, aiding early diagnosis. AI also assists in image acquisition by optimising scanner settings in real time, reducing scan time and motion artifacts.

AI-based post-processing platforms such as Arterys Cardio AI and Circle CVI's cvi42® have FDA clearance and are widely adopted in cardiac MRI analysis. These tools automate left and right ventricular segmentation, calculate ejection fraction and detect fibrosis via late gadolinium enhancement (LGE) maps.

Arterys Cardio AI, in particular, uses cloud-based deep learning models to significantly reduce reporting time and variability between readers. There are studies showing that AI can rapidly segment heart structures to allow analysis and interpretation, with reporting time reduced from 30 minutes to under five minutes [19]. AI modules can also analyse strain patterns and detect diffuse myocardial disease with higher sensitivity than conventional techniques.

AI-based post-processing platforms like Arterys Cardio AI and Circle CVI automate the segmentation of cardiac chambers, quantification of ventricular function, and fibrosis detection. These tools significantly reduce analysis time while maintaining high accuracy [20]

8.3.5 Coronary Intervention: AI in Invasive Angiography and Intravascular Imaging

In PCI, AI supports a range of functions from procedural planning to real-time decision-making. Automated vessel delineation tools, powered by computer vision, provide precise measurements of coronary artery dimensions. AI also enables the characterisation of plaque morphology, differentiating between calcified, fibrotic, and lipid-rich plaques using inputs from coronary angiography, intravascular ultrasound (IVUS), and optical coherence tomography (OCT).

AI in interventional cardiology includes tools like Ultreon™ 1.0 Software (Abbott), an AI-powered IVUS and OCT platform that automatically analyses lesion morphology, lumen dimensions, and calcium depth. This facilitates accurate stent sizing and deployment.

8.3.6 Intravascular Ultrasound and Optical Coherence Tomography

In IVUS specifically, AI algorithms help quantify vessel area, plaque burden, and calcium thickness, which are critical for determining appropriate stent sizing and placement. This improves outcomes by reducing under- or over-expansion of the stent, a known risk factor for restenosis and thrombosis.

AI automates the interpretation of IVUS/OCT images to assess plaque characteristics. Philips' IntelliSpace Cardiovascular integrates AI to evaluate lumen dimensions, detect calcifications, and assist in stent deployment.

8.3.7 Invasive Cardiology: Electrophysiological Mapping and AI-Guided Treatment

In electrophysiology (EP), AI has revolutionised the interpretation and real-time guidance of invasive studies. AI algorithms assist in mapping complex arrhythmogenic substrates by integrating multi-channel electrogram data and high-resolution imaging to identify arrhythmia foci. AI-driven systems can now provide potential maps of electrical activity, highlighting regions of conduction block or slow conduction in AF or ventricular tachycardia. Furthermore, AI helps track catheter movement with increased spatial resolution and suggest ablation targets, thereby shortening procedure time and enhancing accuracy in lesion deployment. These tools are especially useful in complex ablation procedures, where human interpretation alone can be time-consuming and error-prone. The study by Fox et al. [21] illustrates that the use of the forward-solution mapping algorithm based on AI was associated with a 22.6% reduction in total procedure duration versus control cases (233 ± 51 minutes vs. 301 ± 83 min). Evaluating procedure duration by arrhythmia type demonstrated a consistent trend for all arrhythmia types with adequate cases to allow statistical comparison. A reduction in procedure duration was 28.2% for AF, 25.2% for ventricular tachycardia (VT), 25.0% for focal atrial tachycardia (AT), and 20.3% for premature ventricular contractions (PVC) cases. More importantly, the use of the algorithm was associated with a 43.7% reduction in fluoroscopy use, which exposes patients to ionising radiation, versus controls (18.7 ± 13.3 minutes vs. 33.2 ± 18.0 min) [21]. Analysis of fluoroscopy use by arrhythmia type demonstrated a consistent trend toward reduced fluoroscopy use for all arrhythmias with adequate sample size to allow statistical comparison. Reductions in fluoroscopy were recorded as 58.7% for AF, 75.2% for focal AT, 35.8% for VT, and 13.4% for PVC cases.

AI is enhancing catheter ablation procedures by improving substrate mapping and ablation planning. One such FDA-cleared system is the EnSite X™ EP System with EnSite™ AutoMap Module (Abbott), which uses advanced algorithms to automate the collection and annotation of electroanatomical maps. These maps help identify arrhythmogenic regions with high precision. Another notable tool is CardioInsight™ (Medtronic), a non-invasive mapping system that uses AI to reconstruct 3D electroanatomic maps from body-surface ECGs, guiding targeted ablation without intracardiac catheters.

These systems are particularly helpful in AF and VT cases, where electrical complexity demands a combination of real-time imaging, signal analysis, and precise localisation.

AI-guided electrophysiological mapping is used in procedures such as catheter ablation for AF. AI systems like AcQMap (Acutus Medical) provide real-time, high-resolution electroanatomical maps using machine learning algorithms. These maps enhance procedural precision by characterising atrial substrates and guiding ablation strategies [22].

8.4 WEARABLES AND REMOTE MONITORING

The integration of AI into wearable devices, such as smartwatches and biosensors, enables continuous patient monitoring outside the clinic. AI algorithms process large volumes of data from these devices, alerting clinicians to events like paroxysmal atrial fibrillation, heart rate variability anomalies, or fluid retention suggestive of worsening heart failure. In daily practice, this supports earlier intervention and more personalised management. Wearable technologies are transforming ambulatory cardiac care through continuous monitoring. The Apple Watch (series 4 and above), which has FDA clearance for atrial fibrillation detection via ECG, uses onboard AI to analyse rhythm patterns. Similarly, Fitbit and Samsung Galaxy Watch models have incorporated FDA-approved ECG functionality.

The prospective, real-world study by Mannhart et al. focused on assessment of devices widely used by the general population [23]. Five commercially available wearable smart devices—Apple Watch 6, Samsung Galaxy Watch 3, Withings ScanWatch, Fitbit Sense, and AliveCor KardiaMobile— were tested to assess their ability to diagnose AF. A 12-lead ECG read by a doctor served as the baseline to confirm the diagnostic accuracy of these wearable devices. Among the 201 individuals enrolled, 31% had AF. Sensitivity and specificity varied between devices, with the Apple Watch 6 and Samsung Galaxy Watch 3 achieving the highest sensitivity (85%), while the Withings ScanWatch had the lowest (58%). Notably, equivocal tracings requiring manual physician review occurred in up to 26% of cases, decreasing overall diagnostic accuracy. Despite these limitations, manual interpretation of smart device tracings yielded a diagnostic accuracy ranging from 98% to 100%, demonstrating the potential of these technologies for AF screening when combined with expert assessment.

BioIntelliSense's BioSticker™ and iRhythm's Zio XT Patch are FDA-approved continuous monitoring devices that use AI for arrhythmia detection, including AF, bradycardia (slow heart rate), and pauses. Pauses occur due to the disease of the conduction system of the heart, that can be life-threatening. The presence of pauses longer than two to three seconds requires pacemaker implantation to regulate the heart rate. Continuous monitoring devices analyse multi-day ECG recordings and generate structured reports that assist in early diagnosis and treatment optimisation. Reports from those devices can be downloaded remotely via the secure cloud based network to the healthcare providers' database and it can be analysed and interpreted in real time.

These FDA-approved solutions represent just a fraction of the AI ecosystem available to cardiologists today. Importantly, many of them are already integrated seamlessly into electronic health record systems or imaging platforms, enhancing usability in busy clinical settings.

8.5 DATA ANALYTICS AND USE OF AI TO LOOK FOR ACTIONABLE INSIGHTS FROM ELECTRONIC HEALTH RECORDS

The introduction and adoption of electronic health records (EHRs) has initiated widespread interest and created opportunities for translational research with respect to cardiovascular health data [24]. It is reported that the healthcare sector generates 30% of the digital data worldwide [25]. Hence, the use of digital clinical data has the potential to transform healthcare systems into "self-learning health systems" [26, 27]. In contrast to clinical trials, observational cohort studies based on extracts from digital data and EHR do not exclude real-world patients, such as elderly and frail individuals with multiple co-morbidities [28]. Research utilising secondary health data can give valuable insights into the patient pathway, change clinical practice, and improve patient outcomes especially for cohorts of patients who would not have been recruited to clinical trials. The currently available registries of patients presenting with a particular clinical problem pose a unique opportunity to monitor the disease progression and learn about patient outcomes. The wide variety of registries serve as a source of data that can be accessed and mined by researchers as well as commercial organisations developing AI tools. A perfect example of a population-based registry includes the UK Biobank [29], which can be used to improve the understanding of population health.

Governments and policymakers increasingly recognise that the healthcare sector is a field where valuable insights can now be uncovered through big data analytics [30]. As identified by McKinsey et al. countries such as Finland, Germany, UK, Israel, China, and the United States are investing in AI research and developing strategies for the implementation of AI in healthcare sector [30]. The UK government published a series of policy papers [31–34] with a number of overarching goals focused on ensuring (i) that NHS data cannot be monopolised, (ii) that data should be made accessible to trusted organisations through data access platforms, (iii) that legislation should be put in place that would ensure transparency and accountability over how the data is used, and (iv) most importantly that the NHS workforce becomes data literate and skilled in using ML and AI in order to deliver highest-quality healthcare to the UK.

The potential benefits of applying advanced analytics and ML to healthcare data are numerous, including improving patient outcomes, reducing costs, and identifying new therapies e.g. new antibiotics [35]. One area in which advanced analytics and ML can have a significant impact is the identification of patients at high risk for certain diseases or health conditions. By analysing large datasets, ML algorithms can identify patterns and risk factors that may not be apparent to human experts. This can enable healthcare providers to intervene earlier, potentially preventing the development of more serious conditions and saving lives. Another promising application of advanced analytics and ML in healthcare is in the development of personalised treatment plans. By analysing patient data, including genetic information, medical history, and lifestyle factors, ML algorithms can help healthcare providers develop targeted treatment plans that are better suited to individual patients. This can lead to better outcomes, lower costs, and improved quality of life for patients.

The process of learning from healthcare data is tedious and requires time for data preparation, formatting, and cleansing. Figure 8.1 illustrates the stages of the ML pipeline and highlights the main issues that can affect each stage.

Challenges of working with **raw healthcare data, data access, and exploration** can be executed by involving multiple stakeholders in the process of data access and data anonymisation. **Data curation** has to be carefully planned and undertaken in stages, which overlap and run in parallel. Accessing real-world healthcare data provides an opportunity to access very detailed and granular data. Accessing the aggregated open source data available from government websites and statistics offices does not provide enough granularity to mine for clinically meaningful correlations; nevertheless it gives an opportunity to draw conclusion on a wider cohort of patients. The numeric and text data (strings of characters) can be presented in a structured and unstructured format. When numerical data are presented in tabular format, it is easier to preprocess the data. There is, however, a need to extract the information about the numerical value from free text format, and only after this process the numeric value could be tabulated.

Data diversity can be overcome by selecting a limited number of data types, for example, the numeric and text data only, leaving the image and the signal data out of the particular project. The challenge of **data preprocessing** can be overcome by the involvement of domain experts. The lack **of domain specific algorithms** and the use of generic statistics and ML toolboxes are available in commercially available software like MATLAB; the specialist domain knowledge allows effective feature extraction, feature selection, and feature engineering by using generic tools.

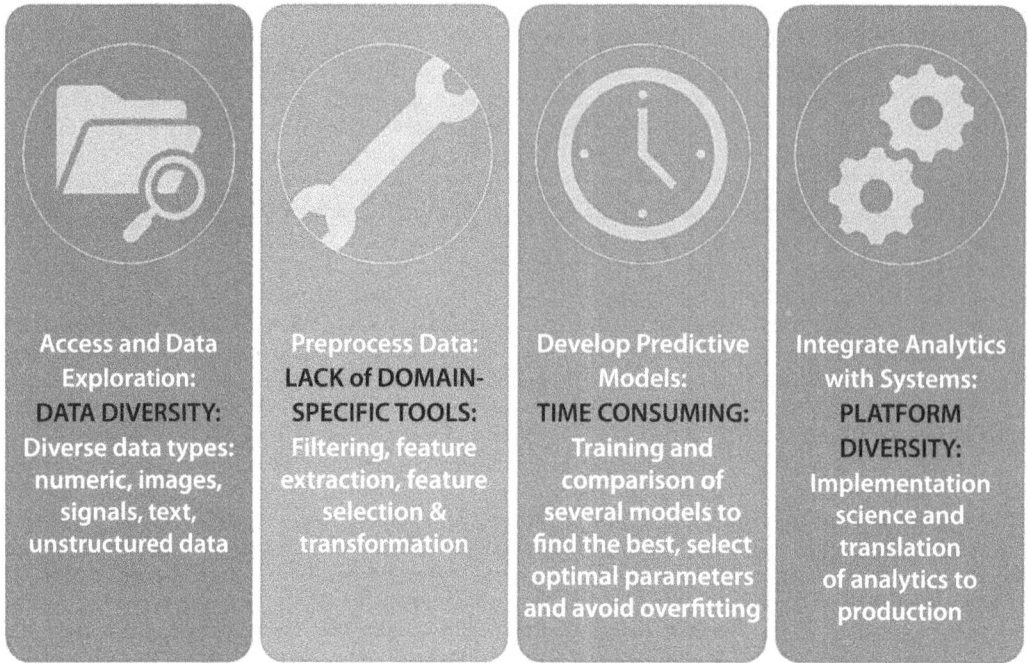

Figure 8.1 Challenges of developing a machine learning pipeline in healthcare.

Developing predictive models is **time consuming**; however, it is not as time-consuming as data exploration and data preprocessing. Over the course of developing the model there is a need to monitor algorithms on an ongoing basis and evaluate how performance will be validated, enabled by cyclical auditing. This process can be replicated in the future and the challenges can be overcome by bringing clinical, research, and technological teams together in order to benefit from the multidisciplinary team involvement in the data mining process. Creating an environment that enables and encourages experimentation will lead to enhancing innovation. An algorithm implemented into practice requires evidence for clinical use. The challenge of analytics integration, science implementation, and translation into production was addressed by examining two approaches to unsupervised ML.

8.5.1 Decision Trees

Supervised ML methods have been widely used to predict the mortality of patients with various cardiovascular conditions. A study on a large administrative heart failure (HF) database showed only marginal improvement in the accuracy of ML predictive models over traditional methods such as logistic regression (LR) [36]. However, the recent review by Shin et al. [37] showed that ML methods outperformed conventional statistical methods in HF mortality prediction in 20 selected studies. The rationale for developing yet another predictive model is to identify predictors of high importance and to explore the role of chronological age of the patient in mortality prediction.

Decision trees are one of the unsupervised ML methods that can be used on large datasets to predict mortality of patients from a trained cohort of patients and the variables of interest. Figure 8.2 illustrates the weight of the importance assigned to the individual patient variable by the decision tree algorithm.

The algorithm executes a decision based on the occurrence of each variable and the importance associated with it as illustrated in Figure 8.3.

Figure 8.3 illustrates each step that the algorithm executes in a decision tree.

8.5.2 Unsupervised ML

K-means clustering is an unsupervised ML method that is commonly used to assign members of the studied group into clusters characterised by distinctive features. This method has been widely used and applied to large EHR datasets. High-quality clustering generates several clusters with high within-cluster similarity but significant between-cluster dissimilarity. The goal of high within-cluster similarity while preserving significant between-cluster dissimilarity is especially challenging

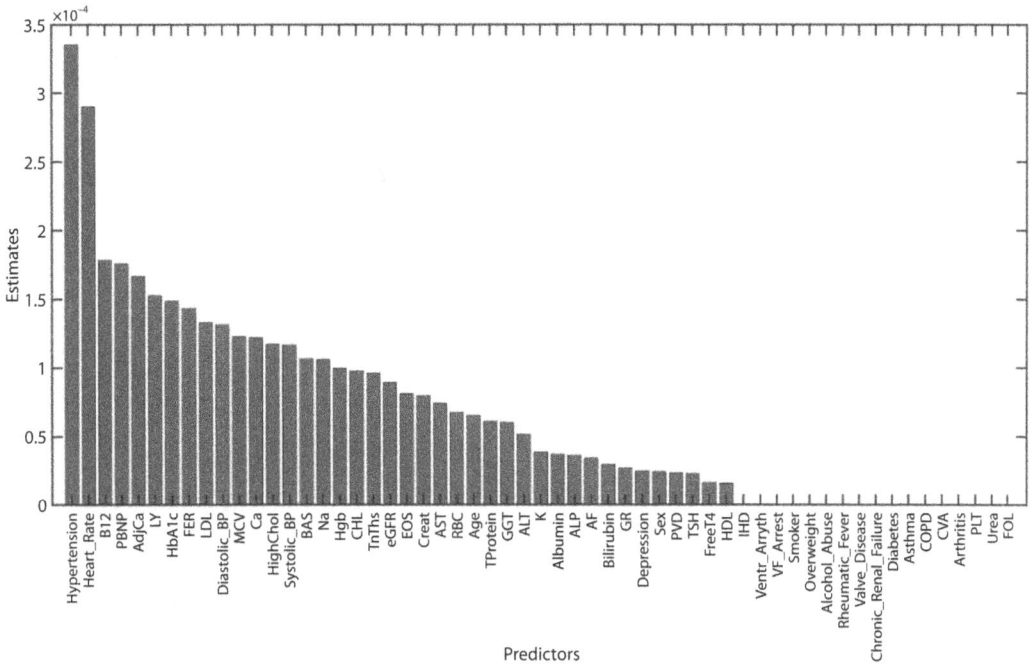

Figure 8.2 Intrinsic predictor of the importance of all variables in a fine tree.

to attain when using clustering on a large dataset. Figure 8.4 shows the example of clusters derived from a dataset of 2008 patient cases of patients with heart failure from the Sichuan Hospital in China, which served as the location for the data collection, which took place between 2016 and 2019 [38].

Clustering methods can aid the redesign the healthcare services in order to improve the detection of the health state in certain groups of patients [38]. They can be used for the purposes of clinical auditing, tracking the quality of care, impact on quality of life, comorbidities, and mortality statistics of specific cohorts of patients, with frequently occurring health problems and with specific health needs. This would serve as evidence for quality improvement interventions, clinical pathways streaming, and service re-design.

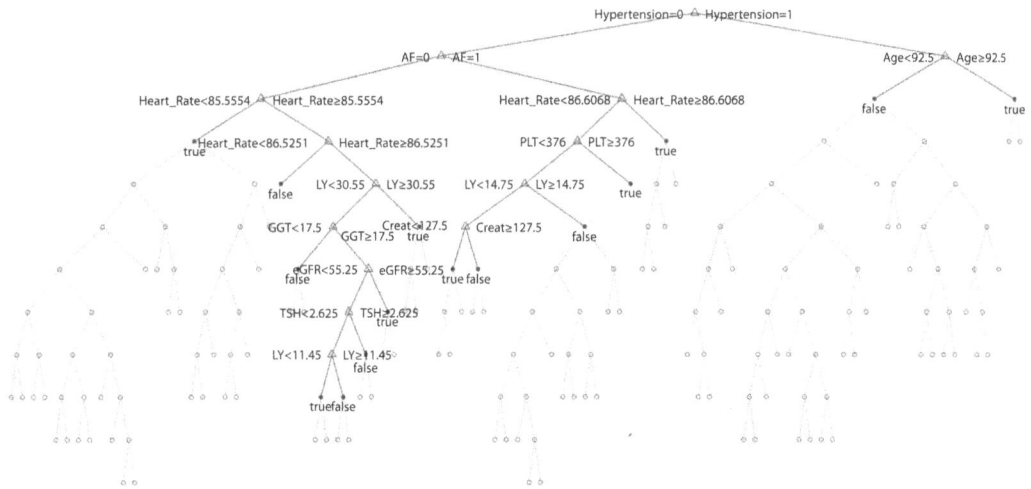

Figure 8.3 Graph of the decision tree using all variables/predictors listed in the Figure 8.2 fine tree. For the purpose of better visualisation, the decision tree has been pruned to node 11.

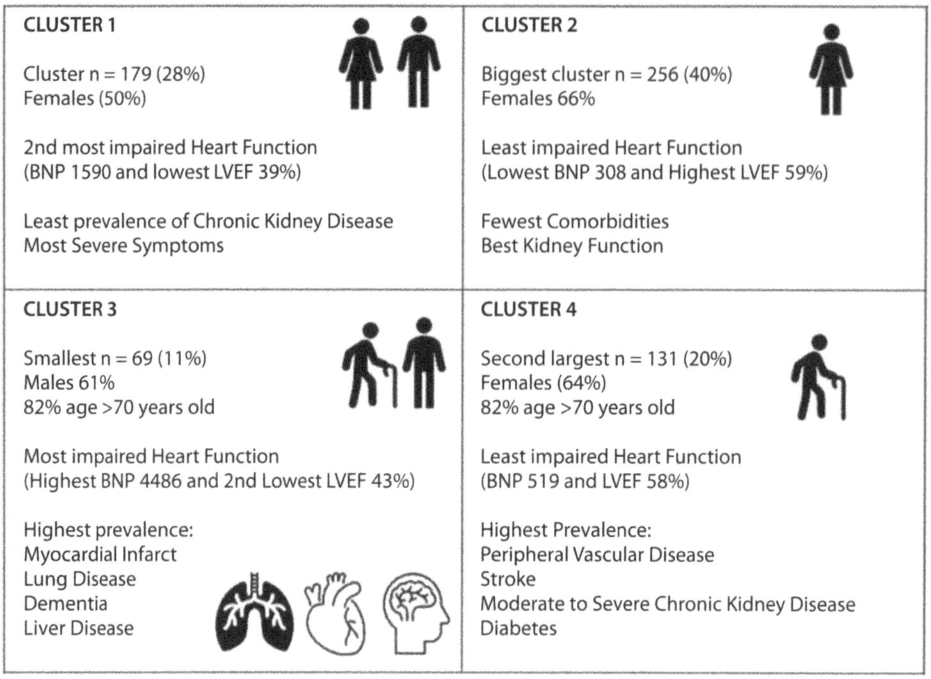

Figure 8.4 Domain-led approach to k-means clustering. Summary of most distinctive features in each cluster [38].

8.6 SUMMARY OF CLINICAL BENEFITS AND OUTCOMES OF AI IN CARDIOLOGY

The clinical integration of AI in cardiology has demonstrated measurable improvements across diagnostics, therapeutic decision-making, and patient management. Examples include the following:

Enhanced diagnostic accuracy: AI tools enhance diagnostic accuracy by detecting subtle imaging patterns or ECG abnormalities that may be overlooked by human reviewers. For instance, AI-assisted ECG interpretation systems have achieved sensitivity and specificity levels over 90% in detecting AF and left ventricular dysfunction [39]. In contrast, a study looking at the accuracy of the ECG assessment by emergency physicians showed lower sensitivity in identification of major ECG abnormalities, with sensitivity of 79% in recognition of AF. In a study where a total of 905 ECGs were analysed, 705 (78%) resulted in a similar interpretation between emergency physicians and cardiologists/expert. However, the interpretations of emergency physicians and cardiologists for the identification of major abnormalities coincided in only 66 reports. ECGs were correctly classified by emergency physicians according to their emergency level in 82% of cases. Emergency physicians correctly recognised normal ECGs (sensitivity = 0.91) [40].

Increased efficiency: Another core benefit is workflow efficiency. AI can rapidly segment cardiac structures in MRI and CT images, reducing reporting time from 30 minutes to under 5 minutes [41]. These efficiencies are particularly valuable in high-throughput environments like emergency departments and cardiac catheterisation laboratories.

Early disease detection and prognostication: Predictive models built from longitudinal EHRs can identify high-risk individuals for myocardial infarction or sudden cardiac death even before symptoms emerge [42]. For example, the Mayo Clinic's AI-enhanced ECG model predicts low LVEF with over 90% accuracy, offering a non-invasive screening alternative.

Remote monitoring and telecardiology domain: AI facilitates real-time alerting for arrhythmias or heart failure exacerbations using wearable sensors. This proactive approach by the patient themselves improves outcomes and reduces hospital readmissions [43].

8.7 CHALLENGES AND LIMITATIONS

Despite the advantages, several limitations hinder the universal adoption of AI in cardiology. Data heterogeneity, privacy issues, algorithmic bias, and a lack of explainability in deep learning models remain significant barriers. In particular, the "black box" nature of many neural networks challenges clinicians' trust in the outputs [44]. Regulatory agencies like the FDA continue to refine pathways to evaluate and monitor AI models, especially those with adaptive learning capabilities.

Only after proving safety and positive impact on patients' outcomes could ML and AI tools be deployed to real clinical environments. The UK Medicines and Healthcare Products Regulatory Agency (MHRA) considers AI to be a medical device [45]. MHRA developed a work program to ensure that AI used for screening, diagnosis, treatment, and management of chronic conditions is treated as a medical device and is appropriately evidenced. Main areas of concern are issues of human interpretability (the earlier-mentioned "black box" effect and lack of transparency of AI) and adaptivity (retraining of AI models in real time). Given that AI and ML are considered medical devices, they should be tested under the same rigorous conditions as all implantable and non-implantable medical devices during prospective randomized controlled trials (RCTs). Carefully designed RCTs with ML support decision tools and predictive models in an intervention arm versus standard of practice would allow objective and robust testing of their effectiveness and impact on clinical practice and patients' outcomes. The next step should be careful planning of RCTs where ML-guided practice could be compared to standard of care with clearly defined outcome measures like safety, improvement of diagnostic process in terms of time from presentation to diagnosis, accuracy of classification to treatment groups, and improvement in time where target medication doses are achieved.

8.8 FUTURE DIRECTIONS

Due to the growing global population, there is an inevitable increase in demand for health services. It is estimated that by 2030, there will be approximately 21.7 million new cancer diagnoses and 13 million cancer-related deaths worldwide, according to the International Agency for Research on Cancer (IARC) projections [46]. This means that

- developing new medications takes a significant amount of time. Typically, creating a new drug takes between 12 and 15 years and costs over USD 2 billion to bring to market [47]. The high costs are driven by expenses related to clinical trial recruitment and execution. Approximately 80% of drugs fail before reaching the clinical trial stage [48].

- there are a limited number of experts relative to the increasing demand. For example, there are about 4.7 radiologists per 100,000 people in Europe, and the number is even lower in the UK [49]. Regarding cardiologists, 2023 data suggests that in the UK there is one cardiologist per 41,335 of the population, with significant regional variation, which equates to approximately 24 per million people [50]. More recent 2024 data shows that the UK is still one of the lowest staffed countries with a reported total of 29 cardiologists (per million people) [51]. Comparing workforce data like these to patient need is critical for planning and supply of services and identifying where AI-assisted tools can have most the impact in the future.

- medical data are typically complex and consist of large datasets. Medical images are now multidimensional (2D, 3D, 4D), often comprising hundreds of images per study [52]. Hospitals must process thousands of images daily to deliver efficient services [53]. Due to the increased demand, volume, velocity, and variety of medical data and data processes, there are inevitable delays in results reaching patients and decision-makers such as specialist medical teams, like cardiac teams for example.

Solutions to these challenges are not readily available, however, harnessing what the modern technology has on offer will allow us to address the outlined challenges. Key elements of addressing those challenges are in the training of a healthcare workforce in data analytics, use of AI and learning from the data.

Future trajectories include the development of explainable AI (XAI) to improve transparency, the integration of AI with genomics and multi-omics data for precision cardiology, and the creation of continuous learning models that adapt to local patient populations. Additionally, as wearable devices become more sophisticated, AI will play an increasingly central role in preventive cardiology, telemedicine, and population health strategies [54].

8.9 CONCLUSION

AI is no longer a theoretical concept but a practical tool embedded in the daily work of the cardiologist. From non-invasive EP studies to wearable ECG monitoring, AI augments diagnostic capability, improves efficiency, and enhances patient outcomes. While ethical and practical challenges remain, the cardiology community is actively shaping a future where intelligent systems work alongside clinicians to deliver safer, faster, and more personalised care.

REFERENCES

1. Heart Statistics: The UK in Numbers (2025) https://www.bhf.org.uk/what-we-do/our-research/heart-statistics [accessed 30th June 2025]
2. Johnson, K.W., Soto, J.T., Glicksberg, B.S. et al. (2018) Artificial Intelligence in Cardiology. J Am Coll Cardiol. 71(23): 2668–2679. https://doi.org/10.1016/j.jacc.2018.03.521
3. Macfarlane, P.W., Kennedy, J. (2021) Automated ECG Interpretation—A Brief History from High Expectations to Deepest Networks. Hearts. 2(4):433–448.
4. Esteva, A., Robicquet, A., Ramsundar, B., Kuleshov, V., DePristo, M., Chou, K., Cui, C., Corrado, G., Thrun, S., Dean, J. (2019) A Guide to Deep Learning in Healthcare. Nat Med. 25(1):24–29. https://doi.org/10.1038/s41591-018-0316-z
5. Topol, E. (2019). Deep Medicine: How Artificial Intelligence Can Make Healthcare Human Again. Basic Books, Inc. Division of HarperCollins 10 E. 53rd St. New York, NY.
6. NICE 2023/NICE, KardiaMobile for Detecting Atrial Fibrillation, MTG64 (2023) https://www.nice.org.uk/guidance/mtg64 [accessed 30th June 2025]
7. Ouyang, D., He, B., Ghorbani, A. et al. (2020) Video-Based AI for Beat-to-Beat Assessment of Cardiac Function. Nature. 580(7802):252–256. https://doi.org/10.1038/s41586-020-2145-8
8. Zhang, J., Gajjala, S., Agrawal, P. et al. (2018) Fully Automated Echocardiogram Interpretation in Clinical Practice: Feasibility and Diagnostic Accuracy. Circulation. 138(16):1623–1635. https://doi.org/10.1161/CIRCULATIONAHA.118.034338
9. Knackstedt, C., Bekkers, S., Schummers, G. et al. (2015) Fully Automated Versus Standard Tracking of Left Ventricular Ejection Fraction and Longitudinal Strain: The FAST-EFs Multicenter Study. JACC. 66(13):1456–1466. https://doi.org/10.1016/j.jacc.2015.07.052
10. Narula, S., Shameer, K., Salem, Omar, A. et al. (2016) Machine-Learning Algorithms to Automate Morphological and Functional Assessments in 2D Echocardiography. JACC. 68(21):2287–2295. https://doi.org/10.1016/j.jacc.2016.08.062
11. Knuuti, J., Wijns, W., Saraste, A. et al. (2020) 2019 ESC Guidelines for the Diagnosis and Management of Chronic Coronary Syndromes. Eur Heart J. 41(3): 407–477. https://doi.org/10.1093/eurheartj/ehz425 [accessed 30th June 2025]
12. National Institute for Health and Care Excellence (NICE). (2021) Chest pain of recent onset: assessment and diagnosis [NG185]. Available from: https://www.nice.org.uk/guidance/ng185 [accessed 30th June 2025]
13. Gulati, M., Levy, P.D., Mukherjee, D. et al. (2021) Writing Committee Members, AHA/ACC/AAPA/ACPM/AGS/APhA/ASH/ASPC/NLA/PCNA Guideline for the Evaluation and Diagnosis of Chest Pain. Circulation. 144(22):e368–e454. https://doi.org/10.1161/CIR.0000000000001029
14. Leschka, S., Alkadhi, H., Plass, A. et al. (2005) Accuracy of MSCT Coronary Angiography with 64-Slice Technology: First Experience. Eur Heart J. 26(15):1482–1487. https://doi.org/10.1093/eurheartj/ehi261
15. Mollet, N.R., Cademartiri, F., van, Mieghem, C.A. et al. (2005) High-resolution Spiral Computed Tomography Coronary Angiography in Patients Referred for Diagnostic Conventional Coronary Angiography. Circulation. 112(15):2318–2323. https://doi.org/10.1161/CIRCULATIONAHA.105.533471
16. Pugliese, F., Mollet, N.R., Runza, G. et al. (2006) Diagnostic Accuracy of Non-Invasive 64-Slice CT Coronary Angiography in Patients with Stable Angina Pectoris. Eur Radiol. 16(3):575–582. https://doi.org/10.1007/s00330-005-0041-0
17. Miller, J.M., Rochitte, C.E., Dewey, M. et al. (2008) Diagnostic Performance of Coronary Angiography by 64-Row CT. N Engl J Med. 359(22):2324–2336. https://doi.org/10.1056/NEJMoa0806576
18. Nørgaard, B.L., Leipsic, J., Gaur, S. et al. (2014) NXT Trial Study Group. Diagnostic Performance of Noninvasive Fractional Flow Reserve Derived from Coronary Computed Tomography Angiography in Suspected Coronary Artery Disease: The NXT Trial (Analysis of Coronary Blood Flow Using CT Angiography: Next Steps). J Am Coll Cardiol. 63(12):1145–1155. https://doi.org/10.1016/j.jacc.2013.11.043
19. Dey, D., Slomka, P., Leeson, P. et al. (2019) Artificial Intelligence in Cardiovascular Imaging: JACC State-of-the-Art Review. JACC. 73(11):1317–1335. https://doi.org/10.1016/j.jacc.2018.12.054
20. Chen, C., Qin, C., Qiu, H. et al. (2020) Deep Learning for Cardiac Image Segmentation: A Review. Front Cardiovasc Med. 7:25. https://doi.org/10.3389/fcvm.2020.00025
21. Fox, S.R., Toomu, A., Gu, K. et al. (2024) Impact of Artificial Intelligence Arrhythmia Mapping on Time to First Ablation, Procedure Duration, and Fluoroscopy Use. J Cardiovasc Electrophysiol. 35(5):916–928. https://doi.org/10.1111/jce.16237
22. Zaman, J., Baykaner, T., Narayan, S.M. (2019) Mapping and Ablation of Rotational and Focal Drivers in Atrial Fibrillation. Card Electrophysiol Clin. 11(4):583–595. https://doi.org/10.1016/j.ccep.2019.08.010
23. Mannhart, D., Lischer, M., Knecht, S. et al. (2023) Clinical Validation of 5 Direct-to-Consumer Wearable Smart Devices to Detect Atrial Fibrillation: BASEL Wearable Study. JACC Clin Electrophysiol. 9(2):232–242. https://doi.org/10.1016/j.jacep.2022.09.011
24. Jensen, P.B., Jensen, L.J., Brunak, S. (2012) Mining Electronic Health Records: Towards Better Research Applications and Clinical Care. Nat Rev Genet. 13:395–405. https://doi.org/10.1038/nrg3208
25. Fry, E., Mukharjeem, S. (2018) Tech's Next Big Wave: Big Data Meets Biology 2018. https://fortune.com/2018/03/19/big-data-digital-health-tech/ [accessed 16th July 2025]
26. Friedman, C.P., Wong, A.K., Blumenthal, D. (2010) Achieving a Nationwide Learning Health System. Sci Transl Med. 2:57cm29. https://doi.org/10.1126/scitranslmed.3001456
27. Friedman, C., Rigby, M. (2013) Conceptualising and Creating a Global Learning Health System. Int J Med Inform. 82:e63–e71. https://doi.org/10.1016/j.ijmedinf.2012.05.010

28. Szummer, K., Wallentin, L., Lindhagen, L. et al. (2017) Improved Outcomes in Patients with ST-Elevation Myocardial Infarction During the Last 20 Years Are Related to Implementation of Evidence-Based Treatments: Experiences from the SWEDEHEART Registry 1995–2014. Eur Heart J. 38:3056–3065. https://doi.org/10.1093/eurheartj/ehx515
29. Health Research Data for the World - UK Biobank. (2025). https://www.ukbiobank.ac.uk/ [accessed 15th July 2025]
30. McKinsey. (2020) Transforming healthcare with AI: The impact on the workforce and organisations 2020. https://eithealth.eu/wpcontent/uploads/2020/03/EIT-Health-and-McKinsey-Transforming-Healthcare-with-AI.pdf [accessed 15th July 2025]
31. UK Government. AI Council (2021) AI Roadmap. Available at: https://www.gov.uk/government/publications/ai-road-map [accessed 15th July 2025]
32. Goldacre, B., Morley, J. (2022) Better, Broader, Safer: Using Health Data for Research and Analysis. Department of Health and Social Care [accessed 15th July 2025]
33. Central Digital and Data Office (2022) Roadmap for Digital and Data, 2022 to 2025. Available from https://www.gov.uk/government/publications/roadmap-for-digital-and-data-2022-to-2025 [accessed 10th July 2025]
34. UK Government. UK Digital Strategy UK's Digital Strategy - GOV.UK. (2022) https://www.gov.uk/government/publications/uks-digital-strategy [accessed 17th July 2025]
35. Yang, J.H., Wright, S.N., Hamblin, M. et al. (2019) A White-Box Machine Learning Approach for Revealing Antibiotic Mechanisms of Action. Cell. 177:1649–1661. https://doi.org/10.1016/j.cell.2019.04.016
36. Desai, R.J., Wang, S.V., Vaduganathan, M. et al. (2020) A Comparison of Machine Learning Methods with Traditional Models for Use of Administrative Claims with Electronic Medical Records to Predict Heart Failure Outcomes. JAMA Network Open. 3:e1918962. https://doi.org/10.1001/jamanetworkopen.2019.18962
37. Shin, S., Austin, P.C., Ross, H.J. et al. (2021) Machine Learning vs. Conventional Statistical Models for Predicting Heart Failure Readmission and Mortality. ESC Heart Failure. 8:106–115. https://doi.org/10.1002/ehf2.13073
38. Jasinska-Piadlo, A., Bond, R., Biglarbeigi, P.A. et al. (2023) Data-Driven Versus a Domain-Led Approach to k-Means Clustering on an Open Heart Failure Dataset. Int J Data Sci Anal. 15:49–66. https://doi.org/10.1007/s41060-022-00346-9
39. Attia, Z.I., Noseworthy, P.A., Lopez-Jimenez, F. et al. (2019) An Artificial Intelligence-Enabled ECG Algorithm for the Identification of Patients with Atrial Fibrillation During Sinus Rhythm: a Retrospective Analysis of Outcome Prediction. Lancet. 394(10201):861–867. https://doi.org/10.1016/S0140-6736(19)31721-0
40. Perrichot, A., Vaittinada Ayar, P., Taboulet, P. et al. (2023) Assessment of Real-Time Electrocardiogram Effects on Interpretation Quality by Emergency Physicians. BMC Med Educ. 23(1):677. https://doi.org/10.1186/s12909-023-04670-x
41. Dey, D., Slomka, P.J., Leeson, P. et al. (2019) Artificial Intelligence in Cardiovascular Imaging: JACC State-of-the-Art Review. J Am Coll Cardiol. 73(11):1317–1335. https://doi.org/10.1016/j.jacc.2018.12.054
42. Rajkomar, A., Oren, E., Chen, K. et al. (2018) Scalable and Accurate Deep Learning with Electronic Health Records. NPJ Digit Med. 1:18. https://doi.org/10.1038/s41746-018-0029-1
43. Weng, S.F., Reps, J., Kai, J. et al. (2017) Can Machine-Learning Improve Cardiovascular Risk Prediction Using Routine Clinical Data? PLoS One. 12(4):e0174944. https://doi.org/10.1371/journal.pone.0174944
44. He, J., Baxter, S.L., Xu, J. et al. (2019) The Practical Implementation of Artificial Intelligence Technologies in Medicine. Nat Med. 25(1):30–36. https://doi.org/10.1038/s41591-018-0307-0
45. UK Government. Software and AI as a Medical Device Change Programme [Internet]. 2021. Available from: https://www.gov.uk/government/publications/software-and-ai-as-a-medical-device-change-programme/software-and-ai-as-a-medical-device-change-programme [accessed 30th June 2025]
46. International Agency for Research on Cancer (IARC). (2023) Global Cancer Observatory: Cancer Tomorrow. Lyon [cited 2025 Jul 15]. Available from: https://gco.iarc.fr/tomorrow[accessed 16th July 2025]
47. DiMasi, J.A., Grabowski, H.G., Hansen, R.W. (2016) Innovation in the Pharmaceutical Industry: New Estimates of R&D Costs. J Health Econ. 47:20–33. https://doi.org/10.1016/j.jhealeco.2016.01.012
48. Hay, M., Thomas, D.W., Craighead, J.L. et al. (2014) Clinical Development Success Rates for Investigational Drugs. Nat Biotechnol. 32(1):40–51. https://doi.org/10.1038/nbt.2786
49. Brady, A.P., Paulo, G., Brkljacic, B. et al. (2025) Current Status of Radiologist Staffing, Education and Training in the 27 EU Member States. Insights Imaging. 16:59. https://doi.org/10.1186/s13244-025-01925-7
50. Ray, S., Clarke, S.C. (2023) Getting It Right First Time (GIRFT): Transforming Cardiology Care. Heart. 109(5):344–8. [cited 2025 Jul 15]. Available from: https://www.gettingitrightfirsttime.co.uk/wp-content/uploads/2021/09/Cardiology-Jul21k-NEW.pdf accessed 16th July 2025]
51. European Society of CARDIOLOGY. CHR_CARD_1M_R,Cardiologists (total) (per million people) https://eatlas.escardio.org/Data/Cardiovascular-healthcare-delivery/Cardiological-specialists/chr_card_1m_r-cardiologists-total-per-million-people [accessed 18th July 2025]
52. Litjens, G., Kooi, T., Bejnordi, B.E. et al. (2017) A Survey on Deep Learning in Medical Image Analysis. Med Image Anal. 42:60–88. https://doi.org/10.1016/j.media.2017.07.005
53. Dreyer, K.J., Geis, J.R. (2017) When Machines Think: Radiology's Next Frontier. Radiology. 285(3):713–718. https://doi.org/10.1148/radiol.2017171183
54. Shameer, K., Badgeley, M.A., Miotto, R. et al. (2017) Translational Bioinformatics in the Era of Real-Time Biomedical, Health Care and Wellness Data Streams. Brief Bioinform. 18(1):105–124. https://doi.org/10.1093/bib/bbv118

9 AI in Radiology

Fahad Mohammed and Sarim Ather

9.1 DEFINITION AND NEED

Artificial Intelligence (AI) refers to technology which aims to mimic the process of human under-standing and decision-making [1]. Within radiology, this would refer to algorithms which help interpret medical images or assist radiologists in closely related tasks that typically require human expertise. Specific techniques may utilise various facets of mathematics and computer science depending on the specific solution required.

The global workforce crisis in radiology is well-documented and stems from a growing demand and supply mismatch. Advancements in imaging technology, coupled with a complex ageing medical population have accelerated the number and complexity of images which require interpretation. This is further exacerbated by workforce shortages and clinician burnout. One striking statistic mentions some centres would require a radiologist to interpret one image every four seconds for eight hours straight to service such demand [2]. With the medical imaging market predicted to grow at an annual rate of 5% and generate $50 billion in revenue by 2032, it is no surprise that AI has received a surge of interest due to its potential to generate greater efficiencies [3].

Radiology has become an early and enthusiastic adopter of modern AI systems due to its perfect position to offer large-scale digital data, well-defined tasks and immediate applicability. Images are mostly standardised which lends them to pixel-based analysis, and radiologists routinely produce text reports, which can serve as labels for training algorithms. This abundance of data, coupled with radiology's heavy pattern-recognition work, makes it a prime candidate for early success, and as such, it is often considered at the forefront of medical AI integration [4, 5].

9.1.1 History and Key Breakthroughs

One of the earliest applications of AI in radiology emerged in the 1990s with computer-aided detection (CAD) systems developed to improve breast cancer screening. Contrary to their intended purpose, these provided no overall significant benefit due to high false positive rates, which reduced accuracy and paradoxically increased interpretation times by 20%. Their primitive nature resulted from being hand-crafted with manually implemented expert rules, leading to waning enthusiasm and culminating in an "AI winter". As such, AI lay dormant in radiology until the rise of "deep learning" techniques during the 2010's [6].

Deep learning aims to mimic human learning by using large datasets to train multilayered neural networks that can automatically identify complex features, recognise patterns and make decisions with little human guidance. Neural networks themselves are computational systems where layers of connected units, or "neurons," process data by adjusting weights and applying functions to learn patterns from the data [4].

Radiology is well suited to utilise deep learning due to its reliance on pattern recognition within a data-rich environment. Whilst AI has been around for many decades, the introduction of large language models into the public domain has created a new wave of discourse. It is thus unsurprising that radiology has also witnessed a notable increase in publications exploring its potential applications within the field [5].

Several milestones have since marked the progression of the "third-era" of AI within radiology. Rapid performance gains in image analysis have been achieved from convolutional neural networks (CNN's) – a specific deep learning technique which applies a filter to identify key features and patterns within images.

A watershed moment in computer vision occurred during the 2012 ImageNet Large Scale Visual Recognition Challenge, when one CNN, called AlexNet, substantially outperformed previous models by cutting their error rate in half. This demonstrated the practical effectiveness of deep learning for large-scale image classification, signalling progress toward human-level performance in visual recognition tasks [7].

Radiology has been able to quickly capitalise on these advances, given the availability of large, labelled datasets within decades of stored images in the picture archiving and communication systems (PACS). Another pivotal moment came with the release of a training set by the American National Institute for Health which contained over 100,000 anonymised chest X-rays and associated disease labels. Researchers were able to create a model called CheXNet which, after only a

DOI: 10.1201/9781032709956-9

month of development, learned to detect pneumonia on chest X-rays more accurately than radiologists [8, 9].

By 2018, regulators cleared the first AI tools for clinical use in radiology. Notably, the Food and Drug Administration (FDA) in 2018 authorised an AI-powered stroke detection system called Viz. ai which analyses CT brain scans and automatically alerts neurologists if it detects a large-vessel occlusion [10]. One may consider this a landmark platform as a result of having been the first approved autonomous triage tool for a critical condition.

Lastly, a 2023 Swedish trial demonstrated that an AI-supported mammography screening protocol could detect as many cancers as the traditional method of double reporting by two radiologists. Furthermore, a substantially lower number of images needed human review, thus confirming that such systems could contribute by also significantly reducing workload [11].

9.1.2 Applications within Radiology

Whilst AI platforms have gained notoriety for their strengths in interpretive tasks, they also offer significant efficiencies throughout the entire service from image acquisition and workflow optimisation through to data extraction (including for other uses such as clinical research). To truly appreciate the full scope of benefits, it is perhaps more meaningful to engage in a discourse about how such systems can be applied across the whole breadth of the clinical environment.

9.1.3 Image Acquisition and Reconstruction

Advancements in imaging modalities such as computed tomography (CT) and magnetic resonance imaging (MRI) have relied on traditional physics-based methods to produce higher-quality images with faster acquisition times and reduced radiation doses. Furthermore, whilst complex techniques such as iterative reconstruction have been considered as early as the 1970s, the lack of available computational power restricted their use within the research domain [12]. Similarly, well-established algorithms already optimise image quality and radiation dose through automatic exposure control systems or reduce contrast use by timing acquisition at the point of maximal enhancement. Furthermore, the use of post-processing filters enhances images by reducing noise and artefacts such that diagnostic clarity is preserved, even at a fraction of the usual radiation dose [13].

MRI is inherently slow due to its prolonged acquisition times, which causes greater susceptibility to motion artefacts, reduces patient tolerance and increases the relative marginal cost per scan. These factors reduce the overall accessibility to an already scarce resource. Traditional techniques such as parallel imaging and compressed sensing tackle such challenges but are computationally heavy and time-consuming as a result.

Modern deep learning techniques use training data to learn the most optimal reconstruction process and provide images quicker, even without full data acquisition. For example, robust artificial neural networks for k-space interpolation (RAKI) utilises neural networks to interpolate missing data within "k-space" (a mathematical matrix used for data storage before conversion into visual information). Similarly, cardiac MRI is particularly challenging due to inherent motion and the need for very high image resolution. One approach applies "variational networks" to allow image reconstruction whilst compensating for normal breathing, in turn negating the necessity for gated acquisition [14].

9.1.4 Automated Detection and Diagnosis

AI has gained publicity due to its ability to provide automatic detection of any potentially visualised pathology. Its strength in particular lies within its ability to consistently detect subtle patterns at a large scale.

For example, within the field of oncology, AI models can identify tumours and characterise them to ascertain whether they require follow-up. Similarly, there is wide recognition for its efficacy within breast cancer screening, where it can highlight suspicious calcifications or masses. AI-supported mammography screening has been shown to achieve cancer detection rates comparable to the usual standard of double reporting whilst reducing workload by as much as 40%. These studies validate the safety and effectiveness of AI-supported screening programmes to improve patient throughput without causing suboptimal care [11, 15].

At the other end of the healthcare spectrum, AI has also been used to provide quick analysis of critical conditions. As previously mentioned, Viz.ai applies AI to enhance the provision of care within critical settings such as strokes and pulmonary embolism which often carry significant mortality and morbidity.

FDA-approved algorithms for detecting such conditions, having been implemented in over 1,600 hospitals within the United States and Europe. Furthermore, Viz.ai seamlessly integrates its findings into an early-warning platform which alerts specialists of critical findings where delays might otherwise impact outcomes negatively [10].

Previous studies have shown that missed fractures within the emergency department account for a disproportionate number of diagnostic errors, perhaps due to large patient volumes. As such, the UK's National Institute for Health and Care Excellence has recently approved four AI platforms to assist in the reduction of errors and diagnostic delay. One meta-analysis has validated the non-inferior diagnostic performance of AI, comparable to that of clinicians [16–18].

9.2 WORKFLOW OPTIMISATION AND TRIAGE

In addition to image analysis, AI is increasingly being used to streamline and optimise radiology workflows such as triaging urgent cases. For instance, it may highlight potential red flags, emphasise critical findings and ensure they receive prompt attention. When integrated within a worklist management system, AI can automatically update and prioritise studies based on their severity, pushing those with suspected life-threatening conditions to the top of the list, thereby minimising delays in care. One practical example may be a system which scans inbound chest X-rays for signs of a pneumothorax. If detected, the system could flag the case as urgent, prompting both the radiologist and requesting clinician to review it immediately. Early trials of these triage systems have shown promising results, and regulatory bodies have established pathways for their approval as computer-aided triage and notification" devices [10].

Many repetitive administrative tasks are also ripe for transformation using AI platforms. For example, they may automatically categorise exams by type and retrieve relevant prior studies or ensure that requests adhere to clinical guidelines. They can also provide real-time monitoring to detect sub-optimal imaging and prompt immediate rescanning without the need for reattendance. Other platforms may optimise appointment scheduling, predict non-attendances and estimate scan duration based on historical data, thus offering optimisation of resource allocation.

Perhaps most pertinent to the radiologist is the use of AI-powered virtual assistants in automating parts of the reporting process. For example, integration within PACS may allow image annotation and consequently pre-populate reports with tumour dimensions, saving time and improving inter-observer variability. Furthermore, these agents can improve the dictation process to transcribe reports and automatically initiate any necessary follow up procedures such as interval scanning [19–21].

9.3 AI-ASSISTED DECISION SUPPORT

There is much speculation about AI systems replacing the radiologist; however, it is perhaps best considered as a decision support tool for clinicians. For example, a liver lesion may draw on imaging features and large medical knowledge banks to prompt the generation of differential diagnoses to be considered by the clinician. Furthermore, AI excels in tracking subtle changes across serial studies and therefore might be able to assess progression more sensitively than the clinician. This might be particularly important when gauging treatment responses, as often happens within oncology [22, 23].

Most importantly, the support provided by AI may extend towards patient-facing applications. For instance, "generative" AI has gained widespread recognition for its ability to produce visually striking content through platforms such as Sora and MidJourney. These technologies can also translate complex technical reports into clear and accessible language, thereby enhancing patient understanding whilst alleviating any concerns [24].

9.3.1 Radiomics and Predictive Analytics

Radiomics extracts quantitative features, such as shape and density, from medical images to predict outcomes such as tumour aggressiveness and treatment response. Unlike analogue interpretation, it utilises data rich scans to reveal patterns beyond human perception. Radiomics has shown strong performance in identifying lymph node metastases in head and neck cancers as well as predicting outcomes within various malignancies. In some cases, genetic data is correlated with imaging features to further enhance capabilities in a field known as radiogenomics [25–29]. Predictive analytics aims to forecast disease progression and the likelihood of clinical sequelae using a combination of imaging and clinical data. For example, it might perform calcium scoring on chest CT scans to predict the likelihood of heart attacks or predict cognitive decline in neuroimaging [30, 31].

9.4 BENEFITS AND KEY CONSIDERATIONS

The integration of AI within radiological practice holds significant promise in offering solutions towards its many challenges. However, realising these benefits depends on addressing critical ethical, legal and practical considerations. For example, mitigating algorithmic bias is essential towards providing equitable care, whilst transparency and responsible use are fundamental in maintaining trust. Clear legal accountability must also be established to support safe and responsible use. By proactively considering these issues, radiology can fully embrace the value of such systems in modernising healthcare.

9.4.1 Benefits

Given the growing gap between demand and supply of radiological services, one of the key advantages of AI integration is the ability to enhance efficiency and improve patient throughput. AI automation provides support across the imaging workflow, from accelerating image reconstruction and prioritising urgent cases through to triaging and streamlining report generation.

For instance, AI-based image reconstruction can significantly reduce scan duration, with one study demonstrating 53% shorter MRI acquisition times, thereby increasing daily patient capacity and improving patient comfort [32]. Additionally, a UK hospital simulation utilised an AI chest X-ray triage system to reduce reporting backlogs significantly, cutting the average turnaround time for critical findings by approximately 75%, from eleven to just under three days. Such tools can also operate continuously, helping to address coverage gaps during nights or weekends [33]. Similarly, automatic anatomical segmentation and lesion measurement provides faster report completion by around 10% which, in aggregate, represents significant overall efficiency gains [34].

Expanding access to radiological services is especially important given its wide geographical discrepancy, especially within remote areas, where there may be a lack of experienced radiologists [35–37]. One Google-funded deep learning system has managed to match radiologists' performance in detecting tuberculosis across over 165,000 images from high-burden countries. The immediate analysis provided allows health workers in rural clinics to quickly assess patients, with studies suggesting an 80% reduction in cost per patient, thus improving scarce resource allocation in poorly funded areas [38].

Beyond efficiency gains, AI can also augment human potential with regards to diagnostic accuracy and report consistency. For example, studies have shown that AI-supported radiologists have an improved sensitivity of detecting pneumothorax and lung nodules [34]. Likewise, AI-assisted wrist fracture detection increases radiologists' sensitivity by nearly 5% without losing specificity [39]. A notable lung cancer screening study demonstrated that a deep learning model reduced false positives by 11% and false negatives by 5% [40]. Natural language processing further enhances reporting accuracy by proactively identifying potential errors, such as laterality discrepancies or omissions of critical findings. Draft-reporting systems can also facilitate quicker writing and serve as automated secondary reviewers, thus improving consistency and promoting uniform interpretation across services [34, 41, 42].

AI has also enabled the integration of clinical data for a more comprehensive and personalised approach to patient care. As previously discussed, AI-driven radiomics can extract detailed image features to predict disease characteristics and outcomes that are challenging for human interpretation alone. One MRI-based radiomics model has accurately predicted complete responses in rectal cancer patients undergoing chemoradiotherapy, outperforming experienced radiologists. This capability facilitates personalised treatment decisions, such as identifying patients who could safely avoid surgery [43].

Constant innovation has broadened radiology's capabilities, including the emergence of "virtual biopsies". One previous investigation has demonstrated accurate identification of mutation status in brain cancer with over 91% accuracy using routine preoperative CT scans, thus closely approaching the performance of traditional genetic testing. This non-invasive approach is clinically significant, enabling earlier prognostic insight and treatment planning without the risks associated with biopsies, particularly in sensitive areas such as the brain [44]. Further studies have integrated imaging with clinical and genomic data to enhance risk stratification beyond conventional methods. One combined AI model used CT radiomic features with clinical variables to more accurately predict five-year disease progression in head and neck cancer than traditional tumour, node, metastasis (TNM) staging alone. Such enhanced predictive power supports more personalised care by identifying high-risk patients who may benefit from intensified treatment or closer monitoring [45]. Researchers have also applied deep learning models to predict future chronic obstructive pulmonary disease (COPD) exacerbations and lung function decline, outperforming traditional risk models. This approach can help clinicians proactively tailor treatment plans, monitor disease progression more effectively and intervene earlier to prevent severe outcomes [46].

9.4.2 Considerations

AI holds tremendous potential to transform radiology, but without responsible implementation and careful attention to ethical and legal considerations, it also carries a serious risk of harm. Such risks may arise at various points within its development and application, which include data acquisition, model training, validation, deployment and clinical integration.

Firstly, the development of AI models is heavily reliant on "training data", which may not be representative of the patient population. It may underrepresent certain characteristics such as race and gender, which could result in sub-optimal performance when applied to these groups. Variable performance amongst health services due to differences in patient demographics or imaging protocols is well demonstrated within the setting of using AI to detect chest infections [47]. Furthermore, AI may demonstrate apparent capacity for intelligent analysis by detecting patterns in confounding data whilst failing to perform the task as intended. One study gained notoriety by highlighting this issue, where a model appeared to accurately classify malignant skin lesions but had learned to associate the presence of rulers with malignancy. This confounding pattern arose because malignant lesions were more often photographed with rulers, leading the model to rely on irrelevant visual cues [48]. More strikingly, a recent study found that some AI models could predict patient race from medical images with over 90% accuracy, despite no identifiable racial features being visible to human experts. The underlying mechanism remains unclear, raising concerns that AI systems may incorporate race as a proxy in clinical decision-making and potentially contribute to biased outcomes [49]. Addressing such biases require diverse, well-curated training data and ongoing monitoring of AI performance across subpopulations. As a result, many organisations now emphasise the need for "fairness" testing as part of their validation process.

Another key challenge with many deep learning models is their inherent "black box" nature. Many models suffer from opaque decision-making processes due to their highly complex architectures using many millions of parameters to perform non-linear computations. Thus, whilst inputs and outputs may be observed, the specific logic used to produce a result may remain unclear. In radiology, this lack of interpretability is especially problematic as clinicians must be able to assess whether a model's conclusions are based on clinically relevant features or irrelevant artefacts [50]. The need for such "explainability" has led to the development of tools such as "heat maps" which highlight specific parts of an image that have influenced the system's decision tree. One instance might be highlighting a specific region on a chest X-ray, which led to the diagnosis of pneumonia.

Lack of explainability can also undermine trust and ultimately lead to failure of adoption [51]. The European Union has signalled the importance of transparency within its proposed AI Act by including requirements for interpretable outputs in high-risk AI systems [13, 52]. Until these solutions become more advanced and reliable, many implementations will likely remain in an assistive mode where a human remains "in the loop" to interpret results within the clinical context. However, this setup can hinder rather than help the radiologist by adding complexity and cognitive load instead of streamlining the diagnostic process [53].

Regardless of how perfectly a system is developed, issues surrounding accountability and legal liability may persist. This contention is perhaps most important within healthcare, where one of the founding principles is to "first do no harm". Furthermore, culpability for the standard of care usually places responsibility on the attending physician; however, these lines may become blurred as AI systems become increasingly autonomous. Professional bodies have suggested that radiologists must understand the limitations of any platform they use and are responsible for its final interpretation, as with any diagnostic tool. In the UK, for example, National Institute for Clinical Excellence (NICE) guidelines on AI use emphasise that these tools do not override the clinician's judgement, and appropriate governance structures must be implemented to ensure sound oversight [54]. Appropriate actions may include decision mapping with the creation of robust audit trails. Moreover, regulatory approval processes require stringent criteria to provide optimal quality assurance for both safety and performance [55]. The continuous learning processes AI utilise also suffer from "performance drift", which may lead to unexpected outcomes. Thus, inherent within these systems is the requirement for continual monitoring and correction to ensure they function as originally intended [56].

9.4.3 Challenges

Integrating AI within radiology presents significant challenges due to the complexity of existing IT systems which include components such as PACS, reporting information systems (RISs) and electronic medical records. Seamless interoperability between these and proposed AI platforms is essential but currently hindered by the lack of universal standards. Although initiatives such as "Integrating the Healthcare Enterprise" are working towards standardisation, many AI solutions still rely on proprietary interfaces, which complicates integration. This is especially true when multiple AI platforms may be utilised within a service [5, 57].

From a cybersecurity and data governance perspective, AI adoption raises additional concerns. Many tools depend on cloud computing, which require hospitals to transmit patient data externally and in turn conflict with existing privacy regulations such as the General Data Protection Regulation (GDPR). As a result, institutions often prefer local deployments or secure private networks, which increases complexity and cost. Furthermore, AI platforms depend on access to large volumes of high-quality data, but obtaining and managing this data carries its own problems. Many models may be trained on retrospective and de-identified images; however, concerns still exist with regards to patient privacy and consent, especially as AI platforms may be developed with intrinsic commercial interest [58].

Another major hurdle is the need for well-annotated datasets. Although PACS archives are extensive, they often contain inconsistencies or reporting errors which make them unreliable for training without extensive cleaning. Creating curated datasets with radiologist-verified labels is both time-consuming and expensive. National initiatives and public competitions such as RSNA AI training and evaluation challenges represent key steps in addressing this, but data scarcity remains a problem for rare conditions [59].

The adoption of AI is often justified by its potential to improve diagnostic accuracy and operational efficiency. However, a significant barrier to implementation is the need for clear evidence to prove its cost-effectiveness. AI tools typically involve substantial costs with regards to both their development and on-going maintenance. Such systems also consume large amounts of energy, which hinders efforts towards environmental sustainability [60]. Thus, these systems represent a large opportunity cost, especially as empirical evidence for potential savings remain limited. Furthermore, any efficiencies gained may be offset by increased detection rates, which can lead to a rise in clinically unnecessary tests, which diminishes any cost savings and potentially increases patient anxiety. Traditional economic evaluation models struggle to account for such externalities, and so specific health technology assessment frameworks have been developed to standardise evaluation and reporting, such as NICE's "CHEERS-AI" [61]. Ultimately, successful integration is dependent on demonstrating tangible health economic value and initiatives such as the NHS AI Diagnostic Fund, which reflects growing support for deployments that address clearly defined clinical needs [62].

9.5 CONCLUSION

The continual development of AI within radiology represents both a transformative opportunity and a complex challenge for modern healthcare delivery. Whilst such systems offer remarkable potential to address key challenges facing the speciality, such as its global workforce crisis, its successful implementation requires careful navigation to prevent patient care from becoming compromised. Further research is required to overcome the technical obstacles previously described, and there must be a concerted effort to increase the discourse on AI's ethical and legal complexities. Moving forward, the field must balance innovation with responsibility, ensuring that AI tools are not only powerful but also equitable, explainable and economically viable. By carefully considering such issues, radiology will be able to exploit the benefits of AI whilst minimising the potential for any complications to result from its use.

9.6 EDITORS' COMMENTS

It is abundantly evident that the availability of digital datasets within radiology have been key to application of developing and developed AI systems along with neural networks and now travelling towards large language models. The chapter identifies the positives and limitations of AI in the field and is clear in its consideration of where technical, legal and ethical components contribute to issues in the medical specialisation. Most importantly it is clear that although image reading and taking pressure from the reporter was initially identified as the main gain, acknowledging that medical imaging/radiology service demand is growing continuously, there are other aspects of the service than can also benefit from AI systems. That said, being able to explain to patients and colleagues how machine-supported decisions have come about and ensuring that fair application occurs across the whole population no matter the background of the service user are potential stumbling blocks that may delay the outlined benefits. If these challenges are dealt with as outlined by the authors, then the benefits will exceed any limitations for improved service to patients, referrers for imaging and the team in the imaging department itself.

REFERENCES

1. Stryker, C., Kavlakoglu, E. (2024) What is Artificial Intelligence (AI)? IBM. https://www.ibm.com/think/topics/artificial-intelligence
2. Everlightradiology.com. (2025) Everlight Radiology – The Global Radiologist Report 2025. https://www.everlightradiology.com/global-radiologist-report-2025
3. Marketus. (2023) Medical Imaging Market. https://market.us/report/medical-imaging-market/ (accessed April 21, 2025).
4. Hosny, A., Parmar, C., Quackenbush, J. et al. (2018) Artificial Intelligence in Radiology. Nature Reviews Cancer 18:500–10. https://doi.org/10.1038/s41568-018-0016-5
5. Kotter, E., Ranschaert, E. (2020) Challenges and Solutions for Introducing Artificial Intelligence (AI) in Daily Clinical Workflow. European Radiology 31:5–7. https://doi.org/10.1007/s00330-020-07148-2
6. Oakden-Rayner, L. (2019) The Rebirth of CAD: How Is Modern AI Different from the CAD We Know? Radiology: Artificial Intelligence 1:e180089. https://doi.org/10.1148/ryai.2019180089
7. Krizhevsky, A., Sutskever, A., Hinton, I. (2012) GE. ImageNet Classification with Deep Convolutional Neural Networks. Communications of the ACM 60:84–90.
8. Wang, X., Peng, Y., Lu, L. et al. (2017) Chest X-Ray Database and Benchmarks on Weakly-Supervised Classification and Localization of Common Thorax Diseases. 2017 IEEE Conference on Computer Vision and Pattern Recognition (CVPR):3462–71. https://doi.org/10.1109/cvpr.2017.369
9. Rajpurkar, P., Irvin, J., Zhu, K. et al. (2017) CheXNet: Radiologist-Level Pneumonia Detection on Chest X-Rays with Deep Learning. ArXiv (Cornell University). https://doi.org/10.48550/arxiv.1711.05225
10. Office of the Commissioner. (2019) FDA Permits Marketing of Clinical Decision Support Software for Alerting Providers of a Potential Stroke in Patients. US Food and Drug Administration. https://www.fda.gov/news-events/press-announcements/fda-permits-marketing-clinical-decision-support-software-alerting-providers-potential-stroke (accessed December 23, 2019).
11. Lång, K., Josefsson, V., Larsson, A.-M. et al. (2023) Artificial Intelligence-Supported Screen Reading Versus Standard Double Reading in the Mammography Screening with Artificial Intelligence Trial (MASAI): A Clinical Safety Analysis of a Randomised, Controlled, non-Inferiority, Single-Blinded, Screening Accuracy Study. Lancet Oncology 24:936–44. https://doi.org/10.1016/s1470-2045(23)00298-x
12. Willemink, M.J., Noël, P.B. (2019) The Evolution of Image Reconstruction for CT—from Filtered Back Projection to Artificial Intelligence. European Radiology 29:2185–95. https://doi.org/10.1007/s00330-018-5810-7
13. Melazzini, L., Bortolotto, C., Brizzi, L. et al. (2025) AI for Image Quality and Patient Safety in CT and MRI. European Radiology Experimental 9. https://doi.org/10.1186/s41747-025-00562-5
14. Lin, D.J., Johnson, P.M., Knoll, F. et al. (2020) Artificial Intelligence for MR Image Reconstruction: An Overview for Clinicians. Journal of Magnetic Resonance Imaging 53:1015–28. https://doi.org/10.1002/jmri.27078
15. Hernström, V., Josefsson, V., Sartor, H. et al. (2025) Screening Performance and Characteristics of Breast Cancer Detected in the Mammography Screening with Artificial Intelligence Trial (MASAI): A Randomised, Controlled, Parallel-Group, Non-Inferiority, Single-Blinded, Screening Accuracy Study. The Lancet Digital Health 7. https://doi.org/10.1016/s2589-7500(24)00267-x
16. Hussain, F., Cooper, A., Carson-Stevens, A. et al. (2019) Diagnostic Error in the Emergency Department: Learning from National Patient Safety Incident Report Analysis. BMC Emergency Medicine 19. https://doi.org/10.1186/s12873-019-0289-3
17. Nice.org.uk. (2025) Overview | Artificial Intelligence Technologies to Help Detect Fractures on X-Rays in Urgent Care: Early Value Assessment | Guidance | NICE. https://www.nice.org.uk/guidance/hte20 (accessed April 12, 2025).
18. Kuo, R.Y.L., Harrison, C., Curran, T.-A. et al. (2022) Artificial Intelligence in Fracture Detection: A Systematic Review and Meta-Analysis. Radiology 304. https://doi.org/10.1148/radiol.211785
19. Dargan, R. (2020) Integrating AI with PACS Key to Improving Workflow Efficiency. www.rsna.org. https://www.rsna.org/news/2020/march/integrating-ai-with-pacs (accessed April 18, 2021).
20. Radai.com. (2025) Revolutionize Workflows with Powerful Radiology AI. https://www.radai.com
21. NHS. (2023) Using an AI-Driven Dictation Platform to Free up Clinicians' Time. NHS Transformation Directorate n.d. Using an AI-Driven Dictation Platform to Free up Clinicians' Time – Gastroenterology Digital Playbook – NHS Transformation Directorate. (accessed June, 2025).
22. Bizzo, B.C., Almeida, R.R., Michalski, M.H. et al. (2019) Artificial Intelligence and Clinical Decision Support for Radiologists and Referring Providers. Journal of the American College of Radiology 16:1351–6. https://doi.org/10.1016/j.jacr.2019.06.010
23. Farič, N., Hinder, S., Williams, R., et al. (2023) Early Experiences of Integrating an Artificial Intelligence-Based Diagnostic Decision Support System into Radiology Settings: A Qualitative Study. Journal of the American Medical Informatics Association 31. https://doi.org/10.1093/jamia/ocad191
24. Park, J., Oh, K., Han, K. et al. (2024) Patient-Centered Radiology Reports with Generative Artificial Intelligence: Adding Value to Radiology Reporting. Scientific Reports 14:13218. https://doi.org/10.1038/s41598-024-63824-z
25. Mayerhoefer, M.E., Materka, A., Langs, G. et al. (2020) Introduction to Radiomics. Journal of Nuclear Medicine 61:488–95. https://doi.org/10.2967/jnumed.118.222893
26. Valizadeh, P., Jannatdoust, P., Pahlevan-Fallahy, M.-T. et al. (2024) Diagnostic Accuracy of Radiomics and Artificial Intelligence Models in Diagnosing Lymph Node Metastasis in Head and Neck Cancers: A Systematic Review and Meta-Analysis. Neuroradiology 67:449–67. https://doi.org/10.1007/s00234-024-03485-x

27. Corredor, G., Bharadwaj, S., Pathak, T. et al. (2023) A Review of AI-Based Radiomics and Computational Pathology Approaches in Triple-Negative Breast Cancer: Current Applications and Perspectives. Clinical Breast Cancer 23:800–12. https://doi.org/10.1016/j.clbc.2023.06.004

28. Adili, D., Mohetaer, A., Zhang, W. (2023) Diagnostic Accuracy of Radiomics-Based Machine Learning for Neoadjuvant Chemotherapy Response and Survival Prediction in Gastric Cancer Patients: A Systematic Review and Meta-Analysis. European Journal of Radiology 173:111249–9. https://doi.org/10.1016/j.ejrad.2023.111249

29. Gillies, R.J., Kinahan, P.E., Hricak, H. (2016) Radiomics: Images Are More than Pictures, They Are Data. Radiology 278:563–77. https://doi.org/10.1148/radiol.2015151169

30. Lin, A., Kolossváry, M., Motwani, M. et al. (2021) Artificial Intelligence in Cardiovascular Imaging for Risk Stratification in Coronary Artery Disease. Radiology: Cardiothoracic Imaging 3:e200512. https://doi.org/10.1148/ryct.2021200512

31. Rudroff, T., Rainio, O., Klén, R. (2024) AI for the Prediction of Early Stages of Alzheimer's Disease from Neuroimaging Biomarkers – A Narrative Review of a Growing Field. Neurological Sciences 45:5117–27. https://doi.org/10.1007/s10072-024-07649-8

32. Yang, A., Finkelstein, M., Koo, C. et al. (2024) Impact of Deep Learning Image Reconstruction Methods on MRI Throughput. Radiology Artificial Intelligence 6. https://doi.org/10.1148/ryai.230181

33. Annarumma, M., Withey, S.J., Bakewell, R.J. et al. (2019) Automated Triaging of Adult Chest Radiographs with Deep Artificial Neural Networks. Radiology 291: 196–202. https://doi.org/10.1148/radiol.2018180921

34. Ahn, J.S., Ebrahimian, S., McDermott, S. et al. (2022) Association of Artificial Intelligence–Aided Chest Radiograph Interpretation with Reader Performance and Efficiency. JAMA Network Open 5:e2229289. https://doi.org/10.1001/jamanetworkopen.2022.29289

35. Sachdev, R., Sivanushanthan, S., Ring, N. et al. (2021) Global Health Radiology Planning Using Geographic Information Systems to Identify Populations with Decreased Access to Care. Journal of Global Health 11. https://doi.org/10.7189/jogh.11.04073

36. Khurana, A., Patel, B., Sharpe, R. (2022) Geographic Variations in Growth of Radiologists and Medicare Enrollees From 2012 to 2019. Journal of the American College of Radiology 19:1006–14. https://doi.org/10.1016/j.jacr.2022.06.009

37. Mollura, D., Culp, M., Lungren, M. (2019) Radiology in Global Health. Cham: Springer International Publishing. https://doi.org/10.1007/978-3-319-98485-8

38. Kazemzadeh, S., Yu, J., Jamshy, S. et al. (2022) Deep Learning Detection of Active Pulmonary Tuberculosis at Chest Radiography Matched the Clinical Performance of Radiologists. Radiology 306:124–37. https://doi.org/10.1148/radiol.212213

39. Jacques, T., Cardot, N., Ventre, J. et al. (2023) Commercially-Available AI Algorithm Improves Radiologists' Sensitivity for Wrist and Hand Fracture Detection on X-Ray, Compared to a CT-Based Ground Truth. European Radiology 34:2885–94. https://doi.org/10.1007/s00330-023-10380-1

40. Ardila, D., Kiraly, A.P., Bharadwaj, S. et al. (2019) End-to-End Lung Cancer Screening with Three-Dimensional Deep Learning on Low-Dose Chest Computed Tomography. Nature Medicine 25:954–61. https://doi.org/10.1038/s41591-019-0447-x

41. Acosta, J.N., Dogra, S., Adithan, S. et al. (2024) The Impact of AI Assistance on Radiology Reporting: A Pilot Study Using Simulated AI Draft Reports. ArXiv (Cornell University). https://doi.org/10.48550/arxiv.2412.12042

42. Joskowicz, L., Cohen, D., Caplan, N. et al. (2018) Inter-Observer Variability of Manual Contour Delineation of Structures in CT. European Radiology 29:1391–9. https://doi.org/10.1007/s00330-018-5695-5

43. Shin, J., Seo, N., Baek, S.-E. et al. (2022) MRI Radiomics Model Predicts Pathologic Complete Response of Rectal Cancer Following Chemoradiotherapy. Radiology 303:351–8. https://doi.org/10.1148/radiol.211986

44. Musigmann, M., Bilgin, M., Bilgin, S.S. et al. (2024) Completely Non-Invasive Prediction of IDH Mutation Status Based on Preoperative Native CT Images. Scientific Reports 14. https://doi.org/10.1038/s41598-024-77789-6

45. Bruixola, G., Dualde-Beltrán, D., Jimenez-Pastor, A. et al. (2024) CT-Based Clinical-Radiomics Model to Predict Progression and Drive Clinical Applicability in Locally Advanced Head and Neck Cancer. European Radiology. https://doi.org/10.1007/s00330-024-11301-6

46. Wu, J., Lu, Y., Dong, S. et al. (2024) Predicting COPD Exacerbations Based on Quantitative CT Analysis: An External Validation Study. Frontiers in Medicine 11. https://doi.org/10.3389/fmed.2024.1370917

47. Zech, J.R., Badgeley, M.A., Liu, M. et al. (2018) Variable Generalization Performance of a Deep Learning Model to Detect Pneumonia in Chest Radiographs: A Cross-Sectional Study. PLoS Medicine 15:e1002683. https://doi.org/10.1371/journal.pmed.1002683

48. Narla, A., Krupel, B., Sarin, K. et al. (2018) Automated Classification of Skin Lesions: From Pixels to Practice. Journal of Investigative Dermatology 138:2108–10. https://doi.org/10.1016/j.jid.2018.06.175

49. Gichoya, J.W., Banerjee, I., Bhimireddy, A.R. et al. (2022) AI Recognition of Patient Race in Medical Imaging: A Modelling Study. The Lancet Digital Health 4. https://doi.org/10.1016/S2589-7500(22)00063-2

50. Marey, A., Parisa Arjmand, P., Sabe, D.M. et al. (2024) Explainability, Transparency and Black Box Challenges of AI in Radiology: Impact on Patient Care in Cardiovascular Radiology. The Egyptian Journal of Radiology and Nuclear Medicine 55. https://doi.org/10.1186/s43055-024-01356-2

51. Awasthi, A., Le, N., Deng, Z. et al. (2024) Bridging Human and Machine Intelligence: Reverse-Engineering Radiologist Intentions for Clinical Trust and Adoption. Computational and Structural Biotechnology Journal 24:711–23. https://doi.org/10.1016/j.csbj.2024.11.012

52. European Parliament. (2025) EU AI Act: First Regulation on Artificial Intelligence. European Parliament. https://www.europarl.europa.eu/topics/en/article/20230601STO93804/eu-ai-act-first-regulation-on-artificial-intelligence (accessed June, 2025).

53. Yu, F., Moehring, A., Banerjee, O. et al. (2024) Heterogeneity and Predictors of the Effects of AI Assistance on Radiologists. Nature Medicine 30:837–49. https://doi.org/10.1038/s41591-024-02850-w

54. NICE. (2023) Overview | Artificial intelligence-derived Software to Analyse Chest X-rays for Suspected Lung Cancer in Primary Care referrals: Early Value Assessment | Guidance | https://www.nice.org.uk/guidance/hte12

55. Impact of AI on the Regulation of Medical Products. (2024) Implementing the AI White Paper principles. Medicines & Healthcare Products Regulatory Agency.

56. Sahiner, B., Chen, W., Samala, R.K. et al. (2023) Data Drift in Medical Machine Learning: Implications and Potential Remedies. British Journal of Radiology 96. https://doi.org/10.1259/bjr.20220878

57. Integrating the Healthcare Enterprise (IHE). (n.d.) IHE International. https://www.ihe.net

58. Sartor, G. and Lagioia, F. (2020) The Impact of the General Data Protection Regulation (GDPR) on Artificial Intelligence. European Parliament. https://dx.doi.org/10.2861/293

59. Viewed on rsna.org (2025) AI Challenges. https://www.rsna.org/rsnai/ai-image-challenge (accessed June, 2025).

60. AI. (2025) Executive Summary – Energy and AI – Analysis – IEA. IEA https://www.iea.org/reports/energy-and-ai/executive-summary (accessed June, 2025).

61. Elvidge, J., Hawksworth, C., Avşar, T.S. et al. (2024) Consolidated Health Economic Evaluation Reporting Standards for Interventions That Use Artificial Intelligence (CHEERS-AI). Value in Health: The Journal of the International Society for Pharmacoeconomics and Outcomes Research 27:1196–205. https://doi.org/10.1016/j.jval.2024.05.006

62. NHS England. (2023) AI Diagnostic Fund. NHS Transformation Directorate. https://digital.nhs.uk/services/ai-knowledge-repository/develop-ai Please add this in at this reference

10 Artificial Intelligence in Onco-Radiology

From Promise to Practice, Industry to Implementation

Christopher McKee

10.1 INTRODUCTION

The year is 2025. The prevailing technological trend is artificial intelligence (AI). Nearly every innovation is marketed with some form of AI integration, reflecting its growing influence across multiple industries, including health and medicine. Yet, despite its recent 'rise to fame' amongst everyday consumers, the concept of AI has been around for more than half a century since John McCarthy coined the term 'AI' in 1956 during the Dartmouth Summer Research Project on Artificial Intelligence [1]. The issue back in the mid-20th century, as is often the case with novel concepts, was that application of AI was highly limited due to available technology at the time. However, following the advent of large neural networks (LNNs), advanced data centres with the latest graphic processing unit (GPU) capabilities, and deep learning techniques, these limitations are no longer an issue. Indeed, the commercial opportunities are vast for utilising this technology within health and medicine. In particular, the past decade has shown a boom in AI solutions being applied to the field of radiology, which has become a clear-use case for AI in medicine.

The American Food and Drug Administration (FDA) approved the first medical device utilising AI in healthcare in 2017, and its application was in radiology. The Arterys medical imaging platform was approved for aiding diagnoses of underlying heart problems. In the same year the first Conformité Européenne (CE)–marked product was also made available on the European market by Aidoc, to comprehensively detect abnormalities in imaging of both the head and neck. Clearly the potential applications of these technologies are extensive, covering essentially every specialty in radiology [2].

Despite significant progress in terms of technological development and market-approved solutions, clinical implementation of these remains far fewer than predictions would have had us believe in the mid-2010s. This section aims to summarise the reasons for this and offer potential avenues to overcome the hurdles to clinical adoption with a consideration for the commercial parties involved as well as the clinical.

By focusing only on applications of AI diagnostic imaging in radiology in oncology services (consequently termed onco-radiology) many of the concepts described are applicable for a wide range of radiology services.

10.2 BARRIERS TO AI ADOPTION IN ONCO-RADIOLOGY

A key question should be asked: 'If AI technology is readily available and everyone agrees on its potential to improve healthcare services why have so few solutions been routinely adopted to date?' The answer is multi-faceted without one particular solution to resolve it.

First and foremost, the field of AI in health and medicine is moving with unprecedented rapidity, which healthcare institutions are struggling to keep up with. This was seen with the introduction of computer aided diagnosis and detection (CAD) software in the late 20th century, so it should be no surprise to see similar issues with AI today. The infrastructure and capability to adopt such technologies remain variable from site to site. Consequently, many hospitals globally are not set up to utilise AI in any impactful manner, often having to default to other, more advanced, hospitals to provide services on their behalf. This ultimately creates a 'postcode/zipcode lottery' where those in more rural settings or less developed economies will be left behind, unless more investment occurs there. Over time this will decline, but currently many sites are simply not able to adopt AI into routine workflow [3].

For those with infrastructure in place, additional challenges exist. Governance, data protection and integration bottlenecks all contribute to delays in AI adoption, even amongst those institutions with the relevant infrastructure in place [3–5]. However, arguably the biggest hurdle to date is the underlying hesitancy to adopt AI-based technology by healthcare professionals themselves. The fear that AI may add work rather than alleviate it, especially when flagging non-critical or incidental findings, further adds to this hesitancy [6].

Further components adding to the challenges of initiating AI include the following:

- **Governance and regulation:** Healthcare institutions must navigate strict regulatory requirements regarding patient data, safety and clinical governance, which often lag behind technological capabilities.

DOI: 10.1201/9781032709956-10

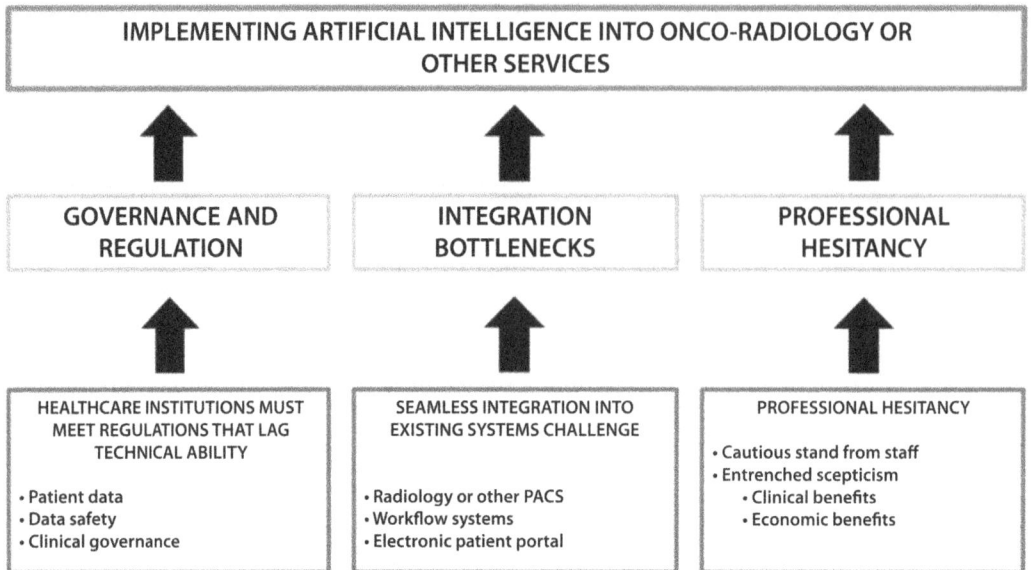

Figure 10.1 The relationship between the challenges of adopting artificial intelligence in onco-radiology.

- **Integration bottlenecks:** Seamless incorporation into existing radiology systems and picture archiving and communication systems (PACS) is not trivial.

- **Professional hesitancy:** Perhaps the most underestimated factor is the cautious stance of healthcare professionals themselves. There is an entrenched scepticism about the clinical and economic benefits of AI tools.

These principles are demonstrated in Figure 10.1.

When we look deeper into this issue of adoption, the story becomes clearer. More recent publications have highlighted a lack of substantial evidence of economic benefit from use of AI in onco-radiology to date. In a recent European Society of Radiologists (ESR) statement [4], AI algorithms were summarised as being used for a large spectrum of use-case scenarios in clinical radiology in Europe. These include

- assistance with interpretive tasks

- image post-processing

- prioritisation in the workflow

Only a minority of users experienced a reduction in the workload of the radiological medical staff due to the AI algorithms. Interestingly, most AI algorithms were found to be generally reliable, with no major problems with the technology itself or its ability to integrate into routine practice. The American College of Radiology (ACR) 2020 survey by Allen et al. (2021) asked whether respondents (radiologists and service representatives) intended to acquire a certified AI-based algorithm. Of 1427 respondents, only a minority (13.3%) answered yes, whereas the majority answered no (52.6%) [7]. The same trend can be seen when assessing devices approved by the FDA in the USA as, even though more than 200 commercial radiology AI products are now approved and available, limited adoption has occurred [7, 8]. This indicates that substantial obstacles must still be overcome before widespread successful clinical use of these products is recognised.

10.3 REAL-WORLD APPLICATIONS: LEADING-USE CASES

Although yet to be routinely adopted, AI tools have demonstrated tangible benefits in onco-radiology, especially in high-prevalence cancers. These use cases are at the forefront of highlighting the advantages to integrating AI into existing clinical pathways and are the ones most often referred to.

Consider lung cancer, a leading cause of cancer-related death globally. Timely detection can be lifesaving, and this is where AI tools are beginning to prove their value. In national lung screening programs, algorithms from companies like Optellum, Annalise and Aidence (acquired recently by DeepHealth) have been integrated to detect pulmonary nodules on computed tomography (CT) scans. These tools don't just scan and report, they assist risk stratification by analysing and comparing nodule characteristics against vast datasets of prior cases. Reports from clinical professionals have stated that these tools appear to show a reduction in false negatives and streamline patient follow-ups. In one UK-based reader study using retrospective chest X-rays, AI assistance led to a measurable increase in early-stage lung cancer detection, particularly at stages I and II, compared to unaided readings [9].

Breast cancer imaging is another major focus of AI diagnostic imaging in oncology. Where density and subtle asymmetries can obscure malignancies on traditional reading methods, AI acts as an additional layer of scrutiny to aid in decision making. iCAD's ProFound AI offers a second read on digital mammograms, providing both a heatmap of suspicious areas and a numerical risk score. This has been particularly helpful for radiologists operating in high-volume settings, offering reassurance or triggering second looks. Studies have shown that such tools improve diagnostic accuracy, especially amongst less-experienced readers, aligning with findings that AI is most helpful when complementing rather than replacing human judgement [10, 11]. Other players continue to emerge in this field such as Lunit and Kheiron medical, which are generating considerable traction in the market for breast cancer applications of AI in imaging.

Finally, prostate cancer diagnostics have also benefited from AI-powered tools to date and are another major focus in the market. Multiparametric magnetic resonance imaging (mpMRI), though powerful, has a steep learning curve and can produce ambiguous results, which is where the use of AI could help to alleviate such difficulties. Once example is Quantib's prostate solution, which leverages machine learning to highlight potentially suspicious regions on MRI and automatically generates structured reports to aid the radiological workflow. Radiologists using machine learning AI applications such as these have reported increased confidence and reduced variability in interpretations, factors crucial in determining patient pathways such as active surveillance versus biopsy [12, 13].

What unites these applications is not just their technical sophistication but their clear real-world impact. Each of these three leading cancers generate a significant burden on global healthcare systems, hence the popularity as commercial and clinical use cases for AI in medical imaging. They serve as proof points that AI can be more than just a research novelty; it can be embedded into routine practice and improve outcomes for patients and healthcare services. Its success, however, has not been acquired overnight. It is predicated on rigorous clinical validation, integration into existing workflows and, perhaps most importantly, clinician trust [14].

10.4 EXPANDING AI'S REACH BEYOND COMMON CANCERS

While early AI applications and adoptions in onco-radiology have predominately focused on the aforementioned cancers (lung, breast and prostate) due to wide ranging availability of data, high incidence rates and clear demand from global healthcare services, there is a crucial need to address other malignancies that are less prevalent but equally lethal. These cancers (detailed below) often suffer from delayed diagnoses and have poorer prognoses for patients as a result. AI's ability to rapidly process and analyse complex imaging data presents an opportunity to make meaningful inroads in these underrepresented domains. Examples of progress in other AI imaging solutions being applied to different cancer types include those listed below and some of the commercial products available on the market currently are listed in Figure 10.2.

- *Liver cancer*: Hepatocellular carcinoma (HCC) remains one of the leading causes of cancer-related deaths globally. Tools developed by Zebra Medical Vision and Arterys (for example) leverage AI to identify liver lesions on CT and MRI scans, enhancing early detection. These tools assist in distinguishing benign from malignant masses, a differentiation that is critical for treatment planning [15].

- *Pancreatic cancer*: Pancreatic adenocarcinoma is notorious for its late presentation and poor prognosis. AI models are currently in early stages for pancreatic cancer use cases and are mostly still in research phases; however, Guerbet's DUOnco Pancreas platform is making progress in this area, having recently been granted breakthrough device status by the FDA [16]. Furthermore, a recent publication from the Mayo Clinic has also shown significant progress in the development of a pancreatic lesion detection model [17]. These applications are showing promise in improving early diagnosis of pancreatic cancer and thus expanding treatment options.

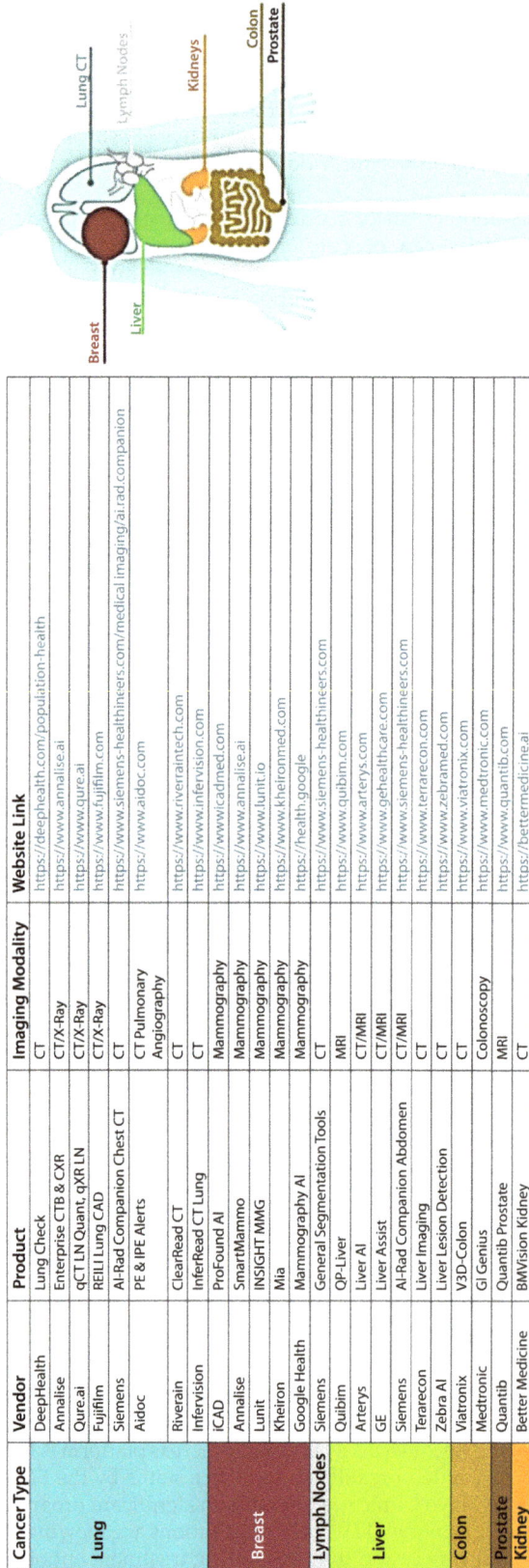

Cancer Type	Vendor	Product	Imaging Modality	Website Link
Lung	DeepHealth	Lung Check	CT	https://deephealth.com/population-health
	Annalise	Enterprise CTB & CXR	CT/X-Ray	https://www.annalise.ai
	Qure.ai	qCT LN Quant, qXR LN	CT/X-Ray	https://www.qure.ai
	Fujifilm	REILI Lung CAD	CT/X-Ray	https://www.fujifilm.com
	Siemens	AI-Rad Companion Chest CT	CT	https://www.siemens-healthineers.com/medical.imaging/ai.rad.companion
	Aidoc	PE & IPE Alerts	CT Pulmonary Angiography	https://www.aidoc.com
	Riverain	ClearRead CT	CT	https://www.riveraintech.com
	Infervision	InferRead CT Lung	CT	https://www.infervision.com
Breast	iCAD	ProFound AI	Mammography	https://www.icadmed.com
	Annalise	SmartMammo	Mammography	https://www.annalise.ai
	Lunit	INSIGHT MMG	Mammography	https://www.lunit.io
	Kheiron	Mia	Mammography	https://www.kheironmed.com
	Google Health	Mammography AI	Mammography	https://health.google
Lymph Nodes	Siemens	General Segmentation Tools	CT	https://www.siemens-healthineers.com
	Quibim	QP-Liver	MRI	https://www.quibim.com
Liver	Arterys	Liver AI	CT/MRI	https://www.arterys.com
	GE	Liver Assist	CT/MRI	https://www.gehealthcare.com
	Siemens	AI-Rad Companion Abdomen	CT/MRI	https://www.siemens-healthineers.com
	Terarecon	Liver Imaging	CT	https://www.terrarecon.com
	Zebra AI	Liver Lesion Detection	CT	https://www.zebramed.com
Colon	Viatronix	V3D-Colon	CT	https://www.viatronix.com
	Medtronic	GI Genius	Colonoscopy	https://www.medtronic.com
Prostate	Quantib	Quantib Prostate	MRI	https://www.quantib.com
Kidney	Better Medicine	BMVision Kidney	CT	https://bettermedicine.ai

Figure 10.2 A non-comprehensive summary of AI imaging solutions in automated cancer detection of lung, breast, lymph node, liver, colon, prostate and kidney applications as of 2025.

- *Kidney cancer*: Better Medicine's BMVision Kidney is the world's first and only clinically validated kidney cancer AI solution and exemplifies the power of AI in detecting incidental kidney tumours. By differentiating between benign and malignant lesions using the Bozniak classification criteria, early identification through non-targeted imaging (i.e., off-view analysis) could lead to improved survival rates [18].

- *Colorectal cancer*: AI has been used predominantly in colonoscopy-based detection, but tools like GI Genius (Medtronic) are being adapted for use in CT colonography [19]. Additionally, a recent publication by Kim et al. highlighted how their AI model could help reduce the frequency of missed colorectal cancers on routine examinations performed for reasons unrelated to colorectal cancer detection [20], further evidencing advancements in this space.

- *Brain tumours*: Rapid detection and characterisation of brain tumours are crucial for timely intervention. Although AI is still predominately in the research phases, recent publications have highlighted the potential for AI imaging solutions to detect brain cancer [21].

10.4.1 Cross-Cutting Tools and Multi-Cancer AI Platforms

Google Health and Butterfly Network are working on AI solutions that span multiple cancer types, supporting early detection across several organ systems. These tools exemplify a shift toward integrated AI models that can work across modalities and indications, increasing efficiency and reach.

The expansion of AI beyond common cancers reflects technological advancements and a greater appreciation for equity in cancer care. Sophisticated deep learning models, more diverse training datasets and federated learning approaches are enabling algorithms to generalise better across populations and imaging settings. Furthermore, as regulatory bodies begin to appreciate the nuances of AI validation, faster approvals and more robust post-market surveillance are anticipated [22].

Continued collaboration amongst academia, industry and clinical institutions is essential to maintain momentum in the discussed under-represented spaces in cancer AI developments. Developing clinically relevant models, supported by robust prospective studies, will be key to ensuring that AI delivers on its promise across all cancer types and will further generate trust that these solutions are as robust (if not more so) than those seen in lung, breast and prostate to date.

10.5 COMMERCIAL AND ECONOMIC CONSIDERATIONS

When discussing AI, we often focus on the clinical perspective; however, commercial viability also remains a sticking point in AI adoption. The market has seen a surge of AI imaging start-ups, many of whom have already been mentioned here, but a significant number of these have faced challenges in securing long-term investment as well as recurring revenue. Without robust economic evidence demonstrating cost-effectiveness, healthcare providers are hesitant to commit to the adoption of imaging AI and insurance-based healthcare systems have not enabled routine reimbursement of said solutions either. While AI systems have demonstrated technical efficacy, the lack of large-scale cost-benefit analyses limits their perceived value to healthcare administrators and policy makers [23].

From a market perspective, healthcare AI is projected to be a multi-billion–dollar industry, with radiology-specific tools forming a substantial subset of AI. However, revenue generation has, to date, been unevenly distributed. Start-up companies face a high failure rate, often relying heavily on venture capital funding without clearly defined paths to profitability. Many of these companies prioritise technological innovation without addressing the critical 'last mile' problems such as regulatory compliance, workflow integration, reimbursement policies and long-term contracting with paying healthcare institutions.

Another key issue is the ability of smaller companies to 'scale at pace'. AI tools validated in a single institution or dataset often underperform when deployed in broader real-world settings, with many experiencing what is known as 'data-set drift' issues. This variability reduces confidence in investment returns within the investor community and either delays or blocks funding for expansion. As a result, larger companies tend to win out as they already have the infrastructure and capital to support long regulatory and implementation processes and thus dominate the market. While their scale ensures stability, it may come at the cost of innovation. It is worth noting that the field of AI in medicine is not alone when it comes to this issue for innovation vs scaling in health technology as a whole.

Health economic modelling provides a possible solution. These models assess the potential return on investment (ROI) by comparing AI-driven workflows against traditional care pathways. In the UK, the National Institute for Health and Care Excellence (NICE) has begun piloting technology assessment frameworks for digital health solutions (including AI), emphasising cost-effectiveness, patient outcomes and workforce impact [24].

The commercialisation challenge is also deeply entwined with reimbursement structures as previously mentioned. Currently, few AI solutions are reimbursed directly by public or private insurers. Payment models such as bundled payments or value-based care initiatives may provide a more natural fit for AI-enabled diagnostics, but this requires careful coordination amongst policymakers, payers and technology developers. To ensure a diverse and competitive AI ecosystem, healthcare systems and investors must prioritise value-based evaluation metrics. These should include not only accuracy and specificity but also real-world efficiency gains, cost reductions, patient outcomes and the ability to scale across diverse healthcare settings [22, 25].

Collaborative funding models, such as public–private partnerships and research consortiums, may also play a critical role in supporting smaller firms. These arrangements help distribute risk, provide access to shared datasets and promote regulatory alignment. By fostering a more equitable innovation landscape, such initiatives could safeguard against market monopolisation and ensure that the most clinically useful tools, not just the most capitalised ones, reach the bedside, where innovation is so crucially needed.

10.6 RETHINKING AI'S ROLE: THE 'OFF-VIEW' APPROACH

In totality it is important to evaluate the trend in AI use cases to date and where they may tend towards in the future. Traditional AI tools in radiology often function as second readers, replicating the human focus on a specific region of interest, such as lung nodules on chest CT or masses in breast mammography. To date this has been the most widely used model seen with AI imaging solutions available on the market. While this 'co-pilot' model has yielded performance improvements and workflow enhancements, it also has inherent limitations. Chief among them is the increased cognitive and operational burden placed on image reporters, who must adjudicate incidental findings that may not have been clinically relevant to the initial imaging intent [26–29].

Now, a promising evolution in AI deployment is emerging which is the concept of 'off-view' or 'off-label' analysis AI tools. This approach expands the scope of AI interpretation beyond the primary diagnostic focus and in doing so acts as both a safety net and triage mechanism for incidental findings of suspicious lesions. For example, in an abdominal CT scan ordered to evaluate appendicitis, an off-view AI tool might flag a previously unnoticed renal mass or early liver lesion. This represents a fundamental shift from redundancy to complementarity in human-AI collaboration [30].

There are many perceived benefits of Off-View AI such as the following:

- *Increased diagnostic yield*: By detecting clinically relevant abnormalities outside the targeted region, off-view tools have the potential to identify incidental but actionable findings.

- *Workflow efficiency*: These tools can prioritize high-risk incidental findings for rapid review while deferring low-risk issues, thereby reducing unnecessary follow-ups.

- *Safety net functionality*: Off-view AI provides a layer of quality assurance, especially valuable in high-volume or time-pressured settings, where even expert radiologists may miss subtle anomalies.

- *Health economic impact*: Early identification of incidental cancers, such as renal cell carcinoma or asymptomatic liver metastases, may significantly reduce downstream treatment costs and improve survival rates [24].

These principles and their relationships are detailed further in Figure 10.3.

It is worth noting that despite the potential advantages listed, implementing 'off-view' AI consideration and understanding when and where to use this approach will be vital to successful implementation of such methodologies. These systems must be rigorously validated to avoid overdiagnosis and to ensure clinical relevance. False positives could lead to patient anxiety and unnecessary diagnostic workups, burdening both the healthcare system and the individual [30].

Integration with existing PACS and radiology information systems (RISs) is another technical hurdle. Workflow interruptions must be minimised to ensure reporter adoption [31]. Additionally, medico-legal frameworks need to evolve to define accountability when 'off-view' AI flags findings that go unaddressed, particularly as the regulatory framework on medical liability when AI is applied is currently inadequate [32]. Several vendors are now stating they are exploring off-view applications of AI in imaging, including Aidoc, Qure.ai and Better Medicine, to name a few.

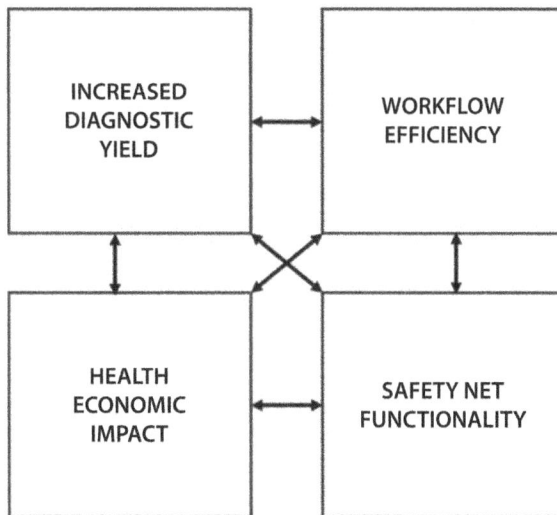

Figure 10.3 The interrelated benefits of 'off-view' AI systems.

Off-view AI represents a new frontier in diagnostic radiology, one that aligns technological capability with clinical intuition and health system priorities. It offers a scalable solution for increasing diagnostic accuracy and efficiency without overburdening reporters and may ultimately shift the paradigm from organ-specific analysis to patient-centred image interpretation, especially when combined with image screening programmes for larger cancer types such as lung, breast and prostate.

10.7 CONCLUSION

Despite a reluctance to adopt AI into routine practice to date, AI is here to stay and will become a vital part of healthcare services within the next decade. Radiology is at the forefront of this revolution, especially within onco-radiology settings. A lack of real-world evidence has delayed the integration of many AI solutions into routine practice, and sadly some innovative commercial start-ups to date, yet the momentum is building. The transition toward more comprehensive AI adoption is likely not a matter of 'if' but 'when' as has been revealed via feedback from the medical community [3].

As AI applications mature, demonstrating not just accuracy but also real-world utility, economic benefit and patient-centred outcomes, health systems will be increasingly incentivised to integrate these tools and reimbursement will be more likely [23]. The future of radiology may no longer be defined by whether AI is used but how effectively it is implemented and in what setting. This transformation will also determine which commercial players survive. While natural market forces may lead to the dominance of well-funded companies and existing large corporations, the clinical community has a role in guiding this evolution and supporting those truly innovative companies towards adoption of AI. By actively engaging with AI developers, validating tools in real-world settings and advocating for evidence-based procurement decisions, clinicians can help ensure that quality, not just capital, determines success and that these tools can end up in routine clinical practice [6].

In the end, successful AI integration will rely on meaningful collaboration amongst healthcare professionals, technology developers (both commercial and academic) and policymakers. Those who champion this interdisciplinary alliance will shape the next chapter in onco-radiology and beyond, where AI becomes the norm in the field of medicine rather than the exception.

10.8 EDITORS' COMMENTS

This chapter has succinctly provided a range of ideas to consider in the eventual wide application of AI in healthcare. Using the onco-radiology focus, it illustrates strengths and limitations and offers examples of where AI can be applied and negotiates the challenges of implementation. Possibly one of the greater challenges is the acceptance of AI as being able to deliver, especially where financial constraints exist. 'Myth busting', which can be delivered only where healthcare staff are prepared to be open about potential and use AI as a positive tool rather than perceiving it as a negative concept, must be attempted to enable health development to continue. After all, it was said that computed tomography was too hard to accomplish in the late 1960s and into the early 1970s for the gains that would be achieved! We are in that development phase now but also need to be mindful of ensuring the most appropriate 'low hanging fruit' is picked to begin with and maintain an eye on the sustainability question in the future – more of which is discussed in Chapter 14.

REFERENCES

1. McCarthy, J. (1956) The Dartmouth Summer Research Project on Artificial Intelligence. http://jmc.stanford.edu/articles/dartmouth/dartmouth.pdf
2. PR Newswire. (2017) Aidoc Receives CE Mark for First Commercial Deep Learning Solution Streamlining Head and Neck Imaging for Radiologists. https://www.prnewswire.com/news-releases/aidoc-receives-ce-mark-for-first-commercial-deep-learning-solution-streamlining-head-and-neck-imaging-for-radiolgists-660261973.html
3. Tapper, J., McKie, R. (2024) NHS cannot Embrace AI Until its Basic IT Systems are up to Scratch. The Guardian, Sunday 15th September. https://www.theguardian.com/society/2024/sep/15/nhs-cannot-embrace-ai-until-its-basic-it-systems-are-up-to-scratch?utm_source=chatgpt.com (accessed June 2025).
4. European Society of Radiology (ESR). (2019) Impact of Artificial Intelligence on Radiology: A EuroAIM Survey among members of the European Society of Radiology. Insights into Imaging, 10, 105.
5. Royal College of Radiologists. (2023). Overcoming Barriers to AI Implementation in Imaging. https://www.rcr.ac.uk/our-services/artificial-intelligence-ai/overcoming-barriers-to-ai-implementation-in-imaging/
6. Topol, E. (2019) Deep Medicine: How Artificial Intelligence Can Make Healthcare Human Again. Basic Books.
7. Allen, B., Agarwal, S., Coombs, L. et al. (2021) 2020 ACR Data Science Institute AI Survey. Journal of the American College of Radiology, 18, 1153–1159.
8. American College of Radiologists. (2022) https://www.acr.org/News-and-PublicationsMore-Than-200-FDA-Cleared-AI-Medical-Imaging-Products-Now-Available
9. Dissez, G., Qureshi, N.R., Chen, Y.Y. et al. (2022). Enhancing Early Lung Cancer Detection on Chest Radiographs with AI-Assistance: A Multi-Reader Study. arXiv, 2208.14742.
10. Rodriguez-Ruiz, A., Lång, K., Gubern-Merida, K. et al. (2019) Stand-Alone Artificial Intelligence for Breast Cancer Detection in Mammography: Comparison with 101 Radiologists. Journal of the National Cancer Institute, 111(9), 916–922.
11. Yala, A., Lehman, C., Schuster, T. et al. (2019) A Deep Learning Mammography-Based Model for Improved Breast Cancer Risk Prediction. Radiology, 292(1), 60–66.
12. Cuocolo, R., Cipullo, M.B. et al. (2020) Machine Learning Applications in Prostate Cancer Magnetic Resonance Imaging. European Radiology Experimental, 4(1), 27.
13. Sun, Z., Wang, K., Kong, Z. et al. (2023) A Multicenter Study of Artificial Intelligence-Aided Software for Detecting Visible Clinically Significant Prostate Cancer on mpMRI. Insights into Imaging, 14, 72.
14. Chen, M., Zhang, B., Cai, Z. et al. (2022) Acceptance of Clinical Artificial Intelligence Among Physicians and Medical Students: A Systematic Review With Cross-Sectional Survey. Frontiers in Medicine, 9, 990604.
15. Zavaleta-Monestel, E., Quesada-Villaseñor, R., Arguedas-Chacón, S. et al. (2024) Revolutionizing Healthcare: Qure.AI's Innovations in Medical Diagnosis and Treatment. Cureus, 16(6), e56247. https://doi.org/10.7759/cureus.61585
16. Guerbets Duonco Pancreas Platform Gets FDA Nod. (2025) https://www.auntminnie.com/clinical-news/ct/article/15740868/guerbet-guerbets-duonco-pancreas-platform-gets-fda-nod
17. Korfiatis, P., Suman, G., Patnam, N.G. et al. (2023) Automated Artificial Intelligence Model Trained on a Large Data Set Can Detect Pancreas Cancer on Diagnostic Computed Tomography Scans as Well as Visually Occult Preinvasive Cancer on Prediagnostic Computed Tomography Scans. Gastroenterology, 165(6), 1533–1546.e4.
18. Better Medicine website for Kidney Cancer. (2025) https://bettermedicine.ai/bmvision/kidney/
19. Biffi, C., Salvagnini, P., Ngo, Dinh, N. et al. (2022) A Novel AI Device for Real-Time Optical Characterization of Colorectal Polyps. NPJ Digital Medicine, 5(1), 84.
20. Kim, S., Seo, H., Choi, K. et al. (2025). Artificial Intelligence Model for Detection of Colorectal Cancer on Routine Abdominopelvic CT Examinations: A Training and External-Testing Study. American Journal of Roentgenology, 224(4).
21. Khalighi, S., Reddy, K., Midya, A. et al. (2024). Artificial Intelligence in Neuro-Oncology: Advances and Challenges in Brain Tumor Diagnosis, Prognosis, and Precision Treatment. NPJ Precision Oncology, 8, Article 80.
22. van Leeuwen, K.G., Schalekamp, S., Rutten, M.J.C.M. et al. (2021) Artificial Intelligence in Radiology: 100 Commercially Available Products and Their Scientific Evidence. European Radiology, 31, 3797–4380.
23. Davenport, T., Kalakota, R. (2019). The Potential for Artificial Intelligence in Healthcare. Future Healthcare Journal, 6(2), 94–98. https://doi.org/10.7861/futurehosp.6-2-94
24. NICE. (2023) Evidence Standards Framework for Digital Health Technologies. National Institute for Health and Care Excellence.
25. Wang F, Casalino LP, Khullar D. Deep Learning in Medicine-Promise, Progress, and Challenges. JAMA Intern Med. 2019 Mar 1;179(3):293–294. doi: 10.1001/jamainternmed.2018.7117.
26. McKinney, S.M., Sieniek, M., Godbole, V. et al. (2020) International Evaluation of an AI System for Breast Cancer Screening. Nature, 577, 89–94.
27. Liu, H., Ding, N., Li, X. et al. (2024) Artificial Intelligence and Radiologist Burnout. JAMA Network Open, 7(11), e2448714.
28. Marka, A.W., Luitjens, J., Gassert, F.T. et al. (2024) Artificial Intelligence Support in MR Imaging of Incidental Renal Masses: An Early Health Technology Assessment. European Radiology, 34(9), 5856–5865. https://doi.org/10.1007/s00330-024-10643-5
29. Pomohaci, M.D., Grasu, M.C., Băicoianu-Nițescu, A.-Ș., Enache, R.M., Lupescu, I.G. (2025) Systematic Review: AI Applications in Liver Imaging With a Focus on Segmentation and Detection. Life, 15(2), 258. https://doi.org/10.3390/life15020258
30. Dudum, R., Asch, S.M. (2023) "Incidentalomas" in the Age of Artificial Intelligence. Journal of General Internal Medicine, 38, 2855–2856.
31. Kotter, E., Ranschaert, E. (2021) Challenges and Solutions for Introducing Artificial Intelligence (AI) in Daily Clinical Workflow. European Radiology, 31(1), 5–7. https://doi.org/10.1007/s00330-020-07148-2 Epub 2020 Aug 14.
32. Cestonaro, C., Delicati, A., Marcante, B. et al. (2023) Defining Medical Liability When Artificial Intelligence Is Applied on Diagnostic Algorithms: A Systematic Review. Frontiers in Medicine, 10, 1305756. https://doi.org/10.3389/fmed.2023.1305756

11 The Application of Artificial Intelligence to Histopathology

Vijay Sharma

11.1 INTRODUCTION

The application of Artificial Intelligence (AI) to histopathological diagnosis is one of the strongest and most promising use cases for the technology in the healthcare setting. Ever since the haematoxylin and eosin stain was first described and applied to human tissues in the 19th century, histopathologists have been accumulating a body of histological knowledge by which the morphological appearances of a pathological process observed at a moment in time can be used to infer how that process will behave in future time. This has been made possible by a century and a half of careful correlation between the morphology and the clinical features, information from other diagnostic modalities, and a vast body of basic and translational science. It works because of the intimate inter-relationship between structure and function that is fundamental to all biological processes. One of the strengths of AI is its ability to identify patterns and make predictions, a strength which aligns well with the process by which histopathological diagnoses are made.

When assessing a case, the pathologist identifies and describes the morphological features (including the macroscopic features in the specimen, not just the microscopic features from the tissue sampled from the specimen), interprets them, and integrates them in the context both of wider knowledge of the disease process and of the specific patient they are presented with. No case is ever assessed in isolation; it is a truism of medicine that any diagnostic effort is flying blind in the absence of knowledge of the wider clinical context, something any diagnostician in receipt of an incompletely filled request form will be only too familiar with. Furthermore, as with all of medicine, cases vary in their difficulty, and pathologists become adept at communicating the level of certainty they can ascribe to their opinion. They also know when a definite answer cannot be given at all and know how to communicate this to the clinical team. In other words, histopathologists, like all diagnosticians, must master the science and the art of using and communicating fuzzy logic. The pathologist's report of a case communicates not simply the result of a test, but a carefully considered professional opinion.

The histopathologist works within a multidisciplinary team. The team, in turn, arrives at a treatment recommendation considered to be in the best interests of the patient. In this endeavour, appreciation of context and nuance is key. Common sense is our best friend. Empathy with the patient is needed, and the outcome – to achieve healing – is ultimately a compassionate exercise. We find ourselves entering into an era in which there is value in articulating these self-evident truths. It is an important frame from which to embark on an exploration of the very real benefits AI can bring to this space, while at the same time appreciating its limitations and its dangers.

11.1.1 The Transition to Digital Pathology

Pathologists are transitioning away from using microscopes and towards using digitised images of slides. This has many advantages. It allows cases to be easily shared between pathologists for consensus opinions, even internationally. With a properly empowered and integrated digital workflow, digital pathology can achieve modest efficiency gains, up to 10%, not least because some tasks, such as measuring the size of lesions or their distance from resection margins, are a lot easier [1, 2]. Finally, of most relevance to this discussion, it opens the way for the application of AI.

A digital workflow needs to have three basic components:

- the scanners which digitise the slides

- the image management system which handles the images

- the laboratory information management system which is the IT system underpinning the entire specimen journey through the laboratory

The digital workflow also requires sufficient bandwidth and processing power to allow a smooth seamless user experience when viewing the images. It also requires copious amounts of storage. Histological digital images are orders of magnitude larger than radiology images, particularly when it comes to 3D imaging using Z-stacking. Consider a loaf of bread; each slice of bread is equivalent to the x and y planes, and the z-axis relates to the entire loaf (Figure 11.1). Healthcare systems need to provide, maintain, and regularly expand this storage.

DOI: 10.1201/9781032709956-11

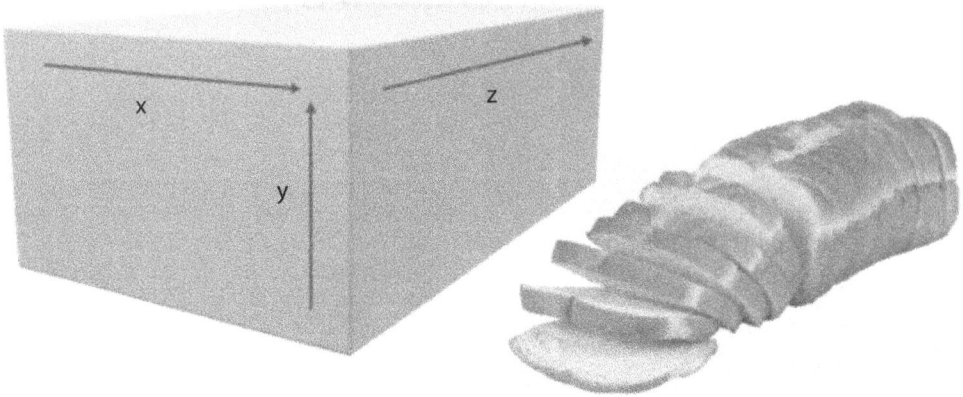

Figure 11.1 Z-stacking analogy: each slice of bread is equivalent to the x and y planes, and the z-axis relates to the entire loaf.

Currently, the transition to digital pathology is gaining momentum but is still incomplete. Internationally there is wide variation in digital maturity and pathologists' experience with the technology. There are two barriers to overcome. The first broadly relates to the investment needed to establish an integrated digital workflow. Without a proper workflow, digital pathology confers no advantage and may even introduce inefficiencies. The second relates to the ability of the users to use digital images instead of the microscope.

The neurophysiological aspect of the latter transition is an interesting one. The image viewed through the microscope is a 3D image. The image viewed on a computer screen is a 2D image. When a pathologist learns their craft on a microscope, all their experience becomes interlinked neurologically with the pathways involved in 3D image interpretation, a process which begins in the visual cortex, but which also involves several other brain regions. The transition to relying solely on a 2D image places the burden of pattern recognition solely on the output of the visual cortex. A period of retraining the brain is needed to achieve this, after which pathologists find they can use digital pathology just as well as their old trusty microscope.

Despite its promise, digital pathology has its blind spots, such as the inability to polarise a slide (an optical trick, much like wearing sunglasses to see fish in a river which would be invisible without the use of sunglasses, that has a variety of uses in visualisation of pathological change) or the loss of subtle morphological features better appreciated in 3D than 2D. For this reason, there will still be cases that require a review of the glass slides. The microscope may find itself relegated to the role of a tool for further investigation, but it is unlikely to disappear completely, at least not until the blind spots are fully addressed. It is also wise to maintain the microscope as a backup to maintain business continuity in the event of a failure of the digital technology.

11.2 AI: SOME TERMS DEFINED

Ideas about the essence of consciousness, human thought, and learning, as well as the foundations of logic, have been considered since the ancient world. From the 1700s, philosophers began to develop theories about the construction of knowledge and whether it can be predicted. A key milestone was the statistical work of Bayes, who in 1763 developed Bayesian reference, a framework for examining the probability of events, which formed the foundation of machine learning.

Some key terms related to AI are defined in Table 11.1 and types of learning approaches are defined in Table 11.2. (See also Chapter 3.) Weak AI is designed and trained to carry out specific tasks, but the learning from these tasks is not generalisable to other tasks.

Strong AI, also known as artificial general intelligence (AGI), would simulate the cognitive capabilities of the human brain. It would be capable of handling fuzzy logic (i.e., dealing with imprecise or uncertain data/information) and autonomously using it to apply knowledge from different domains to find solutions to unfamiliar problems. This kind of AI could be taught histopathological interpretation in the manner that human histopathologists are taught. Strong AI does not exist yet.

AI is expected to evolve through stages. The first stage is of reactive machines which are task-specific machines that have the capacity to react to a situation at hand but have no capacity to learn from past experiences or to make future predictions. IBMs Deep Blue chess computer is a famous

Table 11.1 Definitions of Key Terms

Term	Definition
Machine learning	The subset of AI which uses algorithms to improve performance by learning from data, allowing the algorithms to improve their performance without being explicitly programmed to do so
Deep learning	The subset of machine learning which uses deep neural networks, modelling how the brain works, to identify patterns in large datasets and make predictions.
Generative AI	• A type of AI which uses training data to produce novel outputs which resemble human output • Has the disadvantage of lacking clear quality and validation metrics and is also prone to hallucinations
Foundation models	Large machine learning models trained on a large amount of unlabelled data, forming a scaffold which can then be adapted and fine-tuned with additional training to specific tasks.
Visual language models	A way to cross-train AI between images and language
Vision transformers	• A type of deep learning architecture which supercedes neural networks for image analysis, outperforming neural networks up to four times for accuracy and efficiency • Require larger amounts of data but can be trained faster • Have a self-attention mechanism which means they are more 'aware' than deep learning models
Explainability	The extent to which the method by which the algorithm produces its outputs and predictions can be explained. Most AIs have limited to no explainability, so it is not clear which features of the image are responsible for the prediction made.

Table 11.2 Approaches to Training AI Algorithms

Learning Approach	Definition, Use, Advantages and Disadvantages
Supervised learning	The algorithm is told what an object is and learns to recognise it. • Good for developing AIs for the quantitative evaluation of biomarkers. • Highly explainable • Little room for the generation of novel information • Requires large amounts of annotated data
Unsupervised and weakly supervised learning	The data are unlabelled or loosely labelled (e.g. by clinical outcome) to allow the algorithm to seek and find novel associations. • Good for deriving novel insights from the H+E image, such as predicting the mutation status, prognosis or response to therapy. • Poor explainability
Moderately supervised learning	An intermediate approach between supervised and unsupervised learning. • Good for applications such as spatial multiplex analysis to identify spatial interrelationships in tissues • Poor explainability
Self-supervised learning	A process in which the model learns from the objects themselves through puzzles or pre-set tasks set by the trainers. • Mimics more closely how humans learn

example of such an AI (IBM, 2025) (Deep Blue | IBM https://www.ibm.com/history/deep-blue). Other examples include recommendation engines in online streaming content websites and self-driving cars. The second stage is limited memory, which is the current stage of AI, task-specific machines which can use past experiences to inform future predictions. The third stage is theory of mind, where the AI has artificial social intelligence with the ability to understand emotion. The fourth and final stage is self-awareness, where the AI possesses true consciousness and has become an artificial lifeform.

11.3 ADVANTAGES AND DISADVANTAGES OF AI

AI can compensate for the limitations of the human eye, which is not good at assessing either the intensity of a stain or the proportion of cells showing the stain, and so may well outperform pathologists in quantitative biomarker assessments. It is capable of performing consistently and reliably and can do so 24 hours a day 7 days a week. AI can also put onto a quantitative and objective basis assessments which were previously qualitative and subjective in nature. For this reason, AI can be used to address areas of diagnostic difficulty previously subject to problems of high inter-observer variability [3].

However, when it comes to diagnosis, context is everything, and AI struggles with context. It does not have common sense. The errors it makes are not, for the most part, the kind of errors a human would make. However, the converse is also true, so the combination of a pathologist working together with an AI is powerful, and the published evidence is that the performance of a pathologist and an AI is superior to either alone [4]. Most AI systems have a black-box nature. It is not clear how they produce their outputs. Pathologists, by contrast are able to articulate the reasons for their conclusions, so the combination of AI with a pathologist balances the maximum extraction of information from the image with a degree of explainability in the final professional opinion.

Another crucial point is that the performance of the AI is only as good as the data used to train it. Most AI systems show at least one form of bias, which is one of the most significant concerns in the field and an obstacle to the safe and reliable deployment of the technology (as further discussed in Chapter 5). Going forward, the data must be meticulously curated to eliminate or minimise bias and be fully transparent for appraisal. This will require significant investment in an infrastructure to gather and maintain the vast amounts of data needed to train AI. Current developers have been hampered by the lack of such a resource and have understandably had to rely on what data they can obtain. However, ambitious initiatives in this space are emerging, which is a welcome development (for example, PharosAI).

It is particularly important, when developing an AI algorithm to interpret images, to standardise the images used to train the algorithm as much as possible so that the difference being sought is what the algorithm will be trained on. This is analogous to controlling variables in a scientific experiment or using randomisation to control for confounding factors in a clinical trial. One often-quoted example of what can happen when this is not done concerns an algorithm which was trained to distinguish between huskies and wolves. Because the husky photographs mostly had a snowy background and the wolf photographs did not, the algorithm ended up distinguishing between snow and no snow in the background [5]. Caveat emptor!

11.4 DIGITAL WEATHER AND ALGORITHMIC DRIFT

It is well recognised that variations in the quality and intensity of the staining in particular laboratories as well as the choice of scanner can influence the performance of AI algorithms. It is important for the developers of AI to test their algorithm across a range of laboratories and scanners to account for these effects, and any laboratory deploying AI must do the necessary verification and validation to control for these factors, just as they would for any new chemical assay. In day-to-day work, the use of positive and negative controls can be used to monitor the algorithm's performance. The laboratory should also take steps to minimise any variation in the quality of staining of tissue sections.

The performance of AI algorithms can change because of software updates. The constant updating of computer software can be viewed as a form of 'digital weather'. This is analogous to the way in which the performance of laboratory assays can be affected. The key difference is that chemical assays are explainable, and we have decades of experience in how to troubleshoot problems that arise with them. The phenomenon of digital weather, by contrast, is new to us, and the limited explainability of AI models limits our ability to troubleshoot changes in the AI performance, except by reverting to previous versions once a change is detected. Mitigating the effects of digital weather will require the same quality control methods as are used with chemical assays, such as the use of positive and negative controls and regular participation in quality schemes.

'Algorithmic drift' can also intrinsically alter the performance of algorithms over time. Because algorithms are continuously learning, their performance can and does evolve with time and experience and could lead to emergence. Generative AI is the form of AI which is particularly prone to this. Chat GPT has evolved beyond the initial methods used to train it and is showing an improved ability to generate images from text despite having never been trained on images. In the research setting, this can be a good effect, as it is a way to develop better algorithms. In the clinical setting, however, this drift needs to be controlled so that the standardisation and accuracy of the algorithm is not adversely affected, and to maintain a clear boundary between clinical practice and research. To have our cake and eat it, perhaps the best solution is to have some versions of the algorithm in the research setting which are allowed to learn and evolve, and others in the clinical laboratory which are controlled to maintain laboratory standards. Most companies which have clinically approved AI currently lock down the algorithms to prevent algorithmic drift.

The evidence on the monitoring of AI performance in histopathology is sparse and tends to focus on measures most familiar in the research space for the evaluation of biomarkers and treatments [6]. Such measures, while important, are unlikely to be fully equal on their own to the task of AI monitoring. There are also cautionary studies pointing to the fact that emergent capabilities in AI will be impossible to predict [7], harking back to Alan Turing's original definition of emergent phenomena as being inherently unpredictable, and highlighting the need to lock algorithms down for safe clinical use.

It may be possible to develop AI systems to monitor the function of others. At the time of writing, there are no tools available specifically in the pathology space for AI monitoring of AI performance. Such tools are emerging in other industries, such as Wisecube's Pythia, a hallucination-detection tool which provides real-time monitoring of large language models [8]. However, it is possible to use currently available tools to monitor the quality of the data being inputted into the AI algorithm, such as using monitoring of staining quality with one AI before another AI quantifies the biomarker.

11.5 APPLICATIONS OF AI IN THE LABORATORY WORKFLOW

There are many points in the specimen journey through the laboratory at which AI can be used to improve the efficiency of the workflow:

1. Once a specimen has been dissected, blocks taken, and slides scanned, AI can be used to assess the quality of the slide and any cases showing quality problems reflexed back to have these errors rectified.

2. Cases requiring further blocks to be taken (the rules for which need to be defined specifically for each tissue and pathology) can be reflexed back to the dissection stage for the extra blocks to be taken. This saves time for the pathologist assessing the case.

3. AI can be used to identify when further investigations, including biomarkers, are needed and order these.

4. AI can do automated tumour content assessment for molecular tests, in which knowing the percentage of the specimen that is comprised of tumour is important for the selection of the correct assay [9].

5. AI can monitor the performance of further investigations, such as immunohistochemistry, so that problems can be identified and rectified in real time, as opposed to being identified weeks or months later [10].

6. AI can derive novel predictive and prognostic information to be presented to the pathologist for assessment. At the moment this will complement the use of further tests but with time and experience, it may reduce the need for requesting further tests.

7. AI can provide quantitative assessment of biomarkers, which in turn can reduce the need for further tests. HER-2 assessment in breast cancer is a good example of this application; the confident quantitative assessment of HER-2 by immunohistochemistry can reduce the number of cases that require detection of the HER-2 translocation using in-situ hybridisation, resulting in a significant time and cost saving [11].

8. AI can be used to prioritise cases for reporting and to ensure intelligent and fair case distribution between pathologists. This is particularly valuable in laboratories faced with a backlog as it allows potentially malignant cases to be identified and prioritised for reporting, preventing delays in diagnosis for these patients [12].

Figure 11.2 provides a schematic that outlines the steps (as described above) that AI may be applied within the laboratory setting.

In the era of weak AI, each specific use for each specific tissue type requires its own algorithm. A laboratory employing AI across all of the above steps would be required to procure and maintain a large number of algorithms. There are algorithms in various stages of development across the full range of specimen and tissue types and use cases. The National Pathology Imaging Cooperative (NPIC) of the UK recently launched a first-of-its-kind central register for AI-based pathology tools [13].

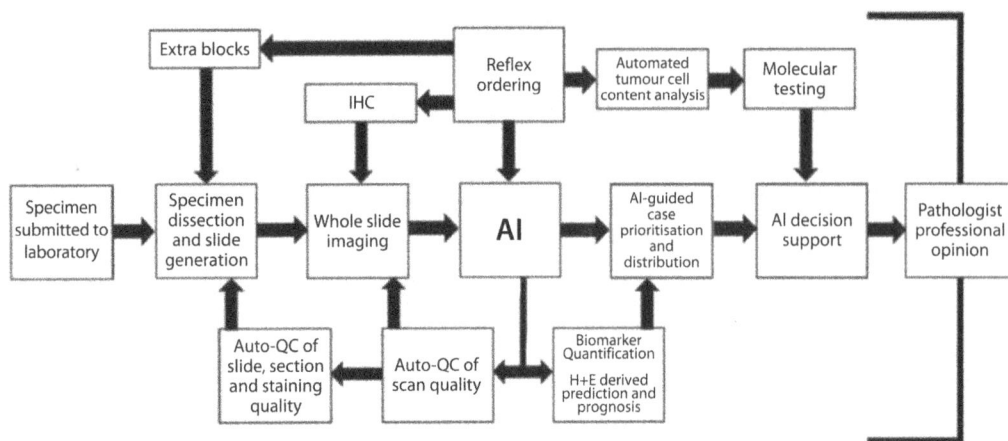

Figure 11.2 Schematic of the laboratory workflow showing the use cases for AI at each stage in the specimen journey. At the final step, the AI-literate pathologist checks and integrates all of the information provided by the AI into their assessment of the case.

11.6 THE VIRTUAL TRAINEE

If a pathology laboratory were to implement AI throughout the workflow as described above, when the case comes to the pathologist, the AI will have minimised the need for the pathologist to go back to the specimen and will have anticipated the more routine additional tests needed, as well as providing additional predictive and prognostic information and a quantitative assessment of the biomarkers. That would be a significant help to the pathologist assessing the case.

AI that has been trained to provide diagnostic information can also be deployed at this stage. Many AIs are in development and a smaller number are available for clinical use [13]. At the time of writing, the AI assessment of prostate cancer shows the best performance [14]. The AI in this setting functions like an experienced pathology trainee, presenting a worked-up case to the consultant for expert assessment. AI has been trained to make diagnoses, assess tumour grade, identify features such as perineural invasion, and so on. As stated above, it is the combination of a pathologist and the AI which is most powerful.

There is also at least one AI which goes a step further, being able to derive from a histological image a description and suggested diagnosis or differential diagnosis, and to refine this based on the results of further investigations [15]. Such decision support is impressive and best regarded as akin to consulting an intelligent textbook, which can also generate customised canned reports for the pathologist to edit.

At present, most of the AIs which are available for clinical use have been approved for second line use, which means that the pathologist must look at the case first and the AI is used to ensure that the pathologist has not missed something. Any other use of such algorithms, including the virtual trainee scenario described above, is, at the time of writing, an off-label use. This needs to be born in mind both by departments implementing AI and by policy makers.

11.7 CRITICAL APPRAISAL OF AI

Many pathologists profess a lack of confidence in their ability to critically appraise AI [16]. It is important to realise that it is not necessary to have a detailed knowledge of programming to be able to appraise AI, although a baseline education should be considered for responsible engagement with clinical AI, as outlined in Chapter 6. Many of the principles are the same as those used to critically appraise the scientific literature. However, AI does introduce additional issues that must be considered.

As with any diagnostic modality, the assessment begins with the context, for example,

■ In what population was the AI developed?

■ Is it relevant to the patients the pathologist is assessing?

- Is there enough transparency to allow the quality of the training data to be assessed? (The answer to this question all too often is no.)

- Have the sensitivity, specificity, and positive and negative predictive values been quoted?

Another key question for AI in particular is, What specifically does the AI get wrong? This is a key question. Currently AI tends to get the rarities wrong, such as misdiagnosing a malignant small round blue cell tumour as inflammation, or struggles with the same diagnostic difficulties pathologists do, such as the assessment of atypia in breast core biopsies. Sometimes it makes mistakes a pathologist would not make, which can be as simple as misinterpreting haemosiderin pigment (a breakdown product of haemoglobin) as positive staining in immuno-histochemistry, something the author has anecdotally observed when assessing algorithms, or as complex as a misclassification born of inherent biases in the algorithm [17]. These errors can be eliminated with more training of the algorithms, and by eliminating bias in AI algorithm development, but they are lurking in the current generation of AI. This is why pathologists must supervise the AIs.

The detailed critical appraisal of AI requires the model to be systematically evaluated for all potential sources of bias. Some key biases will be briefly explored here, but the reader is referred to the checklists and guidelines listed below for a comprehensive discussion (see also Chapter 5). The first question that must be answered is whether there is enough transparency to allow this critical appraisal to be carried out. If the answer to this question is no, that is an immediate red flag. This becomes particularly important for the use of foundation models. In the field of AI, foundation models are becoming a popular way to avoid reinventing the wheel with algorithm development, and they are also likely to be the most feasible way of training algorithms that iron out errors with the rarities. However, this approach risks propagating, and even amplifying, the biases present in the original model. For this reason, key decision-makers in the pathology field, including the European Society of Pathology, have cautioned against the use of foundation models in the current landscape.

There are a number of checklists and guidelines available for the evaluation of AI detailed in Table 11.3. Those relevant to histopathology AI include STARD-AI (for ensuring transparency), TRIPOD AI (reporting guidelines for diagnostic and prognostic models), PROBLAST AI (assessment of the risk of bias in diagnostic and prognostic AI), CONSORT AI (reporting standards for AI in clinical trials), and QUADAS-AI (assessment of the diagnostic accuracy of AI in healthcare).

The FAIR principles state that the data used to train AI should be findable, accessible, interoperable and reusable (for further detail, please see Chapter 5).

Some key biases that can occur in pathology-related AIs include those listed in Table 11.4. The presence of bias in an AI algorithm leads to a lack of generalisability when the algorithm is applied to diverse populations and subjects the under-represented population to the risk of underdiagnosis, overdiagnosis, or misdiagnosis. This in turn risks amplifying existing health inequalities. The mitigation of bias through adherence to the principles outlined in the guidance documents listed above must be a priority going forward.

Table 11.3 Checklists and Guidelines Available for the Evaluation of AI

AI Assessment Tool	Uses	Links
STARD-AI	Ensuring transparency	https://bmjopen.bmj.com/content/11/6/e047709 https://pubmed.ncbi.nlm.nih.gov/32514173/
TRIPOD AI	Guidelines for reporting findings for diagnostic and prognostic models	https://www.tripod-statement.org/ https://www.bmj.com/content/385/bmj-2023-078378
PROBLAST AI	Assessment of the risk of bias in diagnostic and prognostic AI	https://abstracts.cochrane.org/2023-london/probastai-assessing-quality-risk-bias-and-applicability-diagnostic-and-prognostic https://www.bmj.com/content/388/bmj-2024-082505
CONSORT AI	Reporting standards for AI in clinical trials	https://www.nature.com/articles/s41591-020-1034-x
QUADAS-AI	Assessment of the diagnostic accuracy of AI in healthcare	https://www.nature.com/articles/s41591-021-01517-0

Table 11.4 Types of Bias in Histopathology

Type of Bias	Definition and Application
Data bias	The overrepresentation, under-representation or misrepresentation of pathology cases in the training data biases the algorithm. Missing data are a common cause of this bias.
Algorithmic bias	Introduced during algorithmic development when the algorithm becomes skewed in favour of or against certain diagnostic features
Sampling bias	Bias introduced by non-random sampling strategies leading to biased conclusions e.g. erroneous diagnosis of a complete pathological response to neoadjuvant chemotherapy with inadequate sampling of the tumour bed
Measurement bias	Introduced by inaccuracies in the diagnostic tests
Labelling bias	Refers to bias in the assignment of disease labels or classifications. Many subjective areas of pathology are susceptible to this bias, including assessment of the degree of pleomorphism in grading systems or the assessment of atypia in breast biopsies.
Prejudice bias	Arises from preconceptions about certain pathologies or disease groups, such as stereotypical judgements about the likelihood of a certain patient demographic to harbour a particular pathology
Environmental bias	Bias from environmental factors which influence the prevalence of disease and disease outcomes in certain locations. These can be different in urban vs rural settings.
Interaction bias	Introduced by complex interactions between comorbidities, influencing the diagnosis and prediction of the algorithm
Feedback loop bias	When a biased diagnostic decision is used to make further decisions, the effect of the bias is amplified.
Representation bias	Caused by inadequate representation of diverse populations in the data. This frequently manifests with under-representation of ethnic minorities.
Temporal bias	Changes in disease prevalence or diagnostic criteria not accounted for in the historical data included in the dataset
Transfer bias	Arises due to differences in diagnostic practices between central teaching hospitals and community hospitals
Confirmation bias	Introduced when pre-existing beliefs influence the pathologist's interpretation of the case, leading to a failure to consider alternative perspectives or contradictory information.

11.8 ETHICAL AND MEDICOLEGAL CONSIDERATIONS

The pillars of medical ethics are respect for autonomy, beneficence, non-maleficence, justice, and accountability. These pillars place clear responsibilities on the developers and users of AI. Patients must have sufficient control over their interactions with AI. They have a right to know that AI is being used in their diagnosis, how it will be used, and what the benefits and risks are. They have the right to set limits on the use of AI (e.g. requiring that a pathologist also reviews the case) and have the right to refuse to allow AI to be used in their diagnosis. (See also Chapter 2.)

AI developers and users must do all in their power to maximise the benefits of models they develop while minimising the risks and preventing harm. They must also promote equity irrespective of factors such as race, gender, socioeconomic status, or medical condition. They have a responsibility to be accountable, ensuring that the design and implementation of AI are ethical, transparent, and reliable. Potential biases are listed in Table 11.4.

There are grey areas in the use of AI. If the pathologist disagrees with the AI, which should be believed?

There is no single answer to this question. An AI may do better than the pathologist in quantifying a biomarker. However, the pathologist may spot that the AI has misdiagnosed a rare entity. If the pathologist has the final responsibility for the report, then it is the pathologist's call to make.

There is also the question of the medicolegal responsibility for errors resulting from the use of AI. If the pathologist is providing an independent assessment of the case and takes final responsibility for the report, responsibility will continue to sit with the reporting pathologist. However, as AI is increasingly relied on, and particularly when it is trusted to report unsupervised, a greater degree of responsibility must surely be borne by the developers of the AI. The law will be clarified by the test cases which emerge from the deployment of AI in healthcare. There is currently no law which provides for an AI itself to be held liable for medical outcomes.

From a legal perspective, AI poses unique challenges. What is the standard of care for pathologists using AI, which has a degree of autonomy not seen with other medical devices? What information needs to be shared with patients to ensure that they have given informed consent? How does the principle of strict liability apply, where the defendant is held legally responsible for the harm caused in the absence of a finding of fault or negligence? Similarly for vicarious liability, where the principal (the employer) is held liable? Would this discourage the use of AI? Product liability imposes a continuous duty on the manufacturer to warn consumers or the intermediary to the consumers of dangers arising from the use of the product. However, the black-box nature of AI may make it difficult to identify all of the risks inherent in a particular algorithm and to trace the origins of any faults which are detected. Where does the liability fall for effects of digital weather or algorithmic drift?

There is international variation in the legal principles involved. The European Union has passed the Artificial Intelligence Act, which essentially establishes the principle that the operators and developers of AI can be held liable for injuries resulting from the use of AI, and that such liability does not require a finding of fault or negligence. In other words, the plaintiffs under this legislation do not need to prove negligence on the part of the operator or developer, just that harm occurred because of the use of the AI. The USA and Canada do not, at the time of writing, have established legal frameworks governing AI. AI algorithms are likely to be treated and regulated as medical devices, subjecting them to a high level of regulatory scrutiny. (See also Chapter 4.)

11.9 THE FUTURE: WILL AI REPLACE PATHOLOGISTS?

This is a much-asked question. At its present level of performance, it is not advisable for an AI algorithm to be allowed to diagnose cases or generate reports unsupervised by a pathologist, and the current regulatory approvals do not permit this. It is therefore not a panacea for workforce crises in histopathology. However, the ability to use AI will become an essential skill for histopathologists. Pathologists will need to be able to use, prompt, and critically appraise AI and keep pace with the ethical and medicolegal issues it raises.

The performance of AIs will continue to develop and improve, and a threshold will be reached at which the pathology community has sufficient confidence in the technology to consider whether some cases could safely be reported by AI alone. It is inevitable that AI will reach this threshold, and as the technology is developing at exponential speed, this moment is not far away. The question then becomes how to best utilise this diagnostic capability. The regulatory, ethical, and medicolegal frameworks governing AI will need to evolve to be able to deal with the real-world consequences of this emergence.

The first principle that must be observed is that the human pathology workforce must never be allowed to become deskilled in histopathology as a result of AI, no matter how advanced the AI becomes. Histological knowledge must be preserved and passed onto future generations. This is because, ultimately, there will always be a need for a considered, empathic, compassionate, and common-sense opinion, and this remains the domain of the pathologist for the foreseeable future. Strong AI with a theory of mind would shift the calculus on this somewhat, but there is a strong argument to be made that any knowledge that pertains to human healing must be preserved in human hands as well as the AI. This will be of particular importance for difficult cases, where the multidisciplinary discussion is vital. It provides an essential failsafe against the failure or loss of the technology. It also keeps the options of the healthcare systems of the future open. Who knows what unforeseeable challenges may require them to rely more heavily on the human workforce?

The first uses of AI for independent reporting are likely to be to report samples such as endoscopic gastrointestinal biopsies, which are received in huge numbers and many of which are either normal or show benign easily diagnosed features. Even in this scenario, pathologists should continue seeing enough of these cases to maintain their skills. Extending the unsupervised use of AI beyond such uses will need to be done slowly and with careful consideration to the consequences. The ideal pathology department of the future will likely consist of AI-literate pathologists using AI to aid their work and trusting it to unburden them from the more mundane aspects of their job. Pathologists will need to integrate and synthesise larger amounts of more complex information into reports. Attendance at multidisciplinary team meetings will continue, and dissection and autopsy will continue to be tasks performed by pathologists. However, the focus of microscopy reporting will shift and change.

What of the more distant future? Perhaps AI will one day become self-aware. Futurists debate whether this will ever happen. Here is a question that may still be in the domain of science fiction to ask, but worth considering. What happens if the self-aware AI does not want to be a pathologist? In that scenario, pathologists will be right back where they started and will be thankful that they preserved their skills. The practice of pathology itself may well have evolved beyond all recognition by that point, but that is beyond the scope of this chapter to explore.

11.10 CONCLUSION

The use of AI in the setting of histopathological diagnosis is an exciting and important use of the technology. The technology is still in its infancy, particularly with regard to its clinical deployment, but is developing at an exponential rate. The impact of the technology on the delivery of pathology services is likely to be profound, and it raises unique challenges for the infrastructure, regulation, and medicolegal and ethical responsibility of providers of diagnostic services.

Yet for all the complexity that is emerging in this brave new world, the histological slide stained with haematoxylin and eosin remains the keystone of histopathology diagnosis, almost 150 years since it was first described. Simplicity at the heart of complexity. Consistency amid extraordinary transformation: a meeting of the old and the new.

11.11 EDITORS' COMMENTS

Similarities between different services, especially those relying on digitally produced images, have been highlighted here in histopathology practice and demonstrate remarkable alignment with the likes of radiology. As well, considerations of how machines learn, what they learn on, and what the ethical and medicolegal components are to ponder and work towards with surety of digital data safety are also remarkably similar in form and in terms of how they must be negotiated for patient and service safety. It is clear too that wider roles for AI are possible when huge amounts of information are being handled and service demand continues to rise, especially considering the phenomena of digital weather and algorithmic drift and the challenges this can create. Problems of deployment, also outlined in Chapter 10, and those challenges termed 'professional hesitancy' align with pathology, and if not dealt with appropriately, may result in significant delay in system development for the good of service and, more importantly the recipient, i.e. patient and referring practitioner.

REFERENCES

1. Iwuajoku, V., Ekici, K., Haas, A. et al. (2025) An Equivalency and Efficiency Study for One Year Digital Pathology for Clinical Routine Diagnostics in an Accredited Tertiary Academic Center. Virchows Arch. doi: 10.1007/s00428-025-04043-3. Epub ahead of print.
2. Hanna, M.G., Reuter, V.E., Samboy, J. et al. (2019) Implementation of Digital Pathology Offers Clinical and Operational Increase in Efficiency and Cost Savings. Arch Pathol Lab Med. 143(12):1545–1555. doi: 10.5858/arpa.2018-0514-OA. Epub 2019 Jun 11.
3. Huang, W., Randhawa, R., Jain, P. et al. (2021) Development and Validation of an Artificial Intelligence-Powered Platform for Prostate Cancer Grading and Quantification. JAMA Netw Open. 4(11):e2132554. doi: 10.1001/jamanetworkopen.2021.32554.
4. Bulten, W., Balkenhol, M., Belinga, J.A. et al. (2021) Artificial Intelligence Assistance Significantly Improves Gleason Grading of Prostate Biopsies by Pathologists. Mod Pathol. 34(3):660–671. doi: 10.1038/s41379-020-0640-y. Epub 2020 Aug 5.
5. Besse, P., Castets-Renard, C., Garivier, A. et al. (2018). Can Everyday AI Be Ethical? Machine Learning Algorithm Fairness (English Version). doi: 10.13140/RG.2.2.22973.31207.
6. Andersen, E.S., Birk-Korch, J.B., Hansen, R.S. et al. (2024) Monitoring Performance of Clinical Artificial Intelligence in Health Care: A Scoping Review. JBI Evid Synth. 22(12):2423–2446. doi: 10.11124/JBIES-24-00042.
7. Yampolskiy, R.V. (2025) On Monitorability of AI. AI Ethics. 5:689–707. doi: 10.1007/s43681-024-00420-x.
8. Thomas, A., Blidisel, A., Cosmin, P. et al. (2024, August 1). Wisecubeai/Pythia: Open Source AI Hallucination Monitoring. GitHub. https://github.com/wisecubeai/pythia/
9. Hamilton, P.W., Wang, Y., Boyd, C. et al. (2015) Automated Tumor Analysis for Molecular Profiling in Lung Cancer. Oncotarget. 6(29):27938–27952. doi: 10.18632/oncotarget.4391.
10. van Kempen, S., Gerritsen, W.J.G., Nguyen, T.Q. et al. (2025). Monitoring Immunohistochemical Staining Variations by Artificial Intelligence on Standardized Controls. Lab Investig, 105(5), Article104105. doi: 10.1016/j.labinv.2025.104105.
11. Hartage, R., Li, A.C., Hammond, S. et al. (2020) A Validation Study of Human Epidermal Growth Factor Receptor 2 Immunohistochemistry Digital Imaging Analysis and Its Correlation With Human Epidermal Growth Factor Receptor 2 Fluorescence *In Situ* Hybridization Results in Breast Carcinoma. J Pathol Inform. 11:2. doi: 10.4103/jpi.jpi_52_19.
12. White, C.D., Chetty, R., Weldon, J. et al. (2025) A Deep Learning Approach to Case Prioritisation of Colorectal Biopsies. Histopathology. 86(3):373–384. doi: 10.1111/his.15331.
13. Matthews, G.A., McGenity, C., Bansal, D. et al. (2024) Public Evidence on AI Products for Digital Pathology. NPJ Digit Med. 7. doi: 10.1038/s41746-024-01294-3.
14. McGenity, C., Clarke, E.L., Jennings, C. et al. (2024) Artificial Intelligence in Digital Pathology: A Systematic Review and Meta-Analysis of Diagnostic Test Accuracy. NPJ Digit Med. 7(1):114. doi: 10.1038/s41746-024-01106-8.
15. Lu, M.Y., Chen, B., Williamson, D.F.K. et al. (2024) A Multimodal Generative AI Copilot for Human Pathology. Nature. 634(8033):466–473. doi: 10.1038/s41586-024-07618-3 Epub 2024 Jun 12.
16. Vos, S., Hebeda, K., Milota, M. et al. (2025) Making Pathologists Ready for the New Artificial Intelligence Era: Changes in Required Competencies. Modern Pathology, 38(2):100657. doi: 10.1016/j.modpat.2024.100657.
17. Evans, H. and Snead, D. (2024) Understanding the Errors Made by Artificial Intelligence Algorithms in Histopathology in Terms of Patient Impact. NPJ Digit Med. 7(1):89. doi: 10.1038/s41746-024-01093-w.

12 AI in Ophthalmology

Vanessa Otti, Mertcan Sevgi, Rohan Misra, and Pearse Keane

12.1 INTRODUCTION

Artificial Intelligence (AI) is increasingly recognised as a valuable tool in healthcare, and ophthalmology presents a compelling field for its application [1]. This is largely due to the availability of detailed ocular data from imaging modalities such as fundus photographs and optical coherence tomography (OCT).

Ophthalmology is often one of the busiest outpatient specialties in high-income healthcare systems. For example, it accounts for around 10% of the National Health Service waitlist in the United Kingdom [2]. Given these patient volumes, there is a strong impetus to implement efficient models of care. In 2018, the field achieved a milestone when the United States Food and Drug Administration (FDA) permitted the marketing of the first fully autonomous AI system for detecting diabetic retinopathy (DR) without requiring a specialist's confirmation [3].

Global epidemiology data indicate that more than one billion people experience vision impairment [4]. Cataracts and refractive errors remain leading causes of blindness, particularly in adults over 50, while chronic conditions such as diabetic retinopathy, glaucoma, and age-related macular degeneration are becoming more prevalent because of demographic shifts [5–7]. In children, high myopia and retinopathy of prematurity are growing areas of concern [5, 8].

As AI research advances, retinal diseases continue to be a focal point, reflecting both clinical need and the availability of robust imaging datasets [9, 10]. At the same time, there is emerging work in areas like cataracts and corneal opacities, which are significant causes of vision impairment in low- and middle-income countries [11–13]. Challenges remain regarding equitable access to high-quality datasets, and many underserved regions lack the resources to develop or deploy AI solutions [14, 15].

Moving from proof of concept to real-world deployment involves addressing technical, logistical, and financial considerations. This chapter highlights experiences from settings such as Thailand, where AI is being integrated into clinical workflows, and the United States, where reimbursement structures for autonomous AI remain complex. These examples illustrate the multifaceted challenges of implementing AI at scale.

Finally, the chapter explores recent advances in ophthalmic AI, including the emergence of foundation models (FMs). An example is RETFound, which is trained on large collections of fundus and OCT images. Ongoing efforts aim to harness the capabilities of large language models (LLMs) and large multimodal models (LMMs) in ophthalmic care, possibly integrating imaging, textual data, and clinical decision support in the future.

In summary, this chapter shows how the abundant imaging data in ophthalmology underpins AI development. It addresses the epidemiological context, examines implementation case studies, and discusses how foundation models are shaping the trajectory of AI in this field.

12.2 OVERVIEW OF OPHTHALMOLOGICAL DATA

12.2.1 Types of Data in Ophthalmology

Ophthalmology is a data-rich medical field, leveraging diverse data types to diagnose, monitor, and treat a wide range of eye diseases. These data types include imaging, clinical records, and genetic information. While all three categories are essential, imaging data has emerged as the primary focus of AI research in ophthalmology.

12.2.2 The Central Role of Imaging Data in AI Research

Imaging data is the cornerstone of ophthalmic AI research, as it provides a direct window into the structural and functional changes associated with eye diseases. A 2021 study published in *The Lancet* by Khan et al. surveyed global publicly available imaging datasets for ophthalmology, identifying 94 datasets comprising over 500,000 images [15]. The study highlighted the diversity of imaging modalities used in ophthalmology, each tailored to specific diagnostic needs and anatomical regions of the eye. Table 12.1 summarises the key imaging modalities identified in the study, along with their applications and the parts of the eye they examine.

The *Lancet* study underscores the critical role of imaging data in advancing ophthalmic AI research. These datasets enable the development of AI models capable of detecting and diagnosing eye diseases with high accuracy, often matching or exceeding the performance of human experts.

DOI: 10.1201/9781032709956-12

Table 12.1 Imaging Modalities, Applications, and Area of Examination

Imaging Modality	Description	Part of the Eye Examined
Retinal Fundus Photographs	Captures two-dimensional images of the retina, commonly used for diagnosing diabetic retinopathy, AMD, and glaucoma.	Retina
Ultra-Wide Field Fundus Photographs	Captures a larger field of view of the retina compared to standard fundus photography, aiding in diagnosing peripheral retinal pathologies like retinal tears or detachments.	Retina
Fundus Autofluorescence (FAF)	A non-invasive imaging technique that detects autofluorescence emitted by lipofuscin in the retinal pigment epithelium, useful for diagnosing conditions like AMD or inherited retinal diseases.	Retina
OCT	High-resolution, cross-sectional imaging technique that provides detailed views of the retina's layers, vital for diagnosing and monitoring AMD and macular oedema.	Retina
OCT Angiography	Extension of OCT that visualises retinal vasculature, offering insights into diseases affecting blood vessels like diabetic retinopathy and retinal vein occlusion.	Retina
Anterior Segment OCT	Provides detailed imaging of the anterior structures, including the cornea, iris, and angle, to assess conditions like keratoconus or angle-closure glaucoma.	Anterior Segment
External Eye Photographs	Standard clinical photographs of the external structures of the eye, such as eyelids, conjunctiva, and cornea.	External
In Vivo Confocal Microscopy	High-resolution imaging for microscopic examination of living tissue, particularly the cornea, aiding in diagnosing infections, dystrophies, or nerve damage.	Cornea
Scanning Laser Ophthalmoscopy (SLO)	Uses a laser to scan the retina and create detailed, high-contrast images of the retinal layers, often combined with OCT for comprehensive retinal pathology analysis.	Retina
Adaptive Optics-Scanning Laser Ophthalmoscopy	Advanced version of SLO using adaptive optics for ultra-high-resolution images of the retina, enabling visualisation of individual photoreceptor cells and capillaries.	Retina
Fluorescein Angiography (FA)	Involves injecting fluorescein dye into the bloodstream to visualise retinal blood vessels, detecting leakage, blockage, or abnormal growth in diseases like DR or AMD.	Retina
Indocyanine Green Angiography (ICGA)	Imaging technique that uses indocyanine green dye to visualise the choroidal circulation, aiding in diagnosing conditions like polypoidal choroidal vasculopathy or central serous chorioretinopathy.	Retina and Choroid
Slit Lamp Photographs	Detailed images of the anterior segment, including the cornea, iris, lens, and anterior chamber.	Anterior Segment
Phase Contrast Microscopy	Technique to visualise transparent or colourless structures, studying the morphology of cells in the cornea or other transparent eye tissues.	Cornea
Specular Microscopy	Non-invasive imaging to examine the corneal endothelium, providing details about cell shape, size, and density, crucial for diseases like Fuchs' dystrophy.	Cornea
Preocular Tear Film Photograph	Focuses on the tear film coating the eye's surface, assessing stability and distribution for conditions like dry eye syndrome.	Tear Film/External
Videos	Used to record dynamic processes, such as eye movements in strabismus evaluation, blinking patterns, or fluorescein dye flow during angiography.	External and Dynamic Eye Processes

CASE STUDY

INSIGHT- WORLD'S LARGEST OPHTHALMIC BIO-RESOURCE

The transformative potential of large-scale imaging datasets is exemplified by the INSIGHT bio-resource, the world's largest ophthalmic dataset [16]. Established in 2015 through a collaboration between Moorfields Eye Hospital and Google DeepMind, INSIGHT contains over 35 million eye images linked to clinical data. This resource has been instrumental in driving breakthroughs in ophthalmic AI. For instance, in 2018, a study published in *Nature* demonstrated that an AI system trained on data that would later form the basis of the INSIGHT health data research pipeline could recommend the correct referral decision for over 50 eye diseases with 94% accuracy, matching the performance of world-leading eye experts [17]. More recently, in 2023, researchers at Moorfields Eye Hospital and the UCL Institute of Ophthalmology developed the world's first ophthalmology foundation model using INSIGHT data, further highlighting the power of large-scale imaging datasets in training revolutionary AI models.

12.2.3 Clinical and Genetic Data: Complementary Roles

While imaging data dominate AI research in ophthalmology, clinical and genetic data also play vital roles. Clinical data, often stored in electronic health records (EHRs), includes patient history, visual acuity measurements, intraocular pressure readings, and treatment details. These data provide context for imaging findings and enable longitudinal tracking of disease progression and treatment outcomes. Patient-reported outcomes, such as symptoms and quality-of-life assessments, further enrich clinical data by capturing the patient's perspective.

Genetic data are increasingly important, particularly for inherited retinal diseases like retinitis pigmentosa and Leber's congenital amaurosis. Advances in genome-wide association studies (GWAS) and whole-genome sequencing are uncovering genetic risk factors for common diseases like age-related macular degeneration (AMD) and glaucoma. This knowledge paves the way for personalised treatment approaches, where genetic information complements imaging and clinical data to guide therapeutic decisions.

12.2.4 Challenges in Data Collection, Annotation, and Dataset Limitations

Despite the wealth of data available, challenges remain in integrating and standardising diverse data types for AI applications. These challenges, along with the ethical and technical considerations of using large-scale datasets like INSIGHT, will be explored in this section.

12.2.5 Data Collection

The quality and accessibility of ophthalmic data vary significantly across institutions and geographic regions, presenting major challenges for the development of AI systems tailored to diverse global populations. One prominent issue is data accessibility. While some open-access datasets are available, they are often underutilised due to a lack of awareness and discoverability. This limited accessibility can result in biased AI models trained on datasets that fail to adequately represent the diversity of real-world populations.

Representation is another critical challenge. Many datasets lack sufficient samples from underrepresented groups and specific eye diseases. For example, models trained predominantly on data from one demographic may exhibit reduced performance when applied to populations with differing genetic, environmental, or healthcare characteristics. Regional differences in data also reflect varying disease prevalences and health priorities, further complicating efforts to create globally generalisable AI systems. Initiatives such as 'STANDING Together' provide recommendations to tackle bias and promote transparency in health data [18, 19].

In ophthalmology, these issues are exacerbated by disparities in healthcare infrastructure. Low-income regions often lack access to advanced imaging devices, and even when such equipment is available, data collection and systematic integration into usable datasets remain inconsistent. The *Lancet* study [15] highlighted this disparity, revealing that 172 countries – representing 45% of the world's population – do not have any publicly available ophthalmic datasets. This phenomenon, termed health data poverty, creates substantial barriers to leveraging AI for healthcare improvement, particularly in underprivileged areas.

12.2.6 Data Annotation

The quality and performance of AI models hinge on well-annotated datasets, which enable better generalisation and reliability. However, annotating ophthalmic data is uniquely challenging due to its complexity and the specialised expertise required. Tasks such as grading retinal images for diabetic retinopathy or interpreting OCT scans for macular disease often necessitate trained ophthalmologists or retinal specialists. This makes the process both costly and time-consuming.

Inter- and intra-observer variability further complicates the annotation process, as even experienced specialists may disagree on grading or diagnosis. The labour-intensive nature of manual annotation and the current scarcity of well-annotated large datasets present significant barriers to the development of robust AI systems in ophthalmology. One way to mitigate the challenges of data annotation is the development of central reading centres such as MEH (Moorfields Eye Hospital), Stanford and Singapore to help standardise objective grading of anonymised data by trained graders. This can help produce more accurate and unbiased data labels [20].

12.2.7 Synthetic Data and Its Importance

Synthetic data, artificially generated to mimic the statistical properties of real datasets, offer a promising solution to many of these challenges. Techniques such as generative adversarial networks (GANs) and diffusion models can create synthetic retinal images or OCT scans, supplementing real-world datasets and addressing issues of data scarcity, health data poverty, and privacy.

The advantages of synthetic data are manifold:

- Enhanced dataset volume and diversity: Synthetic data expand training datasets without requiring the collection of new real-world samples, making them especially valuable in low-resource settings.

- Bias mitigation: By generating data that represent under-represented populations or rare conditions, synthetic datasets can help counter biases present in existing data.

- Privacy preservation: Synthetic data do not contain identifiable personal health information, thus maintaining patient confidentiality while enabling data sharing and collaboration.

By enabling the creation of large, diverse datasets, synthetic data play a pivotal role in building more robust and generalisable AI models. This is particularly impactful in ophthalmology, where its use can address disparities and improve outcomes for underserved populations globally.

12.3 AI APPLICATIONS IN OPHTHALMOLOGY

12.3.1 Focus of AI Research in Ophthalmology

AI research is advancing across various ophthalmic specialties, with a predominant focus on retinal diseases such as diabetic retinopathy, age-related macular degeneration, and glaucoma [9, 10]. This emphasis is understandable, given the rising prevalence of chronic retinal conditions driven by ageing populations and the global increase in chronic diseases. However, there is also promising AI research targeting other major causes of vision impairment, such as cataracts and corneal opacities, reflecting efforts to address the diverse and evolving needs of populations worldwide.

AI applications in ophthalmology primarily aim to enhance the screening, diagnosis, treatment, and prognosis of eye diseases. For example, AI-based screening tools are being developed to enable early detection and intervention, which are particularly critical for conditions like DR, AMD, and glaucoma, where timely treatment can significantly improve outcomes. Table 12.1 summarises key examples of AI applications in this field. By improving diagnostic accuracy and efficiency, AI has the potential to reduce workloads, minimise misdiagnosis rates, and make eye care more accessible. While AI is not intended to replace ophthalmologists, it serves as a powerful tool to augment their capabilities, ultimately enhancing patient care on a global scale.

12.3.2 Screening and Diagnosis

Currently, the FDA has cleared three algorithms for clinical use: IDx-DR, EyeArt, and AEYE, while the EU has approved additional systems, such as Retmarker, Google's DR detection tool (ARDA), and the Singapore Eye Lesion Analyzer (SELENA) [21]. All these products analyse fundus photography, with a focus on detecting diabetic eye disease [22]. However we are also seeing the emergence of multi-class classifiers such as Retinalzye, which detect multiple diseases such as DR, AMD, and glaucoma. In the case of DR, algorithms carry out specific classification tasks to grade the severity from mild to severe, which can be determined by location and frequency of microaneurysms and

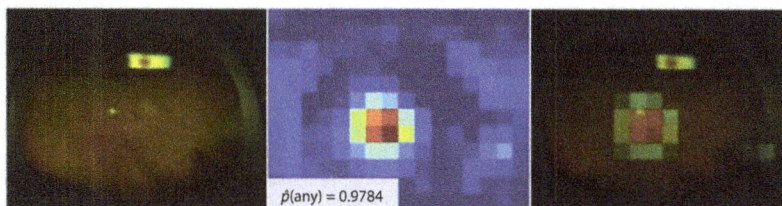

Age: 57 | Sex: M | Dataset labels: Gla
MH:0.055(0)| RP:0.048(0)| AMD:0.039(0)| RVO:0.103(0)| RD:0.053(0)| Gla:0.968(1)| DR:0.079(0)| any:0.978(1)

(a) An example of the model successfully ignoring a reflection artefact and instead attending to the optic disc to correctly detect that the retina is diseased and that the disease in particular is Glaucoma ($\hat{p}(Gla)$ = 0.968).

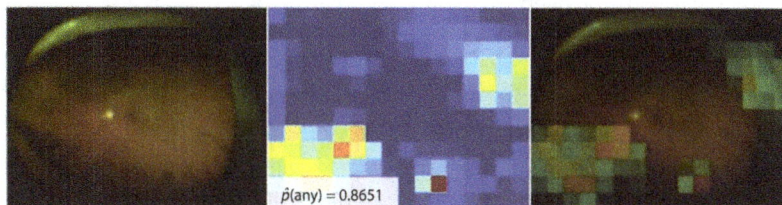

Age: 68 | Sex: M | Dataset labels: Healthy
MH:0.075(0)| RP:0.050(0)| AMD:0.060(0)| RVO:0.080(0)| RD:0.059(0)| Gla:0.231(0)| DR:0.616(0)| any:0.865(0)

(b) An example of the model focusing on artefacts, particularly eyelash artefacts, in the periphery and falsely predicting a high probability of being diseased. The predicted probability of DR is highest ($\hat{p}(DR)$ = 0.616) which could indicate that the model confuses the eyelash artefacts for haemorrhages or microaneurysms. There is also a small bright spot south-west of the optic disc which receives attention and might be interpreted as an exudate.

Figure 12.1 This figure illustrates how AI systems can both succeed and fail in interpreting retinal images. In some cases, the model accurately focuses on clinically relevant features to make the correct diagnosis (a). In others, it is misled by image artefacts, highlighting the importance of model explainability and the need for human oversight in clinical settings (b). Used with permission from Dr Justin Engelmann [24] (Engelmann et al., 2022).

other features in the retina. We are also seeing an emergence of regulated AI that analyses other modalities such as OCT with Retinsight [23]. Retinsight offers two products, fluid monitor and GA monitor. Fluid monitor can visualise retinal fluid types and location, as well as monitor disease progression in neovascular AMD. GA monitor uses segmentation to identify and map progression of GA which is a late form of AMD leading to retinal cell death and ultimately vision loss. Figure 12.1 demonstrates how models may operate to be successful or fail to reject artefacts.

For diabetic eye disease, the aim is screening in the community, outside the secondary and tertiary care setting [25] (Liu et al., 2024) and allowing healthcare providers to screen and refer to secondary care when DR is detected. On a broader scale, national diabetic eye screening programmes (DESPs) exist in only nine high-income countries (HICs), and two upper middle-income countries (MICs) have implemented similar programmes [26]. There is a significant infrastructure requirement for DESPs, and thus one potential solution to lower the barrier to entry is mobile device-based DR screening. The EyeNuk system, which uses the EyeArt software, demonstrated over 95% sensitivity when analysing fundus images captured by smartphones. In addition, SELENA has been trialled for use in Zambia, where the ratio of ophthalmologists to population is 3:1 million (compared to 80:1 million in high-income countries) [27]. It was shown to be a viable and powerful screening tool in developing countries such as Zambia, with future work aiming to increase scope and safe implementation.

AI has also emerged as a transformative tool in the diagnosis and screening of glaucoma. Glaucoma, a leading cause of irreversible blindness worldwide, often goes undiagnosed due to the complexity of its diagnostic process and the reliance on subjective assessments by healthcare providers. In Australia, studies have highlighted the high prevalence of undiagnosed glaucoma, with one population-based study in Victoria revealing that 63% of glaucoma cases were undetected [28]. AI-based tools have achieved sensitivity and specificity rates of up to 96% and 98%, respectively, in identifying glaucomatous optic neuropathy (GON) from fundus images. These algorithms can standardise the interpretation of optic nerve head (ONH) and retinal nerve fibre layer (RNFL) changes, reducing inter-observer variability and improving diagnostic consistency. In Australia, the integration of AI into primary eye care settings has shown promise, with studies indicating that AI-assisted screening models could be cost-effective compared to traditional methods [28].

Other studies have explored the use of AI to diagnose and grade ocular surface diseases and conditions affecting the anterior segment [13]. An exciting use case involves using deep learning (DL) models to classify and assess the severity of cataracts. Traditionally diagnosed and graded subjectively, cataract assessment stands to benefit from AI's ability to provide more objective, standardised criteria. Current grading systems, like the Lens Opacities Classification and Wisconsin Grading System, can be inconsistent [29]. Cataract detection methods range from slit-lamp and external eye photos, including smartphone images, to predictions from fundus photographs [30, 12].

There is also research using handheld cameras to screen for conditions like pterygium [31, 32]. Another interesting use of smartphones is taking photorefractive images in paediatric patients to predict their refractive state by using deep-learning. Chun et al. managed to achieve an accuracy of 81.6%, which shows potential in AI in detecting amblyopia in children, which can lead to long-standing visual impairment if not screened for. These developments offer flexible, affordable solutions for eye care, making it possible to reach patients in remote or underserved regions with limited resources.

12.3.3 Future Directions: Oculomics

There is growing evidence that ocular biomarkers can reveal insights into systemic diseases. [33]. This emerging field is referred to as 'oculomics'. Retinal imaging leads this area of research; however, corneal and anterior segment imaging, along with the analysis of tear fluid, is being used to explore potential connections between ocular biomarkers and systemic diseases. The AlzEye project demonstrates how large-scale data linkage can accelerate these discoveries by combining extensive retinal imaging resources with detailed health records. Figure 12.2 illustrates the process that is supported by the cases discussed below.

CASE STUDY

AlzEye: Building a Large Scale 'Oculomics' Resource

LINKING SYSTEMIC HEALTH RECORDS WITH RETINAL IMAGING

AlzEye is based at Moorfields Eye Hospital in London. It integrates more than six million retinal images from over 350,000 patients with national hospital records, including data on myocardial infarction, stroke, and dementia [35].

Emerging Insights

Although AlzEye includes many potential applications, its main focus is on cardiovascular and neurodegenerative diseases [35]. For example, retinal features of Parkinson's disease could be detected many years before its classic clinical presentation [36]. By drawing on large-scale linked data, AlzEye aims to uncover early biomarkers of these and other systemic conditions, thereby supporting more proactive and preventive approaches to care.

Future Directions

Researchers plan to expand AlzEye's scope by increasing the size of the dataset with additional retinal images, a broader range of systemic health information and newer imaging modalities. This approach will also be adapted for use in community settings, rather than relying solely on hospital-based data [37]. These developments can drive progress in preventive medicine.

Treatment and Prognostication

Besides diagnostics, there is growing research in treatment planning and disease prognosis. In ophthalmic surgery, AI can predict the most appropriate surgical approach based on a patient's unique anatomical features [38]. This is done for eyelid and blepharoplasty with the development of AI-generated 3D models to help surgeons visualise the optimal surgical plan for the best post-operative outcomes [29]. In addition, for keratoplasty, AI models can also predict and anticipate potential complications after surgery, such as predicting the need for rebubbling after Descemet's

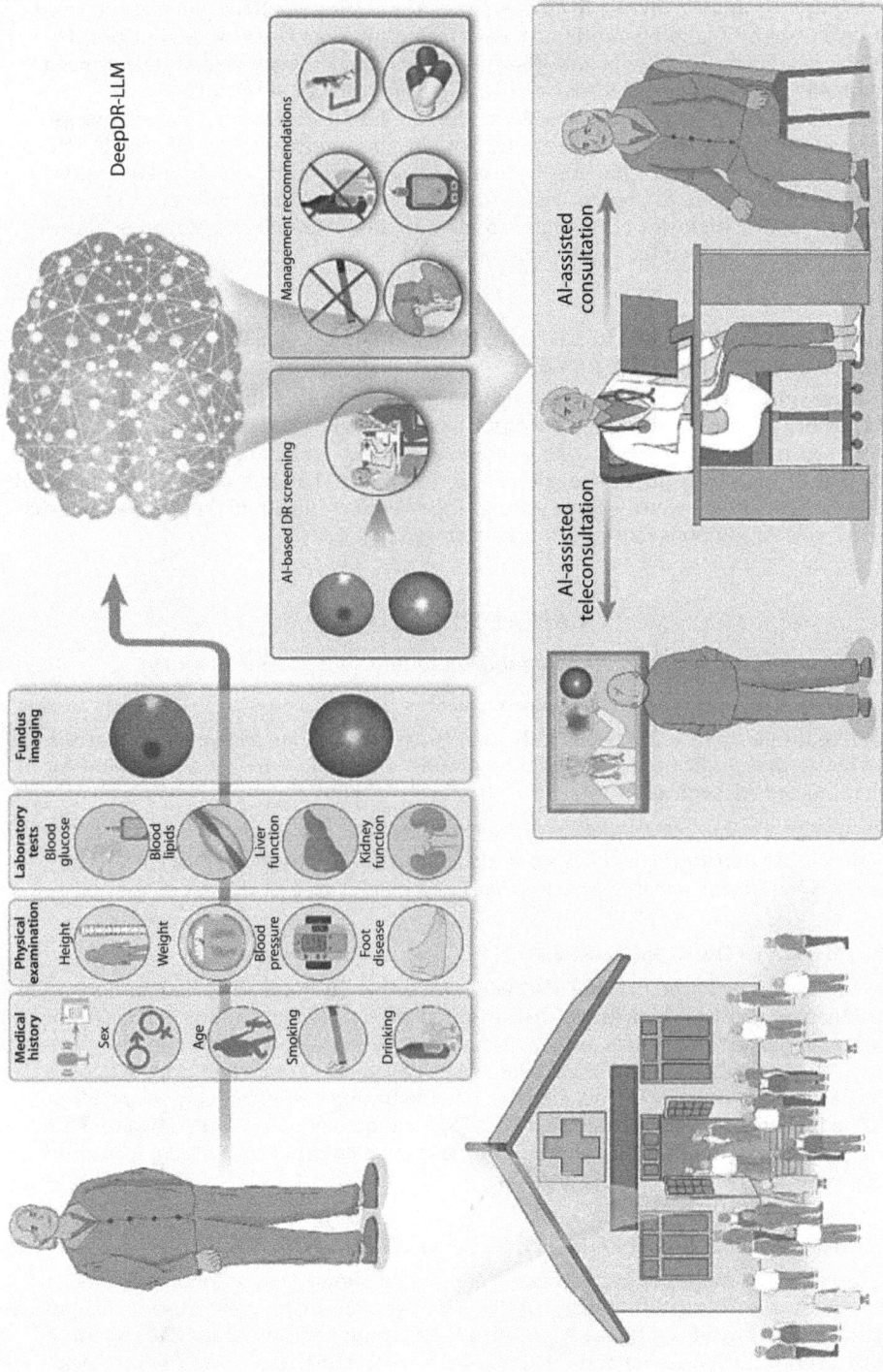

Figure 12.2 Adaptation of the future of clinical integration of the DeepDR-LLM system (multi-modal systems) for the future of primary diabetes care. Patients with diabetes first undergo comprehensive evaluations, including medical history-taking (potentially augmented by automated voice-to-text technology), physical examinations, laboratory assessments, and fundus imaging. Subsequently, the DeepDR-LLM system processes this clinical data to provide concurrent DR screening results and personalised management recommendations for clinicians. Armed with these AI-derived insights, clinicians then deliver treatment guidance and health education to patients, either in person or via teleconsultation [34].

membrane endothelial keratoplasty (DMEK). AI systems can also act as surgical assistants, guiding clinicians through procedures and improving training for ophthalmic surgeons. One example of this is using AI-powered augmented reality (AR) to provide real-time guidance for suture placements to improve surgical precision. Furthermore, AI has the potential to generate personalised treatment plans by analysing multimodal data, including patient history and imaging. For example, AI can predict the number of anti-VEGF injections a patient with wet AMD may need [39], or recommend the most suitable intraocular lens (IOL) for cataract surgery [29].

In addition to predicting treatment plans, AI models are also useful for monitoring disease progression and predicting treatment outcomes. For chronic conditions like DR, AMD, and glaucoma, AI can identify subtle changes in disease status, facilitating timely interventions and adjustments in treatment to prevent vision loss. Another promising application is using AI to identify patients at high risk of rapid progression in conditions like keratoconus, allowing clinicians to prioritise them for closer monitoring [32].

12.4 REAL-WORLD AI FOR DIABETIC RETINOPATHY: TWO CASE STUDIES AND THE CHALLENGES THEY REVEAL

Although AI shows immense promise in detecting and managing DR, bringing these innovations into real-world practice remains challenging. The first case study highlights how the first FDA-cleared autonomous tool secured regulatory approval, reimbursement pathways, and demonstrated health equity benefits. The second, focusing on Google's DR screening in Thailand, reveals the real-world obstacles of deploying AI in a lower-resource setting. Together, they illustrate the diverse considerations needed to create AI solutions that truly work in clinical practice.

CASE STUDY

Autonomous AI for DR: From Regulation to Improving Health Equity

1. REGULATING AI IN OPHTHALMOLOGY (2018)

LumineticsCore (formerly IDx-DR) became the first fully autonomous AI system authorised by the US FDA to detect DR from fundus photographs. This milestone set a precedent for subsequent regulated AI, such as

- *Retinalyze (EU) – Fundus photographs to detect DR, AMD, and glaucoma*
- *Retinsight Fluid Monitor (EU) – OCT segmentation to measure intraretinal fluid*
- *Toku Eyes (EU) – Fundus photos to estimate biological age and cardiovascular risk*

2. PAVING THE WAY FOR REIMBURSEMENT

Regulatory approval is only the first hurdle. As of November 2023, the FDA had authorised over 500 AI-enabled medical devices, yet real-world uptake has lagged. Only a handful of AI solutions, among them tools for coronary artery disease and diabetic retinopathy, have surpassed 10,000 insurance claims in the United States [40]. In this context, LumineticsCore's trajectory is particularly noteworthy: its focus on demonstrating cost-effectiveness and clinical value helped secure a new billing code (CPT 92229) for autonomous DR screening [41]. This reimbursement pathway not only sustains ongoing use but also provides a model for future AI technologies seeking broad clinical adoption.

3. INCREASING ACCESS AND PROMOTING HEALTH EQUITY

Recent evidence from a large integrated healthcare system shows how autonomous AI can measurably boost screening adherence, particularly among historically disadvantaged groups [42]. Compared to sites without AI, those adopting autonomous AI for DR screening saw a greater overall rise in testing and a marked increase in adherence rates among Black/African American patients. Such real-world findings underscore the inclusive potential of well-implemented AI: by making screening more accessible and equitable, it benefits all users and moves healthcare closer to fairness for diverse patient communities.

CASE STUDY

Google's DR Screening in Thailand – Real-World Challenges in Low-Resource Settings

Google's deployment of an AI-based diabetic retinopathy screening tool in Thailand illustrates the complexities of implementing AI in low- and middle-income countries (LMICs) [43]. The project sought to address a shortage of ophthalmologists by introducing a deep learning algorithm for referable DR detection. Although the system showed high accuracy in controlled conditions, several practical hurdles emerged.

KEY CHALLENGES

- *Image quality and environment*: Over 20% of images were deemed ungradable by AI despite being considered acceptable by clinical staff. Limited control over lighting, older fundus cameras, and inconsistent internet connectivity frequently delayed or disrupted the screening process.
- *Workflow integration*: Nurses, already managing heavy patient loads, found the extra steps of uploading images and waiting for AI results added complexity. Internet instability and slow processing times sometimes stalled patient flow, further straining resources.
- *Referral bottlenecks*: Even when the AI system flagged referable DR, travel barriers and limited patient education led to poor follow-up. Nurses were cautious about relying solely on AI-triggered referrals, aware that many patients would struggle to access specialist care.

12.4.1 Lessons Learned

Simply deploying a high-performing AI model is not enough. Contextual factors such as local infrastructure, staffing capacity, and patient adherence are critical. Prospective studies like the ongoing randomised controlled trial (RCT) in Tanzania focus on real-world outcomes, evaluating how immediate AI results and counselling affect follow-up adherence [44]. These insights highlight the ethical imperative to ensure that AI-driven screenings are accompanied by feasible pathways to care, lest they exacerbate rather than mitigate health disparities in resource-limited settings [45].

Within the landscape of large vision models, two key areas of interest are emerging [46]. One involves developing 3D image models that can analyse entire OCT volumes, as current approaches often rely on selected 2D B-scans. Another research direction involves training models on multiple imaging modalities simultaneously, such as OCT, colour fundus photography (CFP), ultrasounds, and slit-lamp images, potentially leading to more comprehensive imaging models.

12.5 FOUNDATION MODELS

The third epoch of AI, characterised by foundation models, represents a fundamentally new approach with distinct applications and scope [47, 48]. Public awareness of this technology has grown significantly thanks to LLMs (see also Table 12.2 for applications). Although medical and ophthalmic uses of these innovations are still in their early stages, we will highlight some of the specific advances currently taking shape in ophthalmology.

RETFound is the first ophthalmology-specific large vision foundation model, trained using self-supervised learning on large sets of unlabelled retinal images [49]. It currently comprises two separate models: one trained on OCT scans and another on CFP, as shown in Figure 12.3. When fine-tuned for downstream tasks, RETFound has been shown to generalise effectively in diagnosis of diseased such as glaucoma and DR; in prognosis of a fellow eye converting to wet-AMD; and in predicting systemic diseases such as heart failure, stroke, myocardial infarction, and Parkinson's disease.

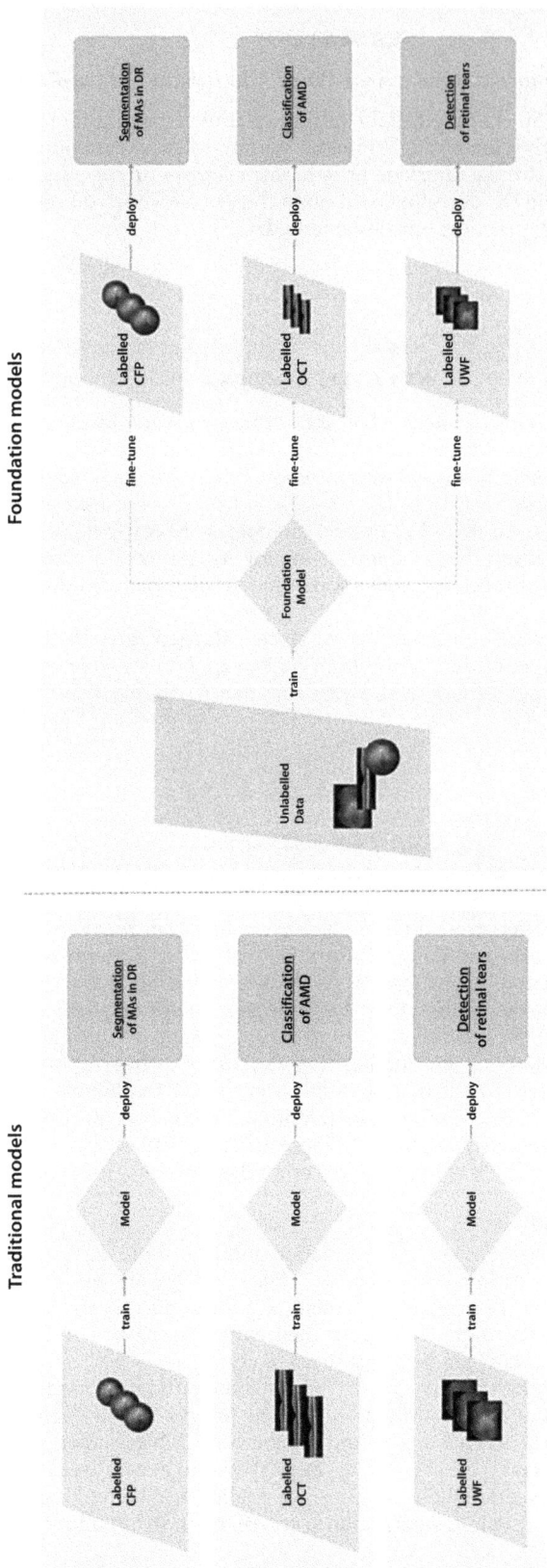

Figure 12.3 This diagram compares how traditional deep learning models and foundation models are trained. Traditional DL models need labelled data and are built for specific tasks. Foundation models, on the other hand, are trained once on large, unlabelled datasets and then fine-tuned for many different tasks, like segmentation, classification, or object detection [46].

Table 12.2 Foundation Models and Their Potential Wider Roles

Model	Task
Large Vision Model RETFound [49].	Ocular disease diagnosis: diabetic retinopathy, glaucoma Ocular disease prognosis: fellow eye converting to wet-AMD Systemic disease prediction: myocardial infarction, heart failure, Parkinson's disease
Large Language Models: ChatGPT [56] Custom GPTs [57]	Ophthalmology specialty exams Q&A Medical education (summaries and teaching of diabetic retinopathy clinical guidelines)
Large Multimodal Models: Med-Gemini [58]	Visual questioning answering for diabetic retinopathy diagnosis and management

In parallel, there has been substantial interest in LLMs. To date, no LLM is regulated in the medical domain [50]. However, various research efforts benchmark these models against medical exam-style questions [51, 52]. Ophthalmology-specific investigations include approaches like AMIE, a patient-facing conversational diagnostic AI. Beyond purely text-based systems, LLMs can be specialised to incorporate images, creating large multimodal models (LMMs) [53, 54]. A notable example is Med-Gemini, which can handle tasks like visual question answering (VQA) using ophthalmic images.

Importantly, developers of these models have introduced evaluation frameworks that consider not only medical correctness but also communication quality and patient-friendliness. While preliminary results are promising, these advances represent early steps toward more generalisable medical AI (GMAI), mirroring how clinicians integrate multiple data sources into their decision-making process [55]. Going forward, it will be essential to conduct clinical trials and address practical considerations for implementation, ensuring that these technologies find meaningful, safe, and effective roles in clinical workflows.

12.6 CONCLUSION

Ophthalmology's wealth of data, from retinal photographs and OCT scans to clinical and genetic records, has positioned the specialty at the forefront of AI innovation. Yet, as this chapter illustrates, a successful transition from proof-of-concept models to tools that truly benefit patients relies on more than data alone. Real-world case studies highlight the realities of implementing AI across different healthcare systems, including regulatory approval, reimbursement pathways, and the need for dedicated infrastructure. Moreover, the concept of 'health data poverty' in many low-resource settings underscores the importance of equitable data sharing and inclusive model development.

Against this backdrop, new directions such as oculomics and foundation models signal a major shift, since ophthalmic imaging can offer insights into both ocular and systemic conditions, potentially reshaping preventive medicine. The emergence of large vision and multimodal models, capable of integrating diverse imaging and textual data, suggests an even broader transformation on the horizon. However, the next phase of progress requires conscientious validation, ethical governance, and context-aware deployment. By addressing these challenges directly, AI can deliver more precise, equitable, and accessible eye care on a global scale.

12.7 EDITORS' COMMENTS

This in-depth chapter gives us great understanding of the role of AI in opthalmic services, particularly screening and surveillance roles for chronic/systemic presentations. As in Chapter 10, an 'off-view' approach could be adopted to contribute more widely than the obvious role that AI was initially conceived to be useful for. The authors have, as in other chapters, identified sources of limitations or bias, areas where care needs to be exercised to ensure the best outcomes are achieved and errors are not in built by not following the basic application/development approaches. In short, it is eminently clear by now that several 'rules' have become apparent in terms of potential pitfalls but also where, through careful application, significant outcomes can be achieved so that care provision is broadened to avoid a post or zipcode lottery situation with respect to service availability. The foundation model discussion has made this clear and is the next exciting potential, building on LLMs in a multimodal approach so that information use is maximised from a test. Consequently, the AI system may detect and highlight more than the obvious role that a test was initially developed for to gain 'more bang for your buck'!

REFERENCES

1. Ting, D. S. W., Pasquale, L. R., Peng, L., et al. (2019). Artificial Intelligence and Deep Learning in Ophthalmology. British Journal of Ophthalmology, 103(2), 167–175.
2. NHS England Digital. (2025). Hospital Outpatient Activity 2023–24. NHS England Digital. https://digital.nhs.uk/data-and-information/publications/statistical/hospital-outpatient-activity/2023-24
3. FDA. (2020, March 24). FDA Permits Marketing of Artificial Intelligence-Based Device to Detect Certain Diabetes-Related Eye Problems. https://www.fda.gov/news-events/press-announcements/fda-permits-marketing-artificial-intelligence-based-device-detect-certain-diabetes-related-eye
4. Bourne, R., Steinmetz, J. D., Flaxman, S., et al. (2021). Trends in Prevalence of Blindness and Distance and Near Vision Impairment Over 30 Years: An Analysis for the Global Burden of Disease Study. The Lancet Global Health, 9(2), e130–e143. https://doi.org/10.1016/S2214-109X(20)30425-3
5. Burton, M. J., Ramke, J., Marques, A. P., et al. (2021). The Lancet Global Health Commission on Global Eye Health: Vision Beyond 2020. Lancet Glob Health, 9(4), e489–e551.
6. Jiang, B., Jiang, C., Li, J., et al. (2023). Trends and Disparities in Disease Burden of Age-Related Macular Degeneration from 1990 to 2019: Results from the Global Burden of Disease Study 2019. Front Public Health, 11, 1138428.
7. Teo, Z. L., Tham, Y.-C., Yu, M., et al. (2021). Global Prevalence of Diabetic Retinopathy and Projection of Burden Through 2045: Systematic Review and Meta-Analysis. Ophthalmology, 128(11), 1580–1591.
8. Wang, D., Duke, R., Chan, R. P., et al. (2019). Retinopathy of Prematurity in Africa: A Systematic Review. Ophthalmic Epidemiology, 26(4), 223–230.
9. Jiang, X., Xie, M., Ma, L., et al. (2023). International Publication Trends in the Application of Artificial Intelligence in Ophthalmology Research: An Updated Bibliometric Analysis. Annals of Translational Medicine, 11(5), 219. https://doi.org/10.21037/atm-22-3773
10. Zhao, J., Lu, Y., Qian, Y., et al. (2022). Emerging Trends and Research Foci in Artificial Intelligence for Retinal Diseases: Bibliometric and Visualization Study. Journal of Medical Internet Research, 24(6), e37532. https://doi.org/10.2196/37532
11. Ting, D. S. J., Foo, V. H., Yang, L. W. Y., et al. (2021). Artificial Intelligence for Anterior Segment Diseases: Emerging Applications in Ophthalmology. British Journal of Ophthalmology, 105(2), 158–168. https://doi.org/10.1136/bjophthalmol-2019-315651
12. Tognetto, D., Giglio, R., Vinciguerra, A. L. et al. (2022). Artificial Intelligence Applications and Cataract Management: A Systematic Review. https://www.surveyophthalmol.com/article/S0039-6257(21)00187-9/fulltext
13. Xu, Z., Xu, J., Shi, C., et al. (2023). Artificial Intelligence for Anterior Segment Diseases: A Review of Potential Developments and Clinical Applications. Ophthalmology and Therapy, 12(3), 1439–1455. https://doi.org/10.1007/s40123-023-00690-4
14. Ibrahim, H., Liu, X., Zariffa, N., et al. (2021). Health Data Poverty: An Assailable Barrier to Equitable Digital Health Care. Lancet Digit Health, 3(4), e260–e265.
15. Khan, S. M., Liu, X., Nath, S., et al. (2021). A Global Review of Publicly Available Datasets for Ophthalmological Imaging: Barriers to Access, Usability, and Generalisability. Lancet Digit Health, 3(1), e51–e66.
16. INSIGHT. (2024). https://www.insight.hdrhub.org/about-insight [Online post]
17. De Fauw, J., Ledsam, J. R., Romera-Paredes, B., et al. (2018). Clinically Applicable Deep Learning for Diagnosis and Referral in Retinal Disease. Nature Medicine, 24(9), 1342–1350. https://doi.org/10.1038/s41591-018-0107-6
18. Alderman, J. E., Palmer, J., Laws, E., et al. (2025a). Tackling Algorithmic Bias and Promoting Transparency in Health Datasets: The STANDING Together Consensus Recommendations. The Lancet Digital Health, 7(1), e64–e88. https://doi.org/10.1016/S2589-7500(24)00224-3
19. Alderman, J. E., Palmer, J., Laws, E., et al. (2025b). Tackling Algorithmic Bias and Promoting Transparency in Health Datasets: The STANDING Together Consensus Recommendations. NEJM AI, 2(1). https://doi.org/10.1056/AIp2401088
20. Tan, C. S., and Sadda, S. R. (2015). The Role of Central Reading Centers—Current Practices and Future Directions. Indian Journal of Ophthalmology, 63(5), 404–405. https://doi.org/10.4103/0301-4738.159866
21. Rajesh, A. E., Davidson, O. Q., Lee, C. S., et al. (2023). Artificial Intelligence and Diabetic Retinopathy: AI Framework, Prospective Studies, Head-to-Head Validation, and Cost- Effectiveness. Diabetes Care, 46(10), 1728–1739. https://doi.org/10.2337/dci23-0032
22. Lim, J. I., Regillo, C. D., Sadda, S. R., et al. (2023). Artificial Intelligence Detection of Diabetic Retinopathy: Subgroup Comparison of the EyeArt System with Ophthalmologists' Dilated Examinations. Ophthalmology Science, 3(1), 100228. https://doi.org/10.1016/j.xops.2022.100228
23. Retinsight. (2024). Viewed on https://www.retinsight.com/ (accessed June 2025).
24. Engelmann, J., McTrusty, A. D., MacCormick, I. J. C., et al. (2022). Detecting Multiple Retinal Diseases in Ultra-Widefield Fundus Imaging and Data-Driven Identification of Informative Regions with Deep Learning. Nature Machine Intelligence, 4(12) 1143–1154. https://doi.org/10.1038/s42256-022-00566-5
25. Liu, J., Xu, X., Li, X. (2024). Interpretation of Expert Consensus on Community Screening of Diabetic Retinopathy. Chinese Journal of Ocular Fundus Diseases, 105–108.
26. Abou Taha, A., Dinesen, S., Vergmann, A. S., et al. (2024). Present and Future Screening Programs for Diabetic Retinopathy: A Narrative Review. International Journal of Retina and Vitreous, 10(1), 14. https://doi.org/10.1186/s40942-024-00534-8
27. Wong, D.C.S., Kiew, G., Jeon, S., et al. (2021). Singapore Eye Lesions Analyzer (SELENA): The Deep Learning System for Retinal Diseases. In A. Grzybowski (Ed.), Artificial Intelligence in Ophthalmology (pp. 177–185). Springer International Publishing. https://doi.org/10.1007/978-3-030-78601-4_13
28. Jan, C., He, M., Vingrys, A., et al. (2024). Diagnosing Glaucoma in Primary Eye Care and the Role of Artificial Intelligence Applications for Reducing the Prevalence of Undetected Glaucoma in Australia. Eye, 38(11), 2003–2013. https://doi.org/10.1038/s41433-024-03026-z
29. Rampat, R., Deshmukh, R., Chen, X., et al. (2021). Artificial Intelligence in Cornea, Refractive Surgery, and Cataract: Basic Principles, Clinical Applications, and Future Directions. Asia-Pacific Journal of Ophthalmology, 10(3), 268–281. https://doi.org/10.1097/APO.0000000000000394

30. Jin, K., Li, Y., Wu, H., et al. (2024). Integration of Smartphone Technology and Artificial Intelligence for Advanced Ophthalmic Care: A Systematic Review. Advances in Ophthalmology Practice and Research, 4(3), 120–127. https://doi.org/10.1016/j.aopr.2024.03.003

31. Nguyen, T., Ong, J., Masalkhi, M. et al. (2024). Artificial Intelligence in Corneal Diseases: A Narrative Review. Contact Lens and Anterior Eye, 47(6), 102284. https://doi.org/10.1016/j.clae.2024.102284

32. Ji, Y., Liu, S., Hong, X. et al. (2022). Advances in Artificial Intelligence Applications for Ocular Surface Diseases Diagnosis. Frontiers in Cell and Developmental Biology, 10, 1107689. https://doi.org/10.3389/fcell.2022.1107689

33. Patterson, E. J., Bounds, A. D., Wagner, S. K., et al. (2024). Oculomics: A Crusade Against the Four Horsemen of Chronic Disease. Ophthalmology and Therapy, 13(6), 1427–1451. https://doi.org/10.1007/s40123-024-00942-x

34. Li, J., Guan, Z., Wang, J., et al. (2024). Integrated Image-Based Deep Learning and Language Models for Primary Diabetes Care. Nature Medicine, 30, 2886–2896. https://doi.org/10.1038/s41591-024-03139-8

35. Wagner, S. K., Hughes, F., Cortina-Borja, M. et al. (2022). AlzEye: Longitudinal Record-Level Linkage of Ophthalmic Imaging and Hospital Admissions of 353 157 Patients in London, UK. BMJ Open, 12(3), e058552. https://doi.org/10.1136/bmjopen-2021-058552

36. Wagner, S. K., Fu, D. J., Faes, L., et al. (2020). Insights into Systemic Disease Through Retinal Imaging-Based Oculomics. Translational Vision Science & Technology, 9(2), 6. https://doi.org/10.1167/tvst.9.2.6

37. Sevgi, M., and Wagner, S. (2024). Strengthening the Signal: Advancing Oculomics Research for Systemic Health Insights. Eye News. https://www.eyenews.uk.com/features/ai- oculomics/post/strengthening-the-signal-advancing-oculomics-research-for-systemic-health-insights

38. Cai, Y., Zhang, X., Cao, J., et al. (2024). Application of Artificial Intelligence in Oculoplastics. Clinics in Dermatology. 42(3):259–267. https://doi.org/10.1016/j.clindermatol.2023.12.019

39. Crincoli, E., Sacconi, R., Querques, L., et al. (2024). Artificial Intelligence in Age-Related Macular Degeneration: State of the Art and Recent Updates. BMC Ophthalmology, 24(1), 121. https://doi.org/10.1186/s12886-024-03381-1

40. Wu, K., Wu, E., Theodorou, B., et al. (2023). Characterizing the Clinical Adoption of Medical AI Devices Through U.S. Insurance Claims. NEJM AI, 1(1). https://doi.org/10.1056/AIoa2300030

41. Abràmoff, M. D., Roehrenbeck, C., Trujillo, S., et al. (2022). A Reimbursement Framework for Artificial Intelligence in Healthcare. NPJ Digital Medicine, 5, 72. https://doi.org/10.1038/s41746-022-00621-w

42. Huang, J. J., Channa, R., Wolf, R. M., et al. (2024). Autonomous Artificial Intelligence for Diabetic Eye Disease Increases Access and Health Equity in Underserved Populations. Npj Digital Medicine, 7(1), 1–6. https://doi.org/10.1038/s41746-024-01197-3

43. Beede, E., Baylor, E., Hersch, F., et al. (2020). A Human-Centered Evaluation of a Deep Learning System Deployed in Clinics for the Detection of Diabetic Retinopathy. Proceedings of the 2020 CHI Conference on Human Factors in Computing Systems, 1–12. https://doi.org/10.1145/3313831.3376718

44. Cleland, C. R., Bascaran, C., Makupa, W., et al. (2024). Artificial Intelligence-Supported Diabetic Retinopathy Screening in Tanzania: Rationale and Design of a Randomised Controlled Trial. BMJ Open, 14(1), e075055.

45. Youssef, A., Nichol, A. A., Martinez-Martin, N., et al. (2024). Ethical Considerations in the Design and Conduct of Clinical Trials of Artificial Intelligence. JAMA Network Open, 7(9), e2432482. https://doi.org/10.1001/jamanetworkopen.2024.32482

46. Sevgi, M., Ruffell, E., Antaki, F., et al. (2025). Foundation Models in Ophthalmology: Opportunities and Challenges. Current Opinion in Ophthalmology, 36(1), 90–98. https://doi.org/10.1097/ICU.0000000000001091

47. Bommasani, R., Hudson, D. A., Adeli, E., et al. (2021, August 16). On the Opportunities and Risks of Foundation Models. arXiv.Org. https://arxiv.org/abs/2108.07258v3

48. Howell, M. D., Corrado, G. S., and DeSalvo, K. B. (2024). Three Epochs of Artificial Intelligence in Health Care. JAMA, 331(3), 242–244. https://doi.org/10.1001/jama.2023.25057

49. Zhou, Y., Chia, M. A., Wagner, S. K., et al. (2023). A foundation model for generalizable disease detection from retinal images. Nature, 622(7981), 156–163.

50. Warraich, H. J., Tazbaz, T., and Califf, R. M. (2024). FDA Perspective on the Regulation of Artificial Intelligence in Health Care and Biomedicine. JAMA. https://doi.org/10.1001/jama.2024.21451

51. Antaki, F., Milad, D., Chia, M. A., et al. (2023). Capabilities of GPT-4 in Ophthalmology: An Analysis of Model Entropy and Progress Towards Human-Level Medical Question Answering. British Journal of Ophthalmology, 108(10), 1371–1378.

52. Singhal, K., Azizi, S., Tu, T., et al. (2023). Large Language Models Encode Clinical Knowledge. Nature, 620(7972), 172–180. https://doi.org/10.1038/s41586-023-06291-2

53. Saab, K., Tu, T., Weng, W.-H., et al. (2024). Capabilities of Gemini Models in Medicine. arXiv [Cs.AI].

54. Tu, T., Palepu, A., Schaekermann, M., et al. (2024). Towards Conversational Diagnostic AI. arXiv [Cs.AI].

55. Tu, T., Shekoofeh, A., Driess D., et al. (2024). Towards Generalist Biomedical AI. NEJM AI, 1(3), AIoa2300138.

56. Antaki, F., Touma, S., Milad, D., et al. (2023). Evaluating the Performance of ChatGPT in Ophthalmology: An Analysis of Its Successes and Shortcomings. Ophthalmology Science, 3(4), 100324. https://doi.org/10.1016/j.xops.2023.100324

57. Sevgi, M., Antaki, F., and Keane, P. A. (2024). Medical education with large language models in ophthalmology: Custom instructions and enhanced retrieval capabilities. The British Journal of Ophthalmology, 108(10), 1354–1361. https://doi.org/10.1136/bjo-2023-325046

58. Yang, L., Xu, S., Sellergren, A., et al. (2024). Advancing Multimodal Medical Capabilities of Gemini (No. arXiv:2405.03162). arXiv. https://doi.org/10.48550/arXiv.2405.03162

13 AI in Dermatology

AI-Enabled Diagnostics in Dermatology – A Case Study in Skin Cancer Devices

Ramsey Hafer, Bhuvanesh Mural, and Kaushik Venkatesh

13.1 INTRODUCTION

Physician shortages across multiple specialties create significant barriers to timely and effective care [1]. Dermatology, in particular, currently faces marked and growing workforce shortages with long waiting times. This in turn is leaving clinicians struggling to meet patient demand. In the United States, workforce projections show a 25% shortage in dermatologists by 2050 [2], highlighting the urgent need and market demand for solutions to improve access to dermatology care. In this context, the field is ripe for innovation with artificial intelligence (AI) to increase efficiency and capacity. AI-driven diagnostic tools are particularly well-positioned to support providers seeing patients with skin disease—both in primary care and specialised dermatology care. Given this projected shortage of dermatologists, AI can help primary care providers (PCPs) identify and triage dermatologic conditions such as acne, bacterial skin infections, and common skin cancers, facilitating timely referrals to specialists while providing adequate care for less complex cases in primary care settings [3].

A notable example of this approach is the ophthalmologic tool IDx-DR, a U.S. Food and Drug Administration (FDA)-approved AI system for detecting diabetic retinopathy, which enables primary care providers to identify the disease early without requiring specialist interpretation. The implementation of this device at Johns Hopkins Hospital in Baltimore, Maryland, led to a substantial increase in screening rates among paediatric patients with diabetes from 49% to 95% and consistently resulted in more patients screened with greater cost savings in most health system scenarios [4, 5]. By integrating AI into primary care workflows, healthcare systems can alleviate bottlenecks, reduce waiting times, and optimise specialist availability for more complex cases. AI-driven solutions in dermatology could have a comparable impact, expanding access to high-quality skin cancer screening and other dermatologic assessments while improving overall healthcare efficiency. Market analysis indicates that the AI-enabled dermatology diagnostics sector is projected to grow at a compound annual growth rate of over 25% globally, increasing from $203 million USD in 2024 to $630 million by 2029 [6].

Among these innovations, DermaSensor serves as a case study in the clinical and regulatory implications of AI-enabled diagnostics in dermatology. Authorised by the FDA in January 2024, DermaSensor became the first AI-enabled device for skin cancer detection intended for use by non-specialists [7]. This milestone underscores the potential of AI to expand diagnostic capabilities beyond traditional specialist settings while also raising critical questions about scope of practice, clinical oversight, and integration into existing workflows. This chapter contextualises DermaSensor's impact by comparing it with similar medical devices and examining the broader implications of AI-driven diagnostics on clinical practice, computational development, and regulatory frameworks in modern healthcare.

13.2 AI-ENABLED SKIN CANCER DETECTION DEVICES AUTHORISED BY THE FOOD AND DRUG ADMINISTRATION

Two major applications of AI in dermatology involve image-based and spectroscopy-based analysis. The former leverages large data sets of high-resolution dermatoscopic images and deep learning models, particularly convolutional neural networks (CNNs, a type of artificial neural network that's used to process and recognise images, mimicking the human visual cortex) that are trained to recognise and classify various skin lesions. AI models can analyse visual features like asymmetry, irregular borders, colour variegation, and structural patterns that may differentiate benign and malignant lesions [8, 9]. Spectroscopic techniques, on the other hand, can provide quantitative data on skin—generating signals that contain characteristic peaks, absorption bands, or scattering distributions that correlate with biochemical properties of tissues. While the machine learning algorithms used by the first AI spectroscopic devices are proprietary and not fully disclosed, the respective technologies and data types suggest the application of classical machine learning techniques such as support vector machines (SVMs) or random forests to model spectral

DOI: 10.1201/9781032709956-13

data [10, 11]. The development of DermaSensor, however, marked a movement towards the application of deep learning in dermatologic AI devices using CNNs to differentiate between benign and malignant spectra. It is important to note that classical machine learning models rely on human-defined features and excel with smaller, more structured datasets, offering greater transparency on its decision-making process. On the other hand, deep learning models, like CNNs, automatically extract complex features from large, unstructured datasets like medical images. This may achieve high accuracy, but it is at the risk of reduced explainability, which can be a challenge in medical AI devices, where clinical transparency is essential [12].

At this point several AI-enabled devices have received FDA authorisation, offering non-invasive methods to assess suspicious skin lesions via spectroscopic information. These technologies vary in their underlying diagnostic methodologies, target user populations, and real-world effectiveness. To better understand this effectiveness when assessing the utility and clinical impact of AI-assisted skin cancer detection tools, two primary performance metrics are considered. Sensitivity, calculated by measuring true positives/(true positives + false positives) refers to a device's ability to correctly identify true positives or cases where cancer is present. A higher sensitivity reduces the risk of missed diagnoses (false negatives), which is critical in skin cancer screening, where early detection improves patient outcomes [13]. Specificity, calculated by measuring true negatives/(true negatives + false positives) refers to a device's ability to correctly identify true negatives or cases where no cancer is present. A higher specificity minimizes false positives, which helps reduce unnecessary biopsies, patient anxiety, and healthcare costs [14]. Currently without AI, the sensitivity and specificity using clinical examination was 76.9% and 89.1% for experienced dermatologists compared with 37.5% and 84.6% for primary care physicians. Using in-person dermoscopy/dermoscopic images, they were 85.7% and 81.3% for experienced dermatologists and 49.5% and 91.3% for PCPs [15].

13.2.1 MelaFind (FDA-Authorized 2011, Discontinued 2017)

Utilising multispectral spectroscopy, MelaFind was the first FDA-authorised dermoscopic device designed exclusively for use by dermatologists in melanoma diagnosis. Multispectral spectroscopy uses multiple wavelengths of light to analyse skin lesion composition based on how different chromophores (molecules like melanin and haemoglobin) absorb and reflect light [16]. It received FDA authorisation via the premarket approval (PMA) pathway. Despite its high sensitivity (98.3%), its specificity (9.9%) was insufficient to minimise unnecessary biopsies and consequently limited adoption. This, in addition to its poor integrability into workflow, led to its discontinuation from the market [17].

13.2.2 Nevisense (Authorised 2017)

Using electrical impedance spectroscopy, Nevisense provides diagnostic support for melanoma, with a high sensitivity (97.0%) and improved specificity (31.3%) to MelaFind. This technique measures electrical currents that pass through skin tissue, capturing changes in cellular structure and membrane integrity that indicate malignancy. Cancerous and non-cancerous cells have distinct electrical properties due to differences in cell membrane composition, water content, and tissue structure [18]. The device's AI algorithm evaluates impedance data to classify lesions. Like MelaFind, it underwent a premarket approval process for high-risk devices by the FDA. Unlike MelaFind, it remains available but is limited to use by dermatologists [18]. However, Nevisense's reliance on electrical impedance spectroscopy, while effective in certain dermatological assessments, limits its applicability beyond melanoma diagnosis. Even though it has a slightly higher specificity than that of DermaSensor, it still warrants concern over unnecessary referral and biopsies.

13.2.3 DermaSensor (Authorised 2024)

Employing elastic scattering spectroscopy, this device is tailored for primary care physicians instead of dermatologists to assess skin lesions for melanoma, squamous cell carcinoma, and basal cell carcinoma. The sensor examines how light scatters when it interacts with tissue, identifying subcellular morphological differences between normal and cancerous cells. Then an AI algorithm based on an expansive databank of spectral scans of various benign and malignant lesions from multiple health care settings is used to categorise the lesion as high or low risk for malignancy as it relates to biopsy-proven sample sets [19]. It was approved via the De Novo pathway, reflecting its low-to-moderate risk. Its sensitivity (96.6%) positions it as a reliable tool for screening, despite a relatively low specificity (21%) [7]. The device's ability to assist in the detection of three common skin cancers provides a broader diagnostic range compared to similar technologies. It is also the only device authorised for use by non-dermatologist providers—a unique development warranting further discussion.

13.3 CONSIDERATIONS FOR DEVICE PERFORMANCE
13.3.1 Access to Representative Training Data

Performance of AI models, especially for classification, is fundamentally defined by the training data set. Models show the highest accuracy for test cases that are within the bounds of the training data but start to deviate in cases on the fringe of the dataset—for example, one-shot and zero-shot learning [20]. One-shot learning refers to the ability of an AI model to accurately classify or make predictions with only a single example of a given class. This approach is particularly useful when training data is limited or expensive to acquire. Meanwhile, zero-shot learning enables a model to generalise to entirely new classes that were not explicitly present in the training dataset by leveraging semantic relationships and prior knowledge.

In dermatology, training the computer vision AI model on diverse datasets is critical to minimising biases. Darker skin tones have been historically under-represented in dermatological AI models resulting in poorer diagnostic performance on darker skin phenotypes [21, 22]. This under-representation risks re-entrenching diagnostic disparities for patients who are already systematically and historically marginalised in dermatology care [21]. Efforts to incorporate balanced datasets are therefore essential for tools like DermaSensor to achieve equitable performance across demographics. In the DERM-SUCCESS pivotal trial, only 13% of patients were from the most pigmented skin types (Fitzpatrick V/VI). Considering this, the FDA had set a post-market surveillance requirement to ensure diverse patient populations are tracked. Guidelines like the Checklist for Evaluation of Image-Based Artificial Intelligence Reports in Dermatology (CLEAR Derm) or the quality assessment of diagnostic accuracy studies (QUADAS-AI) are useful tools to ensure balance among datasets [23, 24].

13.3.2 Additional Modalities of Data

AI-enabled diagnosis in dermatology also has the potential to move beyond computer vision image-based analysis alone. Wearable technologies offer new opportunities for continuous monitoring and diagnostics in dermatology and beyond [25]. Wearables equipped with advanced sensors can monitor skin hydration, temperature, UV exposure, and acidity, in addition to changes in skin texture and colour. Such data can help in early detection of chronic conditions like eczema flares and autoimmune diseases like lupus [26, 27]. Artificial intelligence-enabled wearable sensors with closed-loop haptic feedback have been shown to decrease nocturnal scratch in patients with mild atopic dermatitis in small studies [28]. With the variety of information that AI can interpret, algorithms should be standardised to address variations in diagnostic outputs, ensuring consistent and reliable performance across diverse healthcare environments [29].

Additionally, integrating imaging information with electronic medical record data and patient history may further enhance diagnostic accuracy while also keeping costs lower than more complex multimodal approaches. Using chart-based data, including past diagnoses, lab results, and treatment histories, can complement image-based AI analysis to refine predictions and improve clinical decision-making. This combination of structured and unstructured data can create a more holistic approach to dermatologic care, enabling AI models to provide more patient-specific recommendations while maintaining cost efficiency.

13.4 CONSIDERATIONS FOR IMPLEMENTATION

Rural healthcare workforce shortages particularly impact dermatological care access, with 4.11 dermatologists per 100,000 people in metropolitan areas vs 0.085 in rural areas [30, 31]. AI tools like DermaSensor could play a vital role in bridging these gaps by equipping primary care providers in underserved areas with more advanced diagnostic capabilities, significantly reducing wait times and supporting early detection [32]. However, it is essential to consider the scope of practice and clinical implications of deploying such tools in non-specialist settings. A parallel can be drawn to diabetic retinopathy screening tool, IDx-DR, and the concerns it raised about the role of ophthalmologists in the diagnostic process. The creator of IDx-DR, Michael Abramoff, was labelled the "Retinator" for allegedly disrupting traditional ophthalmology practice, but he actively worked to position AI as a collaborative tool rather than a replacement. By integrating AI into screening workflows rather than direct diagnosis, IDx-DR preserved ophthalmologists' role in interpreting complex cases and guiding patient care.

Similarly, for dermatology, AI-driven tools must be integrated in a way that enhances, rather than diminishes, the role of dermatologists. This could involve leveraging AI for triage and preliminary assessments while ensuring that complex or uncertain cases are still referred to specialists. Additionally, professional organisations could advocate for reimbursement models that recognize dermatologists' oversight of AI-driven diagnostics, ensuring that these advancements do not undermine the sustainability of dermatology practices but instead improve efficiency and expand access. Finding a balance between accessibility and professional integrity will be critical as AI continues to reshape the field.

13.4.1 Facilitating Adoption

Adopting AI-based diagnostic tools in primary care settings presents unique challenges that extend beyond the functionality of any single device. While DermaSensor serves as a useful example of AI-driven skin cancer screening, it also highlights broader concerns surrounding AI adoption in healthcare. A survey by the American Medical Association revealed that physicians are increasingly interested in AI-enabled medical devices, with 66% of respondents reporting AI use in their practices, up from 38% in 2023, yet key adoption concerns included data privacy assurances, seamless integration with EHR systems, adequate training, feedback loops to improve AI tools over time, and increased oversight to address liability and trust issues [33]. Primary care physicians require training to interpret AI-generated outputs effectively, necessitating educational initiatives, transparent performance metrics, and clinical validation. However, these efforts must be balanced with ensuring intuitive user interfaces that minimize cognitive burden for providers and streamline workflow integration [34, 35]. Ensuring that providers receive adequate training on the role and limitations of AI in diagnosis is critical for fostering trust and preventing over-reliance on technology without clinical oversight [21, 34]. For example, to make IDX-DR more explainable despite using CNNs, the creators designed their device to use multiple feature detectors for identifying pathognomonic lesions [36, 37]. A similar approach may be taken with future dermatologic AI devices, categorising key features by individual lesion, allowing for explanation at the disease characteristic level. Additionally, patient education initiatives should clarify AI's function as a support tool rather than a replacement for physician judgement. In the rural setting especially, providers may face greater reluctance due to limited exposure to emerging AI technologies and resource constraints that can hinder access and adoption. Skill gaps among rural healthcare providers may require specialised training programs and targeted educational support to ensure effective utilisation of AI diagnostic tools [38].

Financial incentives and reimbursement models will also play a significant role in determining adoption and utilisation rates [39]. Providers, particularly in low-resource clinical settings, may hesitate to adopt new diagnostic tools without the assurance of sufficient reimbursement. Implementing outcome-based reimbursement plans that reward improved patient outcomes can encourage early adoption and sustained use of AI-driven devices. Aligning financial incentives with clinical benefits will be crucial in ensuring widespread and equitable integration of AI in healthcare.

13.4.2 Quality of Care and Risk of Overutilisation

The promise of AI-assisted diagnostics lies in its ability to improve sensitivity in detecting skin malignancies, thereby facilitating faster patient triage and reducing missed diagnoses. Studies evaluating DermaSensor in real-world primary care settings suggest enhanced sensitivity at 90.0% compared to physician-only assessment at 40.0%. However, this improvement in sensitivity often comes at the cost of lower specificity, leading to a higher rate of false positives. A lower specificity, as seen with DermaSensor's 60.7% compared to primary care clinicians' 84.8%, raises concerns about potential overutilisation of healthcare resources [40].

This phenomenon is not unique to DermaSensor. For example, in the case of SkinVision, a Dutch mobile AI-enabled skin cancer screening app, app users had twice as many biopsies and excisions performed as controls, along with four times the claims for benign skin tumours and nevi (5.9% compared to 1.7%) [39]. The increased benign claims and fewer malignant claims resulted in higher total annual costs for app users (€64.97) vs. controls (€43.09). While improved sensitivity reduces the risk of missed malignancies, the increased burden of unnecessary procedures may elevate healthcare costs and contribute to patient anxiety [41]. A similar pattern contributed to the discontinuation of MelaFind, an earlier AI-powered dermatoscopic tool that faced criticism for overuse and lack of financial sustainability [42, 43]. Overreliance on AI may even inadvertently limit the clinical judgement of providers or introduce overconfidence in AI outputs [44]. These cases highlight the delicate balance between enhancing diagnostic capabilities and avoiding excessive medical interventions that strain healthcare systems and cause undue psychological/physical harm.

13.5 CONSIDERATIONS FOR REGULATION

As AI-driven diagnostic tools become increasingly prevalent in healthcare, regulatory frameworks must evolve to balance innovation with patient safety and equity. One of the most significant recent developments in this space is the FDA's Predetermined Change Control Plan (PCCP), which provides a new approach to regulatory approval, particularly for adaptive AI technologies. The PCCP allows manufacturers to outline predefined modifications to an AI system post-market, ensuring that improvements can be made efficiently while maintaining safety and efficacy [45]. This is especially relevant for tools like DermaSensor, where continuous algorithm optimisation is crucial for improving diagnostic accuracy and addressing biases. Beyond this, the FDA also published its draft guidance for recommendations on marketing submission and lifecycle management in AI-enabled device software. It consolidates insights from existing regulatory guidelines while also introducing new recommendations tailored to AI-specific challenges, highlighting the agency's recognition of the unique regulatory needs for medical devices [46]. The publication of these guidance documents underscores the FDA's commitment to balancing transparency, product safety, and innovation in such a rapidly evolving field.

An equitable access to dermatology services is a critical consideration in all regulatory discussions. Reimbursement models must account not only for the cost of AI devices but also for associated training programs and integration efforts to ensure effective deployment across diverse healthcare settings, including resource-limited environments. Ethical financing and equitable resource allocation are essential to prevent disparities in access and utilisation, making regulatory policies a key driver of AI implementation success [47]. Without careful consideration of resource allocation, there is the risk of exacerbating existing healthcare disparities [48]. These concerns are amplified in settings where limited resources might prevent proper integration of AI technologies or adequate training for providers, thus underscoring the importance of equitable deployment strategies [49].

The importance of diverse and representative training datasets is another crucial aspect of the regulatory process. Ensuring that AI tools are trained on datasets that include a broad range of skin tones, particularly for skin of colour (SOC), is necessary to minimise biases and improve diagnostic accuracy. Frameworks like the PCCP can support this by requiring transparent reporting on model updates and validation methods to ensure that ongoing improvements do not introduce or exacerbate biases. Utilising guidelines such as those from the Coalition for Health AI, and consideration of frameworks like AI nutrition labels may be essential steps in this process. The Coalition for Health AI provides a comprehensive framework focusing on transparency, explainability, and fairness in AI-driven healthcare solutions [29]. Their guidelines emphasise the necessity of continuous monitoring, bias audits, and stakeholder engagement to develop AI systems that do not inadvertently reinforce existing disparities. Meanwhile AI nutrition labels, an emerging concept, provide a standardised way to disclose critical information about AI models, including their intended use, performance metrics across different demographic groups, and potential limitations. These labels serve as a tool for clinicians and policymakers to assess whether a given AI system is suitable for deployment in diverse healthcare settings. Implementing such a structured reporting approach fosters accountability and trust while enabling informed decision-making by healthcare providers and administrators.

Despite its potential, AI in healthcare carries inherent risks that must be carefully managed. Over-reliance on AI-generated diagnoses can lead to clinical complacency, where providers may defer to algorithmic recommendations without critically assessing patient symptoms [50]. Additionally, biased training data or poorly calibrated AI models can reinforce existing healthcare disparities, disproportionately misdiagnosing or over-treating certain populations. Without robust regulatory oversight, there is also the risk that AI systems may prioritize cost-saving measures over patient safety, leading to unintended consequences such as unnecessary biopsies or overtreatment [51]. AI-driven diagnostic tools, when improperly regulated, can contribute to increased healthcare costs and patient anxiety due to excessive medical interventions. Addressing these dangers requires a regulatory framework that ensures AI-driven tools remain transparent, clinically validated, and continuously assessed for bias and efficacy.

Post-market evaluations are pivotal in AI regulation by providing real-world performance monitoring and data validation [52]. These evaluations ensure that AI devices maintain their safety, efficacy, and equity in diverse patient populations. As regulatory bodies adapt to the rapid evolution of AI, continuous oversight mechanisms such as real-time monitoring, periodic reassessments, and structured feedback loops will be essential to ensuring these technologies meet the highest standards of clinical performance. The PCCP's flexibility allows regulators to keep pace with technological advancements while maintaining rigorous safety standards, ultimately setting a precedent for future AI-driven medical technologies.

13.6 CONCLUSION

The development of AI-driven diagnostic tools highlights the evolving role of technology in healthcare, offering new opportunities to improve access and accuracy in medical decision-making. While AI-enabled devices have demonstrated potential in augmenting clinical workflows and expanding diagnostic capabilities, their implementation raises important questions regarding regulation, equitable access, and physician oversight. The case study of DermaSensor serves as an example of these broader trends, emphasising both the possibilities and challenges associated with AI integration. Moving forward, ensuring that AI tools are rigorously validated, transparently regulated, and responsibly deployed will be critical in maximising their benefits while mitigating potential risks. As AI continues to shape the future of medicine, interdisciplinary collaboration among technologists, clinicians, and policymakers will remain essential in guiding its responsible evolution.

13.7 EDITORS' COMMENTS

This chapter discusses the current innovations of AI driven tools in dermatology, which can successfully triage dermatologic conditions, facilitating timely referrals to specialists where required. Less-severe conditions can be diagnosed and treated appropriately in primary care, thereby freeing up specialist centres to deal with more complex cases. There is great scope for future AI-driven innovations to impact service delivery within dermatology, particularly with recognition of the projected staff shortages of the future. As the use of AI-enabled tools continue to develop in capacity and capability, many governance and regulatory frameworks will need to be addressed to ensure safe use outside of specialised dermatology centres.

REFERENCES

1. Pletcher, B.A., Rimsza, M.E., Cull, W.L. et al. (2009) Primary Care Pediatricians' Satisfaction With Subspecialty Care, Perceived Supply, and Barriers to Care. J Pediatr. 156(6):1011–1015. http://doi.org/10.1016/j.jpeds.2009.12.032
2. The Current and Projected Dermatology Workforce in the United States. (2016) J Am Acad Dermatol. 74(5):AB122. http://doi.org/10.1016/j.jaad.2016.02.478
3. Verhoeven, E.W.M., Kraaimaat, F.W., van Weel, C. et al. (2008) Skin Diseases in Family Medicine: Prevalence and Health Care Use. Ann Fam Med. 6(4):349–354. http://doi.org/10.1370/afm.861
4. Ahmed, M., Dai, T., Channa, R. et al. (2025) Cost-Effectiveness of AI for Pediatric Diabetic Eye Exams from a Health System Perspective. Npj Digit Med. 8(1):1–10. http://doi.org/10.1038/s41746-024-01382-4
5. With AI Tool, Johns Hopkins Clinician Boosts Diabetic Retinopathy Screening to 95% Among Pediatric Patients. Accessed February 16, 2025. https://www.hopkinsmedicine.org/news/articles/2023/12/with-ai-tool-johns-hopkins-clinician-boosts-diabetic-retinopathy-screening-to-95-percent-among-pediatric-patients [accessed June 2025]
6. AI In Dermatology Diagnosis Market Trends: Report, 2024 - 2029. Knowledge Sourcing Intelligence LLP. Accessed December 30, 2024. https://www.knowledge-sourcing.com/report/ai-in-dermatology-diagnosis-market [accessed June 2025]
7. Venkatesh, K.P., Kadakia, K.T., Gilbert, S. (2024) Learnings from the First AI-Enabled Skin Cancer Device for Primary Care Authorized by FDA. Npj Digit Med. 7(1):156. http://doi.org/10.1038/s41746-024-01161-1
8. Li, Z., Koban, K.C., Schenck, T.L. et al. (2022) Artificial Intelligence in Dermatology Image Analysis: Current Developments and Future Trends. J Clin Med. 11(22):6826. http://doi.org/10.3390/jcm11226826
9. Musthafa, M.M., Mahesh, T.R., Vinoth, K.V. et al. (2024) Enhanced Skin Cancer Diagnosis Using Optimized CNN Architecture and Checkpoints for Automated Dermatological Lesion Classification. BMC Med Imaging. 24:201. http://doi.org/10.1186/s12880-024-01356-8
10. Szyc, Ł., Hillen, U., Scharlach, C. et al. (2019) Diagnostic Performance of a Support Vector Machine for Dermatofluoroscopic Melanoma Recognition: The Results of the Retrospective Clinical Study on 214 Pigmented Skin Lesions. Diagnostics. 9(3):103. https://doi.org/10.3390/diagnostics9030103
11. Verdel, N., Tanevski, J., Džeroski, S. et al. (2019) A machine-learning model for quantitative characterization of human skin using photothermal radiometry and diffuse reflectance spectroscopy. In: Photonics in Dermatology and Plastic Surgery 2019. Vol 10851. SPIE; 2019:1085107. https://doi.org/10.1117/12.2509691
12. Saranya, A., Subhashini, R. (2023) A Systematic Review of Explainable Artificial Intelligence Models and Applications: Recent Developments and Future Trends. Decis Anal J. 7:100230. http://doi.org/10.1016/j.dajour.2023.100230
13. Stătescu, L., Cojocaru, E., Trandafir, L.M. et al. (2023) Catching Cancer Early: The Importance of Dermato-Oncology Screening. Cancers. 15(12):3066. https://doi.org/10.3390/cancers15123066
14. Wade, J., Rosario, D.J., Macefield, R.C. et al. (2025) Psychological Impact of Prostate Biopsy: Physical Symptoms, Anxiety, and Depression. Journal of Clinical Oncology. https://ascopubs.org/doi/full/10.1200/JCO.2012.45.4801
15. Chen, J.Y., Fernandez, K., Fadadu, R.P. et al. (2024) Skin Cancer Diagnosis by Lesion, Physician, and Examination Type A Systematic Review and Meta-Analysis. JAMA Dermatol. 161(2). https://doi.org/10.1001/jamadermatol.2024.4382
16. Ilişanu, M.A., Moldoveanu, F., Moldoveanu, A. (2023) Multispectral Imaging for Skin Diseases Assessment—State of the Art and Perspectives. https://doi.org/10.3390/s23083888
17. Cukras, A.R. (2013) On the Comparison of Diagnosis and Management of Melanoma Between Dermatologists and MelaFind. JAMA Dermatol. 149(5):622–623. https://doi.org/10.1001/jamadermatol.2013.3405
18. Ollmar, S., Grant, S. (2016) Nevisense: Improving the Accuracy of Diagnosing Melanoma. Melanoma Manag. 3(2):93–96. https://doi.org/10.2217/mmt-2015-0004

19. Manolakos, D., Patrick, G., Geisse, J.K. et al. (2024) Use of an Elastic-Scattering Spectroscopy and Artificial Intelligence Device in the Assessment of Lesions Suggestive of Skin Cancer: A Comparative Effectiveness Study. JAAD Int. 14:52–58. http://doi.org/10.1016/j.jdin.2023.08.019

20. Meshkin, H., Zirkle, J., Arabidarrehdor, G. et al. (2024) Harnessing Large Language models' Zero-Shot and Few-Shot Learning Capabilities for Regulatory Research. Brief Bioinform. 25(5):bbae354. http://doi.org/10.1093/bib/bbae354

21. Narla, S., Heath, C.R., Alexis, A. et al. (2023) Racial Disparities in Dermatology. Arch Dermatol Res. 315(5):1215–1223. https://doi.org/10.1007/s00403-022-02507-z

22. Daneshjou, R., Vodrahalli, K., Novoa, R.A. et al. (2022) Disparities in Dermatology AI Performance on a Diverse, Curated Clinical Image Set. Sci Adv. 8(32):eabq6147. http://doi.org/10.1126/sciadv.abq6147

23. Sounderajah, V., Ashrafian, H., Rose, S. et al. (2021) A Quality Assessment Tool for Artificial Intelligence-Centered Diagnostic Test Accuracy Studies: QUADAS-AI. Nat Med. 27(10):1663–1665. https://doi.org/10.1038/s41591-021-01517-0

24. Daneshjou, R., Barata, C., Betz-Stablein, B. et al. (2022) Checklist for Evaluation of Image-Based Artificial Intelligence Reports in Dermatology: CLEAR Derm Consensus Guidelines From the International Skin Imaging Collaboration Artificial Intelligence Working Group. JAMA Dermatol. 158(1):90–96. http://doi.org/10.1001/jamadermatol.2021.4915

25. King, R.C., Villeneuve, E., White, R.J. et al. (2017) Application of Data Fusion Techniques and Technologies for Wearable Health Monitoring. Med Eng Phys. 42:1–12. https://doi.org/10.1016/j.medengphy.2016.12.011

26. Patel, S., Ershad, F., Zhao, M. et al. (2022) Wearable Electronics for Skin Wound Monitoring and Healing. Soft Sci. 2(2):N/A–N/A. https://doi.org/10.20517/ss.2022.13

27. Frasier, K., Li, V., Sobotka, M. et al. (2024) The Role of Wearable Technology in Real-Time Skin Health Monitoring. JEADV Clin Pract. https://doi.org/10.1002/jvc2.587

28. Yang, A.F., Patel, S., Chun, K.S. et al. (2025) Artificial Intelligence-Enabled Wearable Devices and Nocturnal Scratching in Mild Atopic Dermatitis. JAMA Dermatol. 161(4):e245697. https://doi.org/10.1001/jamadermatol.2024.5697

29. Korfiatis, P., Kline, T.L., Meyer, H.M. et al. (2024) Implementing Artificial Intelligence Algorithms in the Radiology Workflow: Challenges and Considerations. Mayo Clin Proc Digit Health. 3(1):100188. https://doi.org/10.1016/j.mcpdig.2024.100188

30. Feng, H., Berk-Krauss, J., Feng, P.W. et al. (2018) Comparison of Dermatologist Density Between Urban and Rural Counties in the United States. JAMA Dermatol. 154(11):1265–1271. https://doi.org/10.1001/jamadermatol.2018.3022

31. Brumbaugh, B., Goldman, N., Nambudiri, V. et al. (2022) The Resident Physician Shortage Reduction Act: An Opportunity to Address the Rural Dermatology Workforce Deficit. J Am Acad Dermatol. 87(6):1461–1464. https://doi.org/10.1016/j.jaad.2022.06.032

32. Rural Health Policy Documents | National Rural Health Association - NRHA | NRHA. National Rural Health. Accessed December 30, 2024. https://www.ruralhealth.us/advocacy/rural-health-policy-documents [accessed June 2025]

33. 2 in 3 physicians are using health AI—up 78% from 2023. American Medical Association. February 26, 2025. Accessed March 3, 2025. https://www.ama-assn.org/practice-management/digital/2-3-physicians-are-using-health-ai-78-2023 [accessed June 2025]

34. Buck, C., Doctor, E., Hennrich, J. et al. (2022) General Practitioners' Attitudes Toward Artificial Intelligence–Enabled Systems: Interview Study. J Med Internet Res. 24(1):e28916. https://doi.org/10.2196/28916

35. Office AP. HHS shares its Plan for Promoting Responsible Use of Artificial Intelligence in Automated and Algorithmic Systems by State, Local, Tribal, and Territorial Governments in the Administration of Public Benefits. April 29, 2024.

36. Abràmoff, M.D., Leng, T., Ting, D.S.W., Rhee, K., Horton, M.B., Brady, C.J. et al. (2020) Automated and Computer-Assisted Detection, Classification, and Diagnosis of Diabetic Retinopathy. Telemed J E Health. 26(4):544–550. https://doi.org/10.1089/tmj.2020.0008

37. Bienefeld, N., Boss, J.M., Lüthy, R. et al. (2023) Solving the Explainable AI Conundrum by Bridging clinicians' Needs and developers' Goals. NPJ Digit Med. 6(1):94. https://doi.org/10.1038/s41746-023-00837-4

38. Perez, K., Wisniewski, D., Ari, A. et al. (2025) Investigation into Application of AI and Telemedicine in Rural Communities: A Systematic Literature Review. Healthcare. 13(3):324. https://doi.org/10.3390/healthcare13030324

39. Venkatesh, K.P., Raza, M., Kvedar, J. (2023) AI-Based Skin Cancer Detection: the Balance between Access and Overutilization. Npj Digit Med. 6(1):147. https://doi.org/10.1038/s41746-023-00900-0

40. Tepedino, M., Baltazar, D., Hanna, K. et al. (2024) Elastic Scattering Spectroscopy on Patient-Selected Lesions Concerning for Skin Cancer. J Am Board Fam Med. 37(3):427–435. https://doi.org/10.3122/jabfm.2023.230256R2

41. Turani, Z., Fatemizadeh, E., Blumetti, T. et al. (2019) Optical Radiomic Signatures Derived from Optical Coherence Tomography Images Improve Identification of Melanoma. Cancer Res. 79(8):2021–2030. https://doi.org/10.1158/0008-5472.CAN-18-2791

42. Monheit, G., Cognetta, A.B., Ferris, L. et al. (2011) The Performance of MelaFind: A Prospective Multicenter Study. Arch Dermatol. 147(2):188–194. http://doi.org/10.1001/archdermatol.2010.302

43. Ferris, L.K., Harris, R.J. (2012) New Diagnostic Aides for Melanoma. Dermatol Clin. 30(3):535–545. https://doi.org/10.1016/j.det.2012.04.012

44. Ueda, D., Kakinuma, T., Fujita, S. et al. (2024) Fairness of Artificial Intelligence in Healthcare: Review and Recommendations. Jpn J Radiol. 42(1):3–15. https://doi.org/10.1007/s11604-023-01474-3

45. Health C for D and R. Marketing Submission Recommendations for a Predetermined Change Control Plan for Artificial Intelligence-Enabled Device Software Functions. December 3, 2024. https://www.fda.gov/regulatory-information/search-fda-guidance-documents/marketing-submission-recommendations-predetermined-change-control-plan-artificial-intelligence

46. Health C for D and R. Artificial Intelligence-Enabled Device Software Functions: Lifecycle Management and Marketing Submission Recommendations. January 6, 2025. Accessed March 2025. https://www.fda.gov/regulatory-information/search-fda-guidance-documents/artificial-intelligence-enabled-device-software-functions-lifecycle-management-and-marketing

47. Gardner, A., Smith, A.L., Steventon, A. et al. (2022) Ethical Funding for Trustworthy AI: Proposals to Address the Responsibilities of Funders to Ensure That Projects Adhere to Trustworthy AI Practice. Ai Ethics. 2(2):277–291. https://doi.org/10.1007/s43681-021-00069-w

48. Elgin, C.Y., Elgin, C. (2024) Ethical Implications of AI-Driven Clinical Decision Support Systems on Healthcare Resource Allocation: a Qualitative Study of Healthcare professionals' Perspectives. BMC Med Ethics. 25:148. https://doi.org/10.1186/s12910-024-01151-8

49. Chen, J., Yan, A.S. (2025) Hospital Artificial Intelligence/Machine Learning Adoption by Neighborhood Deprivation. Med Care. 63(3):227–233. https://doi.org/10.1097/MLR.0000000000002110

50. Jabbour, S., Fouhey, D., Shepard, S. et al. (2023) Measuring the Impact of AI in the Diagnosis of Hospitalized Patients: A Randomized Clinical Vignette Survey Study. JAMA. 330(23):2275–2284. https://doi.org/10.1001/jama.2023.22295

51. Tighe, P., Mossburg, S., Gale, B. (2024) Artificial Intelligence and Patient Safety: Promise and Challenges. PSNet [internet]. Rockville (MD): Agency for Healthcare Research and Quality, US Department of Health and Human Services. https://psnet.ahrq.gov/perspective/artificial-intelligence-and-patient-safety-promise-and-challenges [accessed 30th June 2025]

52. Yuba, M., Iwasaki, K. (2023) Performance Evaluation Methods for Improvements at Post- Market of Artificial Intelligence/Machine Learning-Based Computer-Aided detection/diagnosis/triage in the United States. PLOS Digit Health. 2(3):e0000209. https://doi.org/10.1371/journal.pdig.0000209

14 Sustainability in Clinical AI

Derrik Nghiem, Siddhant Dogra, and Florence X. Doo

14.1 KEY "SUSTAINABILITY IN CLINICAL AI" CONCEPTS

Healthcare is a major source of greenhouse gas (GHG) emissions, contributing approximately 4.6% of total GHG emissions globally in 2021 [1–3]. In healthcare, artificial intelligence (AI) is an increasingly used technology, with capabilities transforming clinical workflows, diagnostics, treatment planning, and patient management. With AI adoption expected to continue increasing, its role raises potential concerns around the environmental sustainability of AI tools [4–7]. The purpose of this chapter is to guide healthcare professionals, clinical informaticists, and AI developers in making practical, sustainable choices – maximizing AI's clinical benefits while minimizing its environmental footprint. Sustainability in clinical artificial intelligence (AI) requires familiarity with several foundational concepts:

Planetary health emphasizes the interdependence of human and environmental health. Environmental sustainability in healthcare – including in emerging areas like AI – thus becomes a core component of safeguarding human health. Healthcare interventions must improve patient care without undermining environmental systems upon which long-term health relies [8, 9]. Embracing planetary health principles in clinical care and AI means striving for clinical innovation that *adds value to patient care without subtracting value from our environment.* (See Figure 14.1.)

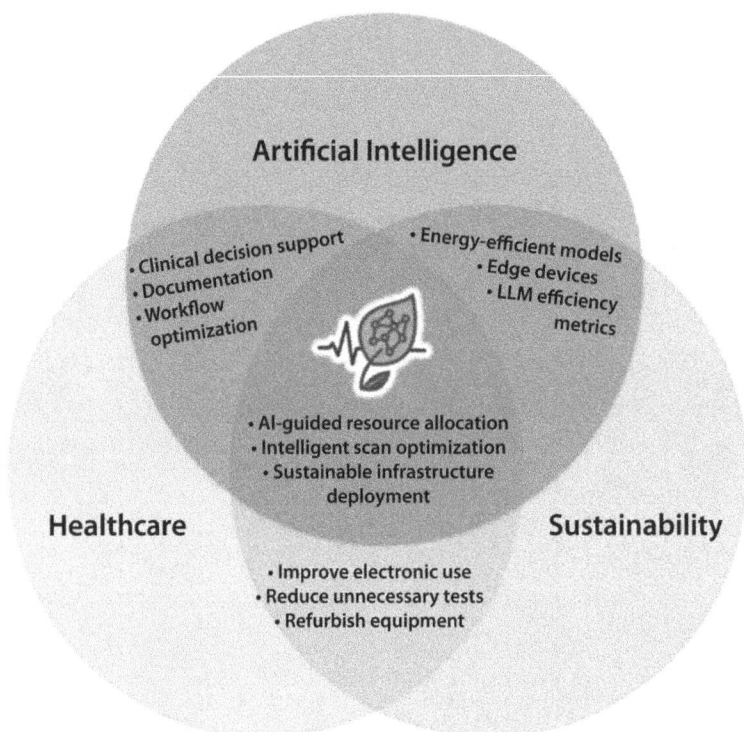

Figure 14.1 Overview Venn diagram, describing the intersection of artificial intelligence, healthcare, and sustainability. Each domain contributes unique levers for improvement: AI offers computational intelligence and automation; healthcare supplies clinical context and patient-centric workflows; and sustainability brings a focus on minimizing environmental impact. Pairing two domains can deliver tangible benefits, e.g., AI-driven clinical decision support and documentation that streamline care, low-power edge models that cut AI carbon cost, and reductions in unnecessary tests that conserve resources. However, the central nexus (combined leaf-AI-health icon) demonstrates how truly integrated solutions such as AI-guided resource allocation, intelligent scan optimization, and climate-conscious infrastructure planning can enhance patient outcomes and operational efficiency while advancing health-system sustainability.

DOI: 10.1201/9781032709956-14

The greenhouse gas (GHG) protocol categorizes emissions into three scopes [10, 11]:

Scope 1: Direct emissions from owned sources (i.e., magnetic resonance imaging [MRI] machines or hospital generators).

Scope 2: Indirect emissions from purchased energy (i.e., electricity from grid).

Scope 3: Indirect emissions from external activities (i.e., vendor-provided cloud services, manufacturing of medical equipment, and devices).

The World Health Organisation and other authorities have urged sectors (like healthcare) to adopt sustainable practices and reduce GHG emissions as average global temperatures rise [2, 12].

Energy and carbon footprint: GHG emissions are typically quantified in terms of *carbon dioxide equivalent (CO_2e)*, which accounts for the different global warming potential of various gases [11]. For example, releasing 1 kg of methane has a much greater warming effect over 100 years than 1 kg of CO_2; CO_2e normalizes such differences into a single metric. In practical terms, the energy consumed by computing hardware is the main driver of AI's carbon footprint, since most energy worldwide is still produced by burning fossil fuels [13]. In healthcare AI, this translates to measuring and managing the carbon cost of model training, data storage, and clinical deployment. Each kWh of electricity used has a certain *carbon intensity* (which depends on the energy source – e.g., coal vs. solar, where renewable energy sources have reduced intensity or impact) [11]. Different metrics to measure these processes and systems individually (or in total), can help estimate carbon footprints.

Lifecycle assessment (LCA) covers all phases of a product or process – from raw material extraction to manufacturing, transport, use, and end-of-life disposal or recycling. LCA is essential for understanding healthcare IT's true carbon footprint. Life cycle assessment can be *attributional* – focusing on attributing the current environmental impacts associated with a product or service, or its share within a defined boundary – or *consequential*, which considers broader system-wide effects (including how choices influence market or behavior changes) [11, 14]. For example, an attributional LCA might calculate the total CO_2e emitted by a CT scanner over 10 years of use, whereas a consequential LCA might also consider how the availability of that scanner leads to more imaging utilization (an indirect effect) and will measure emissions per additional scan. A key insight of LCA is that significant emissions often occur *outside* the use phase. For instance, manufacturing high-end electronics (like GPUs for AI computation or the magnet of an MRI machine) and disposing of e-waste at end-of-life can each carry a substantial carbon burden.

14.2 ENVIRONMENTAL CHALLENGES OF AI IN HEALTHCARE

AI applications generate significant environmental burdens across their lifecycle.

14.2.1 Energy-Intensive Training and Inference

Training a deep learning model often requires running Graphics Processing Units (GPUs) or other accelerators at full tilt for hours, days, or even weeks. This electricity usage has a carbon footprint that depends on the energy source (fossil-fuel vs. renewable). For example, training GPT-3 consumed over 1,200 megawatt-hours (MWh), equal to the annual electricity use of over 100 homes [15]. An often-overlooked environmental impact is the duplication of effort in AI research and development. In academia and industry, many groups might be training similar models from scratch, repeating experiments and thus energy expenditures. A more collaborative approach (data-sharing, using common public models, or federated learning) could reduce the total compute required globally by leveraging one training effort across institutions. Journals and grants are starting to encourage researchers to share models and data openly.

Similarly, within a hospital system, having siloed AI projects that don't coordinate can lead to multiple parallel compute workflows where one well-designed workflow could serve all. Encouraging a platform approach (one robust system that handles multiple AI tasks) can consolidate computing needs and eliminate duplicate hardware. Also, continuously running a clinical AI tool in the "background" could draw substantial power. For example, a German modeling study found that widespread worldwide use of deep learning in pathology would require approximately 86,590 km² (0.22%) of world forest to sequester the annual 16 megatons (Mt) of CO_2e generated [16]. Many AI deployments likely use more computational resources than needed, wasting energy. The challenge is making stakeholders aware of these "invisible" emissions and encouraging optimization.

14.2.2 Infrastructure and Operational Impacts

The hardware used by AI – from high-end GPUs in a server rack to chips on the hospitals' imaging machines – has an *embodied carbon cost* from manufacturing. For instance, producing a data center's worth of servers results in many tons of CO_2e emitted (often scope 3 for the hospital) across the life cycle stages – from extracting raw materials (metals, rare earths), manufacturing in factories, and finally shipping/transportation to hospitals. If AI adoption leads to more hardware procurement (e.g., additional servers or edge devices), it indirectly drives those upstream emissions. Additionally, the rapid pace of AI (with constantly improving hardware) can shorten hardware replacement cycles, contributing to electronic waste.

Also, running AI tools generates heat. In both local server rooms and large data centers, considerable amounts of energy and water are spent on cooling systems. A 1 MW data center might evaporate hundreds of gallons per minute for cooling; some cloud providers build in cooler climates or near renewable energy sources to mitigate both carbon and water impact [17, 20]. In regions facing water scarcity, large IT cooling demands pose an environmental justice issue (data centers competing with local communities for water). By 2027, the global AI demand is projected to account for 4.2–6.6 billion cubic meters of water withdrawal, which is more than half of the United Kingdom's annual water withdrawal [17]. While this is a broader tech industry challenge, it becomes a healthcare challenge as our IT needs grow. AI superimposed on growing telehealth, imaging demands (radiology, ophthalmology, dermatology, pathology, etc.), and growing electronic health records (EHRs) all mean more servers humming away in the background.

14.2.3 Rebound Effect

As AI makes some healthcare processes more efficient or cheaper, overall AI usage increases and potentially cancels out the environmental "gains" – a *rebound effect* (shown in Figure 14.2).

For instance, if AI significantly reduces the time and cost to read certain scans, a hospital might end up doing many more of those scans, thus consuming more energy in scanners and data processing. In radiology, AI could enable imaging in settings that previously lacked it (which is good for patient care, but from a carbon perspective means more machines running). This is not to say we should withhold beneficial diagnostics for the environment's sake, but it means any efficiency

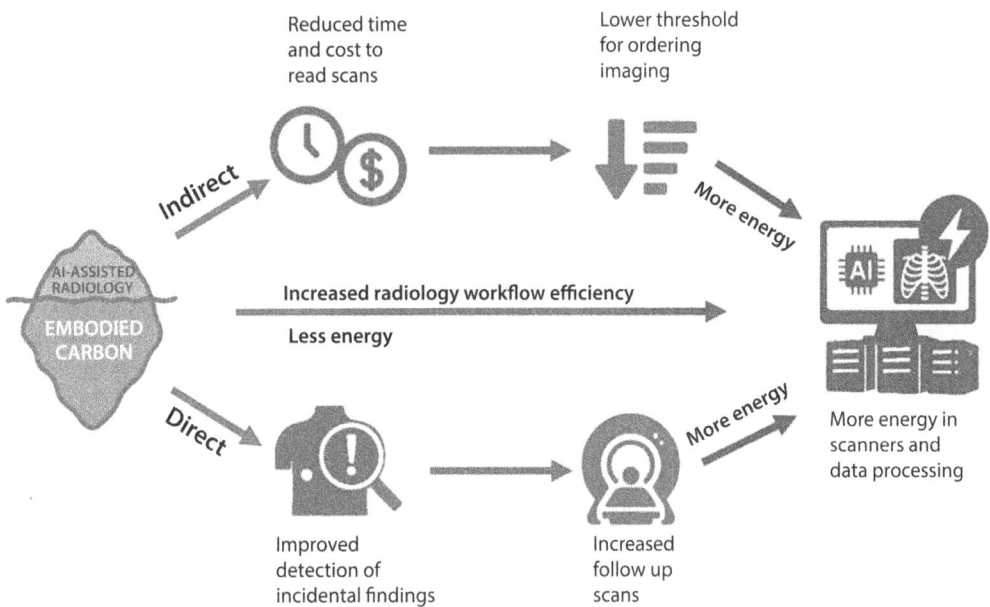

Figure 14.2 The *rebound effect* concept applied to radiology AI. This figure illustrates the rebound effect of AI implementation in radiology. While AI directly enhances efficiency through improved detection of incidental findings and indirectly through reduced time/cost to read scans, this increases follow-up scans and decreases the threshold to order scans, respectively. These changes can drive up total energy used in scanners and data processing.

gains from AI should be coupled with conscious efforts to prevent overutilization. Otherwise, we risk a scenario where AI makes each procedure greener, but the number of procedures rises so much that total emissions still go up. This challenge intersects with healthcare economics and ethics – ensuring AI is used judiciously and for true patient benefit, not just because it's easier to do more. However, some researchers postulate that hardware/software efficiency innovations may, in fact, paradoxically lead to overall improved or balanced environmental impacts, so research remains to be done [21, 22].

In summary, AI's negative environmental impacts mainly stem from hardware requirements, energy use (and its carbon emissions), and systemic factors like duplication and overuse. These challenges reinforce why "sustainable AI" should not be only a buzzword but rather a necessary consideration as we adopt these tools. Recognizing the problems is the first step; next, we will look at how AI can be part of the *solution* and the ways we can harness AI to improve sustainability in healthcare operations.

14.3 STRATEGIES FOR SUSTAINABLE AI IMPLEMENTATION

To align AI development and deployment with sustainability goals, a multipronged strategy is needed. This includes **mitigation strategies** (actions to reduce or prevent GHG emissions and environmental harm from AI and healthcare operations) and **adaptation strategies** (actions to build resilience and prepare for the impacts of climate change on healthcare delivery). Many of these strategies involve technology decisions, clinical practice adjustments, and broader institutional policy shifts. Below, we outline key actionable steps and considerations (Figure 14.3):

As a complement to Figure 14.3, Figure 14.4 presents a checklist that outlines both practical mitigation and adaptation strategies for sustainable AI use in healthcare systems. It serves as a quick-reference guide for local institutions aiming to reduce environmental impact as AI integration evolves.

14.4 TECHNICAL AND OPERATIONAL CONSIDERATIONS: PRACTICAL AI MANAGEMENT

14.4.1 "Green" Design of AI Models and Systems (Mitigation)

From the outset, AI tools should be designed for (energy) efficiency. Developers can adopt the emerging practice of "green AI" – favoring algorithms that achieve required performance with lower computational cost. This might mean using efficient architectures, leveraging transfer learning (so that large training runs are not done from scratch), and using cloud computing instances that are optimized for throughput per watt [23, 24]. If an AI process is running overnight doing batch processing of images, ensure that it is configured to use only the needed resources (e.g., don't use a whole GPU for a lightweight task if it could run on a CPU or smaller accelerator).

Also, larger AI models aren't always superior. Recent research found smaller, clinically fine-tuned AI models (e.g., Vicuna 7B) performed comparably with a medical data labeling task when compared to larger models (Llama 70B) – while consuming significantly less energy [25]. This highlights *algorithmic efficiency* – where choosing a simpler model that is *good enough* for the clinical task. There is little point in deploying a massive 1-trillion parameter model in a clinic if a 13-billion parameter model yields similar patient outcomes; the larger model would only needlessly consume more power and incur more cost. Choosing appropriately sized models can potentially be important for sustainable AI orchestration.

In radiology AI, there is a call to develop transparent efficiency metrics and reporting standards for models, effectively creating an ENERGY STAR-like rating for AI software [11, 26]. This would allow purchasers to compare, say, two picture archiving and communication systems (PACS) AI add-ons based on not just accuracy but also how much energy they consume. One emerging recommendation is for researchers to report the computational resources and energy consumed by their AI models (akin to how we report model performance) to encourage conscious choices about model complexity. Journals and conferences can encourage or mandate code and model sharing (and some already do).

14.4.2 Sustainable Lifecycle Management and Computing Infrastructure (Mitigation)

Many mitigation opportunities come from rethinking equipment lifecycle. *Procurement policies* can prioritize energy-efficient devices (look for ENERGY STAR certified computers, efficient power supplies for PACS storage, etc.) and those from companies with strong sustainability programs. For hardware, consider vendors that offer *refurbished* or remanufactured machines. In radiology, extending the life of scanners delays emissions of manufacturing a new one, and tends to be cost-saving: refurbishing one MRI to use for an extra five years instead of buying new can avoid ~79 tons

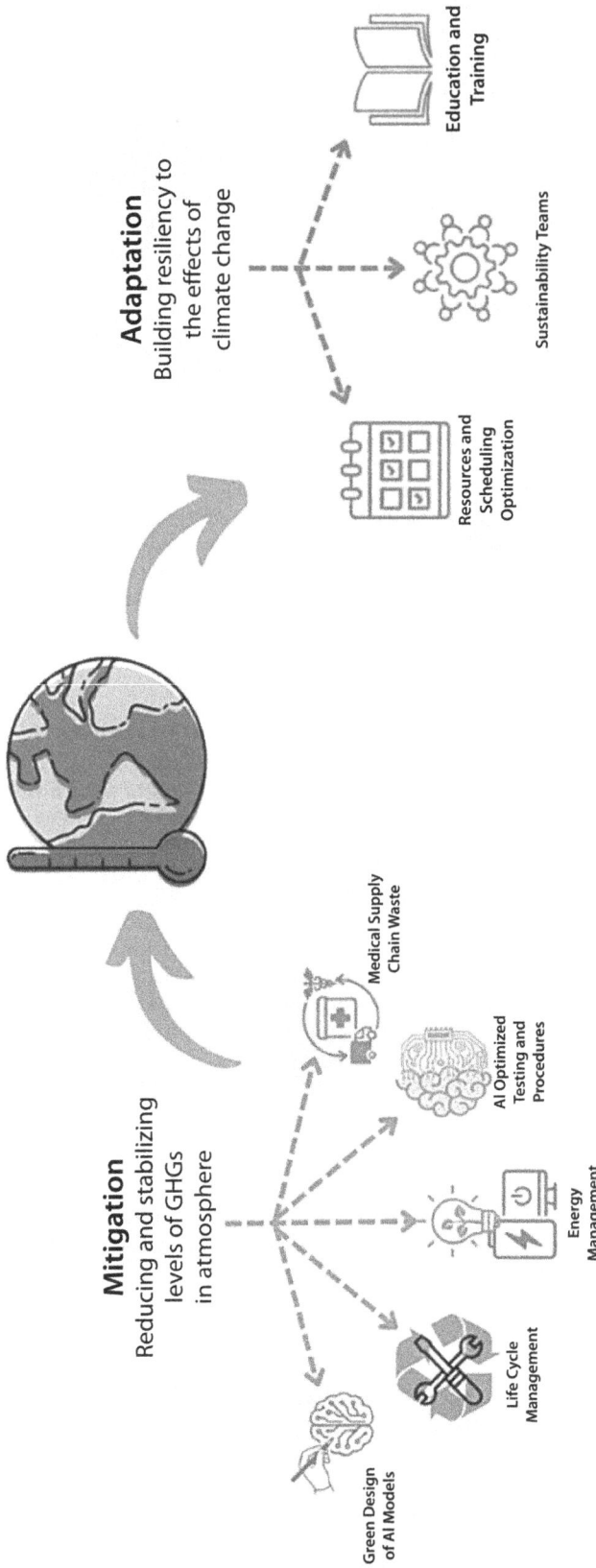

Figure 14.3 Climate action strategies for AI in healthcare. This diagram outlines two complementary climate action strategies in the context of healthcare AI. **Mitigation** efforts aim to reduce and stabilize greenhouse gas emissions through green AI design, life cycle management, energy management, AI optimized testing, and management of medical supply chain waste. **Adaptation** strategies focus on building resilience to climate change through optimizing resource scheduling, forming sustainability teams, and providing climate education and training. Together, these approaches support sustainable integration of radiology AI in healthcare systems. (*Please also refer to the* Figure 14.4 *checklist, which complements this* Figure 14.3.)

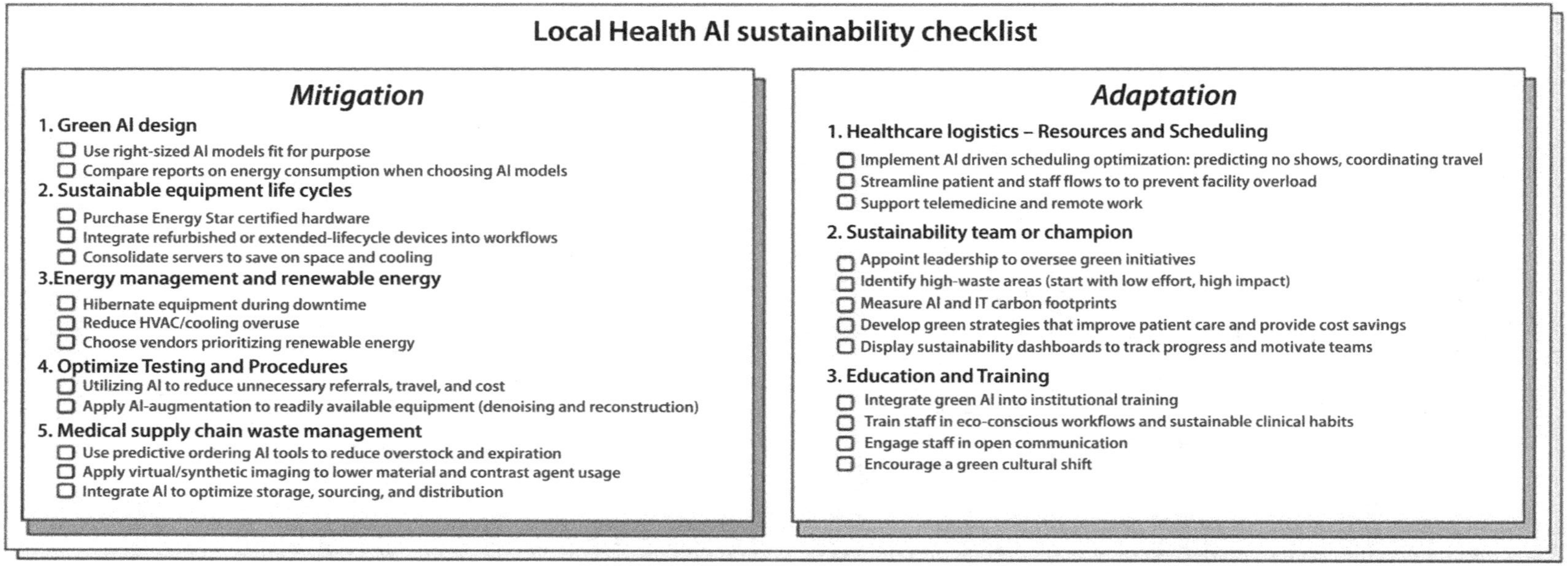

Local Health AI sustainability checklist

Mitigation

1. Green AI design
☐ Use right-sized AI models fit for purpose
☐ Compare reports on energy consumption when choosing AI models

2. Sustainable equipment life cycles
☐ Purchase Energy Star certified hardware
☐ Integrate refurbished or extended-lifecycle devices into workflows
☐ Consolidate servers to save on space and cooling

3. Energy management and renewable energy
☐ Hibernate equipment during downtime
☐ Reduce HVAC/cooling overuse
☐ Choose vendors prioritizing renewable energy

4. Optimize Testing and Procedures
☐ Utilizing AI to reduce unnecessary referrals, travel, and cost
☐ Apply AI-augmentation to readily available equipment (denoising and reconstruction)

5. Medical supply chain waste management
☐ Use predictive ordering AI tools to reduce overstock and expiration
☐ Apply virtual/synthetic imaging to lower material and contrast agent usage
☐ Integrate AI to optimize storage, sourcing, and distribution

Adaptation

1. Healthcare logistics – Resources and Scheduling
☐ Implement AI driven scheduling optimization: predicting no shows, coordinating travel
☐ Streamline patient and staff flows to to prevent facility overload
☐ Support telemedicine and remote work

2. Sustainability team or champion
☐ Appoint leadership to oversee green initiatives
☐ Identify high-waste areas (start with low effort, high impact)
☐ Measure AI and IT carbon footprints
☐ Develop green strategies that improve patient care and provide cost savings
☐ Display sustainability dashboards to track progress and motivate teams

3. Education and Training
☐ Integrate green AI into institutional training
☐ Train staff in eco-conscious workflows and sustainable clinical habits
☐ Engage staff in open communication
☐ Encourage a green cultural shift

Figure 14.4 Local health AI sustainability checklist. (Please also refer to Figure 14.3.)

CO_2e [8, 27]. Departments can establish an upgrade cycle where devices are assessed for potential refurbish rather than automatic replacement. *Reusable supplies* should be favored over single-use when safe and feasible (e.g., storage media). Additionally, request that vendors take back old equipment for proper recycling or disposal – some companies will manage end-of-life of their products, ensuring that precious metals are recycled and toxins contained. Keep an inventory of electronics and have an e-waste recycling program for old workstations, monitors, etc., to prevent them from going to landfill.

Health systems also face critical decisions regarding infrastructure: *cloud solutions* versus on-premises computing. Efficient data storage reduces energy demands significantly. Strategies include deduplication, data compression, and tiered storage systems [28]. On the other hand, cloud services typically offer better energy efficiency due to scale, efficient cooling, and renewable energy usage [23].

Another aspect is software longevity: choose software solutions that can run on existing hardware and don't force hardware upgrades every year. Lightweight AI software that can operate on an average hospital computer is better than one that insists on a brand-new high-power workstation for each healthcare worker. By the same token, choose AI that can integrate into existing infrastructure (for example, on the cloud or on a shared server) rather than requiring a dedicated GPU box installed in every reading room.

14.4.3 Energy Management and Renewable Energy (Mitigation)

Use less energy and use cleaner energy. To use less, implement robust *power management policies*: turn off or hibernate servers when not in use (and potentially use AI to predict usage patterns); turn off idle monitors, workstations, and ancillary electronics after hours either via IT policies or smart outlets. Use virtualization to consolidate workloads so that you don't have 10 servers half idle but rather five running at higher utilization (the fewer physical machines running, the less base load). *Cooling optimization* is also vital – work with facilities to ensure data rooms aren't over-cooled. (Raising the thermostat a few degrees or using smart climate control can save a lot, as one study noted that nearly half of interventional radiology [IR] suite emissions came from climate control, and relaxing temperature control by 10% saved ~60 tons CO_2e/year.) [29] Another idea is *waste heat recovery* – partnering with facilities to reuse the heat from waste incineration or data center equipment to warm other parts of the hospital or pre-heat water, which can save 5–30% of energy [30, 31].

On the supply side, healthcare systems can invest in renewables: solar panels on hospital roofs, geothermal heating/cooling systems, or green power from utilities. If AI is running in the cloud, choose cloud providers or data center regions that use renewable energy. At minimum, offsetting emissions via renewable energy credits or carbon offsets is an option, though direct reduction is preferable. A forward-looking strategy is to incorporate renewable energy and carbon impact clauses into vendor contracts – e.g., when signing a deal for a cloud PACS archive, specifying that the vendor must use (or offset) 100% renewable energy for the service by a certain date. This pushes the industry toward greener operations.

14.5 CLINICAL PRACTICE: AI AS AN ASSISTIVE SUSTAINABILITY TOOL

AI also offers opportunities to enhance environmental sustainability in healthcare, and several promising use cases have emerged for "smarter" care delivery:

14.5.1 Optimized Testing and Procedures (Mitigation)

AI-based *clinical decision support* can reduce unnecessary procedures, lowering both emissions and healthcare costs – and importantly, avoiding steps that provide little benefit to patient outcomes. For instance, decision-support algorithms in frontline settings have successfully reduced advanced imaging volume by up to 8.2% and potentially can also reduce unnecessary specialist referrals, improving resource allocation [32–34]. This is a scenario where doing *less* is better – and AI can ensure that "less" happens in a safe, patient-centered way by providing an evidence-based second check on orders [35]. Importantly, fewer scans mean less energy but also less consumption of contrast media, laundry waste, and less data to store – a cascade of sustainability benefits. Also, an Australian study recommended ordering low-impact imaging (X-ray and ultrasound) in place of high-impact MRI and CT when clinically appropriate to do so (17.5 kg CO_2e/scan for MRI; 9.2 kg CO_2e/scan for CT; 0.5 kg CO_2e/scan for mobile chest radiograph, and 0.5 kg/scan for ultrasound) [14].

On the other hand, *AI-enabled opportunistic screening* is an unrealized resource. AI systems already analyzing routine clinical data or images can further detect additional diseases, enhancing preventive care without extra resource use. For example, primary care clinics using AI to screen for diabetic retinopathy from routine eye exams have reduced specialist referrals, minimizing patient visits, travel emissions, and healthcare costs [36–38].

AI can also augment existing technologies. AI algorithms, especially for long-duration exams (like MRI and positron emission tomography [PET]), can help accelerate imaging acquisition time, adjust protocols, and minimize re-scans. Since the energy consumption of an imaging exam is roughly proportional to scan duration (the machine draws power throughout the scan), shorter scans mean less energy per exam. This has the dual benefit of reducing energy use and improving the patient experience (less time in the scanner and increased appointment access). Techniques like AI-based reconstruction and denoising allow high-quality images to be obtained from faster or lower-dose scans today, without loss of diagnostic quality, by filling in gaps in data [31]. AI can also automate parts of image acquisition, such as positioning and protocol selection, to avoid wasted sequences or repeats. Furthermore, AI can analyze how imaging parameters (like X-ray tube current, MRI pulse sequences) correlate with energy use, potentially leading to protocols that are energy-optimized.

14.5.2 Medical Supply Chain Waste (Mitigation)

AI tools predict precise resource needs, minimizing waste. Influence should be given at the procurement stage to select sustainable vendors or stipulate the requirement for sustainability disclosures in contracts.

In inventory and supply chain, AI predictions could ensure that imaging departments order only what they need in terms of supplies (films, contrast, etc.), reducing waste from expired or excess stock. For instance, hospital-wide AI-driven predictive ordering tools can reduce unnecessary blood transfusions or reduce waste for perishable platelets, significantly lowering waste and associated environmental burdens [39, 40], and may be an emerging field to apply large language models [41]. Furthermore, AI can help find the closest and fastest (omnichannel) blood supply, addressing underlying global supply and demand imbalances in the supply chain [42].

Some imaging modalities use contrast agents (like iodine, gadolinium, or specialized agents for ultrasound) which have environmental implications. Reducing contrast use lowers direct material consumption and cost. It also avoids the environmental downstream effects of contrast media production (nonrenewable resources) and disposal (where it may end up in wastewater). Certain agents are potent greenhouse gases themselves if released into the atmosphere, such as sulphur hexafluoride microbubbles in ultrasound contrast, which has a global warming potential of 23,500 tons of CO_2 [43–45]. While amounts used in patients are small, improper disposal or leaks could have outsized effects. Additionally, gadolinium-based MRI contrast can accumulate in water bodies and ecosystems if waste is not handled properly [46–50]. AI can help by optimizing contrast usage – determining when contrast is truly needed and even by creating virtual synthetic contrast images [51, 52]. Overall, this reduces the need to administer actual contrast agents. AI might also predict the minimum dose of contrast needed for a given patient or scan to achieve adequate imaging, preventing the common practice of using a one-size-fits-all dose. This is a win for both patient safety (avoiding contrast when not needed avoids any risk of side effects) and planetary health.

14.5.3 Healthcare Logistics – Resources and Scheduling (Adaptation)

AI-driven optimization of scheduling and treatment planning reduces patient (and staff) travel emissions, with similar patient outcomes [53–55].

Efficient scheduling means fewer idle scanner hours (less waste of keeping it powered on) and can also reduce the total number of days patients need to travel. *No-show prediction models* (which predict the likelihood a patient will miss an appointment) allow staff to proactively reschedule or double-book slots [56]. AI can further optimize by routing staff or patients by capacity needs, or by minimizing after-hours scans that might require extra energy (lighting; heating, ventilation, and air conditioning [HVAC] at odd hours). For example, an AI logistics algorithm implemented at an National Health Service (NHS) elective surgery center effectively coordinated patient transport, significantly reducing unnecessary travel and associated emissions [57, 58]. Furthermore, AI auto-segmentation tools can speed up radiotherapy contouring, reducing wait times by one to two hours per cancer patient [59]. Imagine a system that has this combination, providing automated faster contouring, freeing up more slots, optimizing the schedule for a network of clinics so that patients are given appointments at the location closest to them or combining multiple appointments on the same day to avoid repeat trips.

AI tools can also help support *remote work* and *telemedicine* when appropriate, encourage sustainable transportation, and increase care access for remote communities. In a U.S. study, the impacts of IT usage are negligible compared to the more major impact of switching from working onsite to working from home, which reduces up to 58% of work's carbon footprint [60]. Furthermore, this could improve air pollution affecting human health [61]. If healthcare professionals can work from home some days, that cuts commuting, yielding cost and emission benefits – and can also improve work–life balance (potentially reducing burnout).

14.6 EVERYONE: INSTITUTIONAL CULTURE AND POLICIES

Technology alone isn't enough – human factors are key.

14.6.1 Sustainability Team or Champion (Adaptation)

Establish a sustainability team or champion within the health system and/or IT department. At the departmental level, this person (or group) can oversee green initiatives, track progress, and keep sustainability on the agenda. At the institutional level, multidisciplinary sustainability committees can oversee sustainability targets, such as reducing unnecessary diagnostic testing and optimizing resource use. Early on, target "high-impact, easy wins" such as reducing HVAC in empty procedure suites mentioned earlier [29]; if AI systems or servers produce heat, possibly use that heat in the building (with engineering co-solutions). Some interventions, like switching to renewable energy or installing efficient equipment, may require upfront investment – leadership buy-in is key for those. It is important to *engage stakeholders and leadership*, including external partners (like utility companies or local governments, on community energy projects).

Measure AI and IT carbon footprints at departmental or organizational levels using available tools [11]. Consider designing and implementing a *sustainability dashboard.* It can help track metrics like monthly energy use (or CO_2e estimates) of equipment/AI tools, reduction targets, or even beyond these technologies as a broader green survey. Displaying such a dashboard raises awareness and can motivate staff ("what gets measured gets managed").

If "green" practices (AI or non-AI related) can demonstrably improve patient care and save money (co-benefits), one can build a strong case to invest further in sustainability initiatives.

14.6.2 Education and Training (Adaptation)

Reading this textbook is a great start! Educate colleagues about why powering down equipment matters, or how climate change can impact health (to build the case for these efforts). Engage people in identifying wasteful practices, especially those "closest to the ground" who know where inefficiencies lie. For example, technologists might notice that a certain scanner is left on all weekend due to a scheduling quirk; once identified, that can be fixed. Encourage healthcare professionals to consider environmental impact in their decision-making (e.g., when contemplating whether to recommend an immediate follow-up CT scan vs. an alternative). Some institutions have started including AI, as well as climate and health topics in medical education [62–64], which over time will make new clinicians more attuned to these issues.

Throughout our discussion, we have seen that human-AI choices can *enable sustainable healthcare practices.* Many of these solutions yield the so-called co-benefits often sought in public health: they save energy and emissions while simultaneously improving efficiency, reducing costs, or enhancing patient care. It is important to note, however, that realizing these benefits at scale will require human-technical workflow integration – e.g., an AI recommendation to skip an MRI sequence is useful only if the radiologist trusts it and the techs have a workflow to implement it smoothly.

14.7 FUTURE OUTLOOK AND CALL TO ACTION

Looking ahead, aligning AI with environmental sustainability will likely become an expected part of healthcare innovation. To achieve sustainability in healthcare AI at scale, broader policy initiatives are necessary:

- **Research and innovation:** The intersection of AI and sustainability is a budding research field. We can expect more studies in both adaptation and mitigation – quantifying/reducing AI-related emissions in different clinical contexts as well as preparing the health system to deal with climate-impacted care.

- **Standardization and ecolabeling:** As suggested earlier, advocate for clear sustainability metrics (and potential labeling) for healthcare IT products, analogous to the American ENERGY STAR certification [11, 26].

- **Governance and regulatory encouragement:** Push for policies mandating transparency on environmental impacts of healthcare AI tools during procurement and regulatory approvals. For instance, require vendors to disclose their carbon footprint or to have a plan for carbon neutrality.

- **International and interdisciplinary collaboration:** Solving sustainability in AI will involve cross-industry efforts. Engage in local, national, and international sustainability initiatives to exchange best practices and promote collective action [65, 66]. We can make sure that AI technology solutions suit our clinical priorities by voicing healthcare-specific needs (like reliability and privacy requirements and sustainability concerns).

- **Culture shift:** We anticipate a future culture where considering the carbon footprint becomes a normal part of clinical (informatics) operations. Just as radiation dose monitoring is now routine in radiology (with dose index registries, alerts for high dose, etc.), we might see "carbon dose" monitoring become routine – where sustainability will be increasingly baked into how we innovate and practice.

14.8 EDITORS' COMMENTS

By discussing the evolving concepts of sustainability in AI, this chapter has illustrated definitions, addressed the detrimental and positive sustainable aspects of clinical AI, and suggested a spectrum of technical strategies for health professionals to address these challenges. Hopefully developers and medical professionals can co-produce AI into a low-emissions future. The actions we take today, from simple energy-saving measures to advocating for systemic change, will determine whether AI becomes part of the climate solution rather than part of the problem. The ultimate goal is a healthcare system where clinical quality, economic efficiency, and environmental sustainability are achieved together, consequently benefitting patients, providers, and the planet.

REFERENCES

1. Romanello, M., Walawender, M., Hsu, S.C. et al. (2024) The 2024 Report of the Lancet Countdown on Health and Climate Change: Facing Record-Breaking Threats from Delayed Action. The Lancet. 404(10465):1847–1896. https://doi.org/10.1016/S0140-6736(24)01822-1.
2. Rabin, A.S., Pinsky, E.G. (2023) Reducing Health Care's Climate Impact – Mission Critical or Extra Credit? New England Journal of Medicine. Massachusetts Medical Society. 389(7):583–585. https://doi.org/10.1056/NEJMp2305709
3. Eckelman, M.J., Huang, K., Lagasse, R. et al. (2020) Health Care Pollution And Public Health Damage In The United States: An Update. Health Affairs. Health Affairs. 39(12):2071–2079. https://doi.org/10.1377/hlthaff.2020.01247
4. Strubell, E., Ganesh, A., McCallum, A. (2019) Energy and Policy Considerations for Deep Learning in NLP. Proceedings of the 57th Annual Meeting of the Association for Computational Linguistics [Internet]. Florence, Italy: Association for Computational Linguistics; 2019 [cited 2022 Dec 6]. p. 3645–3650. Available from: https://aclanthology.org/P19-1355 [accessed June 2025]
5. Strubell, E., Ganesh, A., McCallum, A. (2020) Energy and Policy Considerations for Modern Deep Learning Research. Proceedings of the AAAI Conference on Artificial Intelligence. 34(09):13693–13696. https://doi.org/10.1609/aaai.v34i09.7123
6. Kaack, L.H., Donti, P.L., Strubell, E. et al. (2022) Aligning Artificial Intelligence with Climate Change Mitigation. Nature Climate Change. 12(6):518–527. https://doi.org/10.1038/s41558-022-01377-7
7. Doo, F.X., Vosshenrich, J., Cook, T.S. et al. (2024) Environmental Sustainability and AI in Radiology: A Double-Edged Sword. Radiology. 310(2):e232030. https://doi.org/10.1148/radiol.232030
8. McKee, H., Brown, M.J., Kim, H.H.R. et al. (2024) Planetary Health and Radiology: Why We Should Care and What We Can Do. Radiology. 311(1):e240219. https://doi.org/10.1148/radiol.240219
9. Doo, F.X., McGinty, G.B. (2023) Building Diversity, Equity, and Inclusion Within Radiology Artificial Intelligence: Representation Matters, from Data to the Workforce. Journal of the American College of Radiology. 20(9):852–856. https://doi.org/10.1016/j.jacr.2023.06.014
10. Singh, H., Eckelman, M., Berwick, D.M. et al. (2022) Mandatory Reporting of Emissions to Achieve Net-Zero Health Care. New England Journal of Medicine. Massachusetts Medical Society. 387(26):2469–2476. https://doi.org/10.1056/NEJMsb2210022
11. Doo, F.X., Parekh, V.S., Kanhere, A. et al. (2024) Evaluation of Climate-Aware Metrics Tools for Radiology Informatics and Artificial Intelligence: Toward a Potential Radiology Ecolabel. Journal of the American College of Radiology. 21(2):239–247. https://doi.org/10.1016/j.jacr.2023.11.019
12. World Health Organization. Climate change and health research: current trends, gaps and perspectives for the future [Internet]. World Health Organization; 2021. Available from: https://apps.who.int/iris/handle/10665/353062 [accessed 30th June 2025]
13. Bashir, N., Irwin, D., Shenoy, P. (2023) On the Promise and Pitfalls of Optimizing Embodied Carbon. Proceedings of the 2nd Workshop on Sustainable Computer Systems [Internet]. New York, NY, USA: Association for Computing Machinery; 2023 [cited 2025 Apr 4]. p. 1–6. Available from: https://dl.acm.org/doi/10.1145/3604930.3605710 [accessed June 2025]
14. McAlister, S., McGain, F., Petersen, M. et al. (2022) The Carbon Footprint of Hospital Diagnostic Imaging in Australia. The Lancet Regional Health - Western Pacific. 24:100459. https://doi.org/10.1016/j.lanwpc.2022.100459
15. Patterson, D., Gonzalez, J., Le, Q. et al. (2021) Carbon Emissions and Large Neural Network Training. arXiv (Preprint) [Internet]. 2021 Apr 23 [cited 2023 Jul 6]; Available from: http://arxiv.org/abs/2104.10350 [accessed June 2025]
16. Sadr, A.V., Bülow, R., von Stillfried, S. et al. (2024) Operational Greenhouse-Gas Emissions of Deep Learning in Digital Pathology: a Modelling Study. The Lancet Digital Health. 6(1):e58–e69. https://doi.org/10.1016/S2589-7500(23)00219-4
17. Li, P., Yang, J., Islam, M.A. et al. (2023) Making AI Less "Thirsty": Uncovering and Addressing the Secret Water Footprint of AI Models. arXiv (Preprint) [Internet]. 2023 Apr 6 [cited 2023 Sep 1]; Available from: http://arxiv.org/abs/2304.03271 [accessed June 2025]

18. Mytton, D. (2021) Data Centre Water Consumption. NPJ Clean Water. 4(1):1–6. https://doi.org/10.1038/s41545-021-00101-w
19. Monserrate, S.G. (2022) The Cloud Is Material: On the Environmental Impacts of Computation and Data Storage. MIT Case Studies in Social and Ethical Responsibilities of Computing [Internet]. MIT Schwarzman College of Computing; 2022 Jan 27 [cited 2023 Oct 3];(Winter 2022). Available from: https://mit-serc.pubpub.org/pub/the-cloud-is-material/release/1 [accessed June 2025]
20. Siddik, M.A.B., Shehabi, A., Marston., L. (2021) The Environmental Footprint of Data Centers in the United States. Environmental Research Letters. 16(6):064017. https://doi.org/10.1088/1748-9326/abfba1
21. Koomey, J., Masanet, E. (2021) Does Not Compute: Avoiding Pitfalls Assessing the Internet's Energy and Carbon Impacts. Joule. 5(7):1625–1628. https://doi.org/10.1016/j.joule.2021.05.007
22. Patterson, D., Gonzalez, J., Hölzle, U. et al. (2022) The Carbon Footprint of Machine Learning Training Will Plateau, Then Shrink. Computer. IEEE Computer Society. 55(07):18–28. https://doi.org/10.48550/arXiv.2204.05149
23. Doo, F.X., Kulkarni, P., Siegel, E.L. et al. (2024) Economic and Environmental Costs of Cloud Technologies for Medical Imaging and Radiology Artificial Intelligence. Journal of the American College of Radiology. 21(2):248–256. https://doi.org/10.1016/j.jacr.2023.11.011
24. Hoffmann, J., Borgeaud, S., Mensch, A. et al. (2022) Training Compute-Optimal Large Language Models. arXiv (Preprint) [Internet]. 2022 Mar 29 [cited 2023 Sep 13]; Available from: http://arxiv.org/abs/2203.15556 [accessed June 2025]
25. Doo, F.X., Savani, D., Kanhere, A. et al. (2024) Optimal Large Language Model Characteristics to Balance Accuracy and Energy Use for Sustainable Medical Applications. Radiology. 312(2):e240320. https://doi.org/10.1148/radiol.240320
26. ENERGY STAR [Internet]. 1992 [cited 2023 May 6]. Available from https://www.energystar.gov/about/how-energy-star-works/history
27. McAlister, S., Barratt, A., Bell, K. et al. (2024) How Many Carbon Emissions Are Saved by Doing One Less MRI? The Lancet Planetary Health. Elsevier. 8(6):e350. https://doi.org/10.1016/S2542-5196(24)00092-5
28. A guide to good practice for digital and data-driven health technologies [Internet]. GOV.UK. [cited 2025 Apr 5]. Available from: https://www.gov.uk/government/publications/code-of-conduct-for-data-driven-health-and-care-technology/initial-code-of-conduct-for-data-driven-health-and-care-technology [accessed June 2025]
29. Chua, A.L.B., Amin, R., Zhang, J. et al. (2021) The Environmental Impact of Interventional Radiology: An Evaluation of Greenhouse Gas Emissions from an Academic Interventional Radiology Practice. Journal of Vascular and Interventional Radiology. 32(6):907–915.e3. https://doi.org/10.1016/j.jvir.2021.03.531
30. Bujak, J.W. (2015) Heat Recovery from Thermal Treatment of Medical Waste. Energy. 90:1721–1732. https://doi.org/10.1016/j.energy.2015.06.124
31. Heye, T., Knoerl, R., Wehrle, T. et al. (2020) The Energy Consumption of Radiology: Energy- and Cost-Saving Opportunities for CT and MRI Operation. Radiology. Radiological Society of North America. 295(3):593–605. https://doi.org/10.1148/radiol.2020192084
32. Sutton, R.T., Pincock, D., Baumgart, D.C. et al. (2020) An Overview of Clinical Decision Support Systems: Benefits, Risks, and Strategies for Success. NPJ Digital Medicine. 3(1):1–10. https://doi.org/10.1038/s41746-020-0221-y
33. Schranz, A.L., Ryan, D.T., David, R. et al. (2024) Impact of Point-of-Care Clinical Decision Support on Referrer Behavior, Imaging Volume, Patient Radiation Dose Exposure, and Sustainability. Insights into Imaging. 15(1):4. https://doi.org/10.1186/s13244-023-01567-7
34. Cunningham, E., Schlicher, J., Yanes, A. et al. (2024) A Physician-Created Platform to Speed Clinical Decision-Making and Referral Workflow. NEJM Catalyst. 5(9):CAT.23.0401. https://doi.org/10.1056/CAT.23.0401
35. Doo, F.X. (2024) Sustainable diagnosis: Environmental impact of imaging AI [Internet]. THIS Space, the annual conference of The Healthcare Improvement Studies (THIS) Institute at the University of Cambridge. 2024 [cited 2025 Apr]. Available from: https://www.thisinstitute.cam.ac.uk/events/this-space-2024-2/ [accessed June 2025]
36. Gulshan, V., Peng, L., Coram, M. et al. (2016) Development and Validation of a Deep Learning Algorithm for Detection of Diabetic Retinopathy in Retinal Fundus Photographs. JAMA. 316(22):2402–2410. https://doi.org/10.1001/jama.2016.17216
37. Ipp, E., Liljenquist, D., Bode, B. et al. (2021) EyeArt Study Group. Pivotal Evaluation of an Artificial Intelligence System for Autonomous Detection of Referrable and Vision-Threatening Diabetic Retinopathy. JAMA Network Open. 4(11):e2134254. https://doi.org/10.1001/jamanetworkopen.2021.34254
38. Zhang, Y., Shi, J., Peng, Y. et al. (2020) Artificial Intelligence-Enabled Screening for Diabetic Retinopathy: A Real-World, Multicenter and Prospective Study. BMJ Open Diabetes Res Care. 8(1):e001596. https://doi.org/10.1136/bmjdrc-2020-001596
39. Kwon, H.J., Park, S., Park, Y.H. et al. (2024) Development of Blood Demand Prediction Model Using Artificial Intelligence Based on National Public Big Data. Digit Health. 10. https://doi.org/10.1177/20552076231224245
40. Schilling, M., Rickmann, L., Hutschenreuter, G. et al. (2022) Reduction of Platelet Outdating and Shortage by Forecasting Demand With Statistical Learning and Deep Neural Networks: Modeling Study. JMIR Medical Informatics. 10(2):e29978. https://doi.org/10.2196/29978
41. Hurley, N.C., Schroeder, K.M., Hess, A.S. (2023) Would Doctors Dream of Electric Blood Bankers? Large Language Model-Based Artificial Intelligence Performs Well in Many Aspects of Transfusion Medicine. Transfusion. 63(10):1833–1840. https://doi.org/10.1111/trf.17526
42. Ghouri, A.M., Khan, H.R., Mani, V. et al. (2023) An Artificial-Intelligence-Based Omnichannel Blood Supply Chain: A Pathway for Sustainable Development. Journal of Business Research. 164:113980. https://doi.org/10.1016/j.jbusres.2023.113980
43. Tang, C., Fang, K., Guo, Y. et al. (2017) Safety of Sulfur Hexafluoride Microbubbles in Sonography of Abdominal and Superficial Organs: Retrospective Analysis of 30,222 Cases. Journal of Ultrasound in Medicine. 36(3):531–538.
44. Zhao, B., Xu, Q., Lu, J. (2024) Recent Advances in Abatement of Methane and Sulfur Hexafluoride non-CO2 Greenhouse Gases Under Dual-Carbon Target. Science of the Total Environment. 948:174992. https://doi.org/10.1016/j.scitotenv.2024.174992
45. Simmonds, P.G., Rigby, M., Manning, A.J. et al. (2020) The Increasing Atmospheric Burden of the Greenhouse Gas Sulfur Hexafluoride (SF6). Atmospheric Chemistry and Physics. 20(12):7271–7290. https://doi.org/10.5194/acp-20-7271-2020
46. Brünjes, R., Hofmann, T. (2020) Anthropogenic Gadolinium in Freshwater and Drinking Water Systems. Water Research. 182:115966. https://doi.org/10.1016/j.watres.2020.115966
47. Kümmerer, K., Helmers, E. (2000) Hospital Effluents as a Source of Gadolinium in the Aquatic Environment. Environmental Science & Technology - ACS. 34(4):573–577. https://doi.org/10.1021/es990633h

48. Laczovics, A., Csige, I., Szabó, S. et al. (2023) Relationship between Gadolinium-Based MRI Contrast Agent Consumption and Anthropogenic Gadolinium in the Influent of a Wastewater Treatment Plant. Science of the Total Environment. 877:162844. https://doi.org/10.1016/j.scitotenv.2023.162844

49. Oluwasola, I.E., Ahmad, A.L., Shoparwe, N.F. et al. (2022) Gadolinium Based Contrast Agents (GBCAs): Uniqueness, Aquatic Toxicity Concerns, and Prospective Remediation. Journal of Contaminant Hydrology. 250:104057. https://pubmed.ncbi.nlm.nih.gov/36130428/#:~:text=doi%3A%2010.1016/j.jconhyd.2022.10405

50. Pereto, C., Lerat-Hardy, A., Baudrimont, M. et al. (2023) European Fluxes of Medical Gadolinium to the Ocean: A Model Based on Healthcare Databases. Environment International. 173:107868. https://doi.org/10.1016/j.envint.2023.107868

51. Cao, K., Xia, Y., Yao, J. et al. (2023) Large-Scale Pancreatic Cancer Detection via non-Contrast CT and Deep Learning. Nature Medicine. 29(12):3033–3043. https://oi.org/10.1038/s41591-023-02640-w

52. Choi, J.W., Cho, Y.J., Ha, J.Y. et al. (2021) Generating Synthetic Contrast Enhancement from non-Contrast Chest Computed Tomography Using a Generative Adversarial Network. Scientific Reports. 11(1):20403. https://doi.org/10.1038/s41598-021-00058-3.

53. Yusuf, H., Gor, R., Saheed, R.M. et al. (2024) Travel-Associated Carbon Emissions of Patients Receiving Cancer Treatment from an Urban Safety Net Hospital. Future Healthcare Journal. 11(4):100174. https://doi.org/10.1016/j.fhj.2024.100174

54. Bryant, A.K., Lewy, J.R., Bressler, R.D. et al. (2024) Projected Environmental and Public Health Benefits of Extended-Interval Dosing: an Analysis of Pembrolizumab Use in a US National Health System. The Lancet Oncology. 25(6):802–810. https://doi.org/10.1016/S1470-2045(24)00200-6

55. Ranschaert, E., Topff, L., Pianykh, O. (2021) Optimization of Radiology Workflow With Artificial Intelligence. Radiologic Clinics of North America. 59(6):955–966. https://doi.org/10.1016/j.rcl.2021.06.006

56. Liu, D., Shin, W.Y., Sprecher, E. et al. (2022) Machine Learning Approaches to Predicting No-Shows in Pediatric Medical Appointment. NPJ Digital Medicine. 5(1):1–11. https://doi.org/10.1038/s41746-022-00594-w.

57. Walsh, A. (2024) How embracing Artificial Intelligence improves the human experience [Internet]. The Health Innovation Network. 2024 [cited 2025 Apr 5]. Available from: https://thehealthinnovationnetwork.co.uk/blogs/how-embracing-artificial-intelligence-improves-the-human-experience/ [accessed June 2025]

58. Sharma, V., Pritchard-Jones, R., Scott, S. et al. (2023) Accuracy of a Tool to Prioritise Patients Awaiting Elective Surgery: an Implementation Report. BMJ Health Care Inform. 30(1):e100687. https://doi.org/10.1136/bmjhci-2022-100687

59. Constantinou, A.D., Hoole, A., Wong, D.C. et al (2025) OSAIRIS: Lessons Learned From the Hospital-Based Implementation and Evaluation of an Open-Source Deep-Learning Model for Radiotherapy Image Segmentation. Clinical Oncology Journal - Royal College Of Radiologists. 37:103660–39522322. https://doi.org/10.1016/j.clon.2024.10.032

60. Tao, Y., Yang, L., Jaffe, S. et al. (2023) Climate mitigation potentials of teleworking are sensitive to changes in lifestyle and workplace rather than ICT usage. Proceedings of the National Academy of Sciences. Proceedings of the National Academy of Sciences; 2023 Sep 26;120(39):e2304099120. https://doi.org/10.1073/pnas.2304099120

61. Stefaniec, A., Brazil, W., Whitney, W. et al. (2024) Examining the Long-Term Reduction in Commuting Emissions from Working from Home. Transportation Research Part D: Transport and Environment. 127:104063. https://doi.org/10.1016/j.trd.2024.104063

62. Brouillette, M. (2024) Medical Schools Are Updating Their Curricula as Climate Change Becomes Impossible to Ignore. JAMA. 332(10):775–776. https://doi.org/10.1001/jama.2024.13506

63. Jowell, A., Lachenauer, A., Lu, J. et al. (2023) A Model for Comprehensive Climate and Medical Education. The Lancet Planetary Health. 7(1):e2–e3. https://doi.org/10.1016/S2542-5196(22)00215-7

64. Succi, M.D., Chang, B.S., Rao, A.S. (2025) Building the AI-Enabled Medical School of the Future. JAMA. https://doi.org/10.1001/jama.2025.2789

65. Schoen, J., McGinty, G.B., Quirk, C. (2021) Radiology in Our Changing Climate: A Call to Action. Journal of the American College of Radiology. 18(7):1041–1043. https://doi.org/10.1016/j.jacr.2021.02.009

66. Rockall, A.G., Allen, B., Brown, M.J. et al. (2025) Sustainability in Radiology: Position Paper and Call to Action from ACR, AOSR, ASR, CAR, CIR, ESR, ESRNM, ISR, IS3R, RANZCR, and RSNA. Radiology. Radiological Society of North America. 314(3). https://doi.org/10.1148/radiol.250325

Case Study A: Practical Implication – How to Integrate AI Responsibly into Life and Personal Health – The Hear Glue Ear Example

Tamsin Browne

A.1 THE PROBLEM

Working as a paediatrician with expertise in hearing and development, I saw a gap in the system for patients with mild, fluctuating, hearing loss caused by congestion from coughs, colds or ear infections. This type of congestion is often called *glue ear* although its medical name is *otitis media* with a fusion, abbreviated to OME.

Whilst most adults have experience of getting congested and not hearing very well during a bad cold, adults are able to understand phrased speech and maintain the gist of sentences even if they miss up to 50% of the what's being said. Adults are not generally learning new words; they can read to mitigate any problems; they have developed a certain amount of lip-reading skills; and they have social skills to be able to explain to others about their hearing and communication needs.

Children, on the other hand, have smaller anatomy and when they get bunged up from coughs and colds, the congestion in the middle ear (fluid building up behind the eardrum) can be more persistent, lasting many weeks and sometimes months. The other problem is that children get so many coughs and colds that parents often comment on constantly streaming noses. This means that glue ear can recur. In fact, 80% of children will experience glue ear in their childhood and around one quarter to one third will experience it more than once. Glue ear tends to cause a fluctuating mild to moderate, unilateral or bilateral hearing loss for a few days, weeks, months or even years. It often self resolves over time and children tend to experience it less as they grow into pre-teens and teenagers.

The medical pathway for managing glue ear often starts with the parents attending an initial visit to a health visitor or family practitioner about their child not listening, saying "Pardon?" or "What?" all the time or turning up the volume on the television. Sometimes the initial concern is around mispronunciations, or speech and language delay. Research suggests that children struggling with reading in the first few years at school could benefit from having a hearing screening test. After the initial presentation the child will be referred for a hearing test, if the first hearing test shows that a child has glue ear, there is a three-month waiting period to see if the condition self-resolves. If the second hearing test three months later also shows hearing loss secondary to glue ear, then the child is referred to an ear specialist or ear, nose and throat (ENT) surgeon, who will consider further management. The ear surgeon may discuss hearing aids or a grommet operation (grommets is a UK term for what are known as tympanostomy tubes or T-tubes in other countries).

The first data collection of 200 patients going through this pathway showed that, on average, children waited around 12 months to get an intervention (from first presenting to a doctor to having a hearing aid or a grommet operation). Twelve months is a long time to have a hearing loss, particularly at such a critical time in development. Twelve months is also a large proportion of a child's life. There is a lot of research indicating the importance of good development in the first five years of life and the impact of hearing loss on development. Yet all the school hearing screening programmes in the UK and across Europe had fairly consistently shown that one in ten children starting school will have glue ear. Hearing support is widely available in high-income countries and yet children routinely waited long periods of time between appointments, with hearing difficulties that risk their development. In paediatric clinics, I would see children who had a history of glue ear, later presenting with concerns around attention, listening, learning, speech and language difficulties, auditory processing difficulties, dyslexia, social communication or autistic features.

It didn't feel like rocket science to be suggesting that children with hearing loss need to be able to hear in a timely way and be supported not to fall behind in their development.

A.2 PERSONAL EXPERIENCE

With five children myself the odds were that one child would have glue ear, and indeed my fourth child had persistent ear infections leading to glue ear which impacted her hearing. She would particularly struggle to hear after any coughs or colds. Her other siblings constantly brought back viruses from school or nursery, and she would pick up frequent upper respiratory tract infections. I sometimes wonder if she had an immunoglobulin A deficiency, which is also associated with glue ear, but she was never tested. Her glue ear was diagnosed as she started school. She found reading challenging and spelling particularly difficult and therefore would shy away from books or writing.

Listening difficulties led to listening fatigue, and therefore school days felt long. Her learning trajectory slowed, and her confidence waned. It also turned out that even if you were a paediatrician and knew all the medical colleagues involved in the National Health Service (NHS) pathways, it still took one year for her to receive an intervention and receive a grommet operation. Complications from grommet operations include postoperative ear infections and a persisting hole in the eardrum, which also happened to her. If an eardrum is discharging pus or has a hole, it cannot perform its function well and therefore the child still has some degree of hearing loss. I tried to find hearing support, but her hearing often fluctuated, which is hard to programme a hearing aid to, and any ear discharge or pus meant she couldn't wear something in her ear anyway. Bone conduction hearing aids were very expensive and not routinely available.

Bone conduction hearing aids can be very useful in glue ear (and in fact many middle-ear conditions) because they turn sound into a vibration and send the vibration across the bones of the skull directly to the inner hearing (known as the cochlea). This means that the sound does not need to travel through the air to the eardrum and can be simply rerouted as a vibration round the eardrum (bypassing any glue ear). However, this type of bone-conduction (BC) hearing aids are costly, often £1000 to £3000, which means that at the time, they were not regularly used – particularly for a condition which affects so many children across the country. Therefore, my initial resolve was to use these bone conduction hearing aids in a study to see if supporting children early with this type of aid would improve hearing while they had glue ear and therefore reduce any resulting speech difficulties, developmental delays or learning problems. However, a trusted colleague pointed out that even if it was proved that BC aids should be used, they were still too costly for the health service or parents to afford them. This is what triggered a journey into innovation.

A.3 THE MISSION – SUPPORT HEARING EARLY AND STOP CHILDREN FROM FALLING BEHIND

I was pretty sure that if a child couldn't see well, we would send them to school with a pair of glasses, and yet we were allowing children to go to school with poor hearing for long periods of time, despite prolific and robust research showing the impact this could potentially have on speech, development and learning. The mission was to help children to hear at an early stage (with a hearing technology or hearing headset) and also to leverage all that time between appointments, where the families could be empowered to support their child at home to develop skills that were frequently affected by glue ear. This included listening skills, auditory processing skills, reading skills, auditory memory as well as speech and language enrichment.

The developmental support could be available via an app (see Figure A.1).

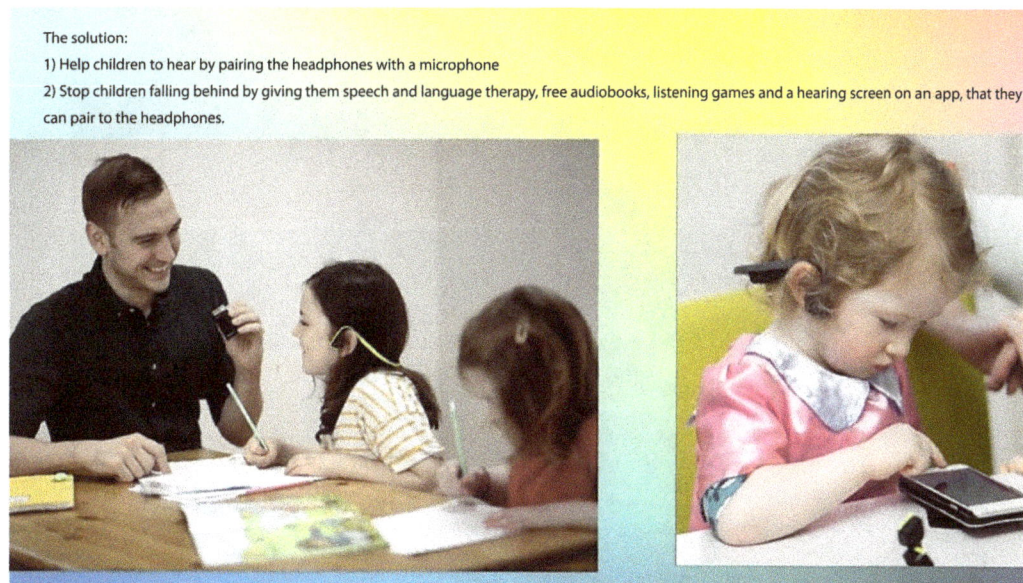

The solution:

1) Help children to hear by pairing the headphones with a microphone

2) Stop children falling behind by giving them speech and language therapy, free audiobooks, listening games and a hearing screen on an app, that they can pair to the headphones.

Figure A.1 The hearing device.

The child could wear simple headphones that use bone conduction technology and could be paired via Bluetooth to a small microphone that could be worn by a teacher or parent or perhaps a speech and language therapist. This would help the child to hear what the teacher, parent or therapist was explaining, particularly over any background noise.

Alternatively, the BC headphones could be paired via Bluetooth to a computer, smart phone or tablet to access an app. The app could help to track the child's hearing at home and provide child-development activities around phonics, rhyming words, reading, listening and processing auditory information.

A.4 THE APP

The app had a speech and language therapy section where videos demonstrate to families how to support a child's speech and language development (Figure A.2). An information section explains further details about glue ear. Songs provide rhyming words so that children can hear the differences between similar-sounding words.

Specially written books can be used as audiobooks (which helps auditory processing and listening skills) and questions at the end of the stories stimulate a child's auditory memory.

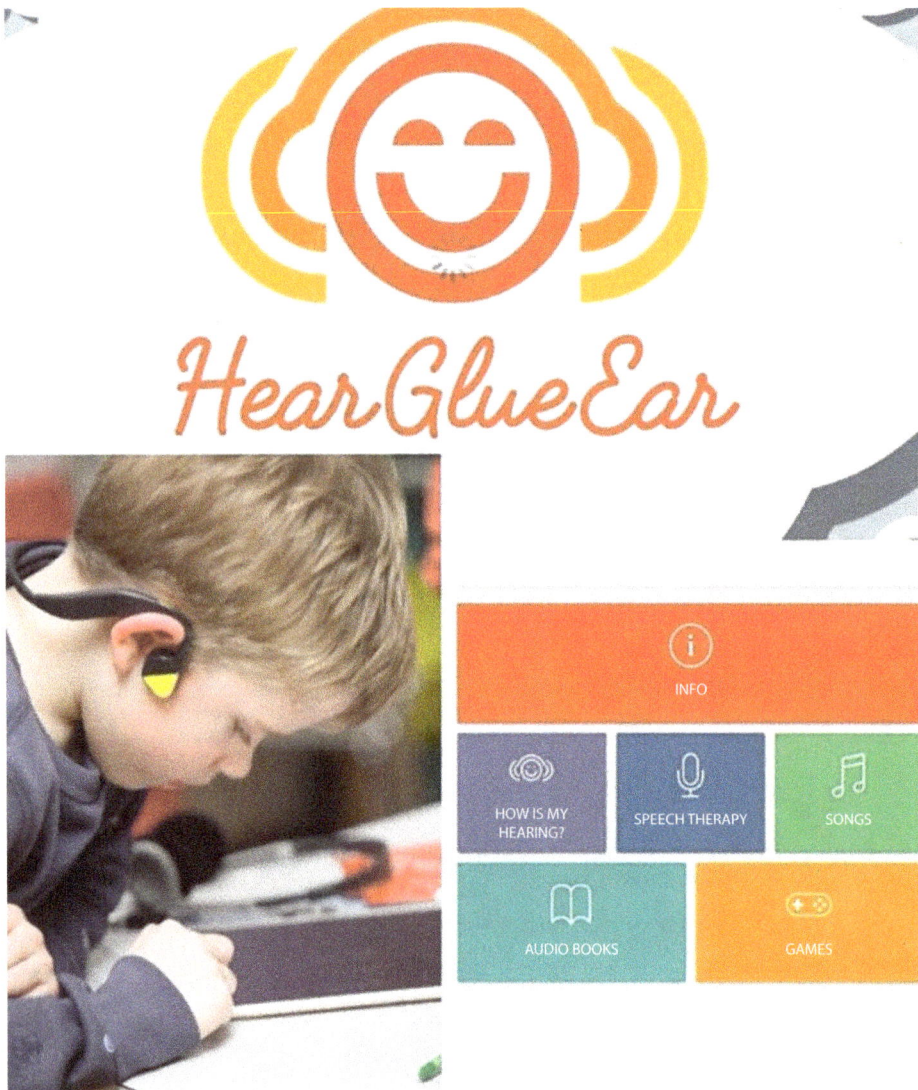

Figure A.2   Hear Glue Ear app.

A.4.1 The Team Around the App

The app was planned with audiologists, teachers of the deaf, sensory support teachers, paediatricians, ENT surgeons, clinical engineers and speech therapists. The multidisciplinary team were clear that the app should be kept simple. The app was designed for two- to eight-year-olds and aimed to appeal to typically developing children as well as children with Down syndrome, as Down syndrome is associated with a higher instance of glue ear.

A.4.2 Patient and Public Involvement, Co-Production and Research

Although I thought we had done well by getting a group of families together in a village hall to discuss their needs around what was needed in an app to support glue ear, I did not manage to keep the same group involved enough. Subsequently, once the app was built, we began a research study which immediately involved children and families pointing out improvements that were needed. Hence the research study had to be stopped, changes needed to be made to the app, and the research study restarted again.

At the time it was difficult to know what outcomes people wanted to see around app use, and many organisations couldn't give any steer on what digital health outcomes were important when evaluating an app.

Additionally, in 2018 there was no patient Wi-Fi available within the hospital, and therefore we were unable to help patients to download the app onto their phone or device with support from the team; instead, they had to go away with a piece of paper and remember to download it at home. Despite this, 73% of families downloaded the app and were still using it a week after the appointment. I telephoned Organisation Reviewing Care and Health Apps (ORCHA) and asked them if 73% was a reasonable number. They were particularly congratulatory since they had noticed this was about the maximum any apps were engaging with patients. Digital exclusion was prevalent, although the gap was closing year on year, and would close significantly over the COVID-19 pandemic which affected the world a year later.

A.4.3 Lack of App Downloads

The app was created in 2018 and by 2019 had been researched, registered as a medical device and obtained high ORCHA patient safety scores. However, no staff were downloading the app. There were multiple barriers to staff engagement: although some staff were complimentary about the app, they felt that they were "not techy" and weren't sure about using apps on their own phones never mind anyone else's, so would rather not recommend apps to others. Digital literacy was variable amongst staff. Many staff had trained in hospitals where mobile phones were not allowed and had remembered notices on the walls banning mobile phone use in clinical areas. The government and medical organisations expected adoption of new digital health solutions, but medical and specialty training was devoid of any digital health education. No staff were trained in digital health. At the time, the majority of medical organisations did not have a digital health committee, with very few hospital-based digital experts who could advise on health apps. Previously patient leaflets had to be approved through hospital reading committees, but there was no hospital committee to review apps. In order to adopt and use one app, staff needed to understand the wider benefits of digital health solutions.

However, paediatric clinics were full of children walking in with devices/phones/iPads/tablets and parents were delighted to distract their child while they talked. Children loved being on devices but some of the time used them to watch questionable material. Screen time was being widely vilified (although this didn't seem to stop children being on devices). Hear Glue Ear studies were mindful of not adding too much screen time and therefore never recommended app use for longer than 15 minutes a day. Prescribing apps was not a common topic and the NHS library, which started with a very small number of apps, later closed down. At the time, a local survey of both medical students and consultants to understand digital health adoption indicated a low level of understanding, similar to that of the general public, with many turning to app store ratings or other social media posts for recommendations. Fortunately, consultants additionally reported that they would recommend only an app that they had looked through themselves and had accessed research papers on. Clinicians had no way of knowing how to include app recommendations in consultations. Indeed, in order to prescribe an app, clinicians needed to take a digital history regarding a patient's digital literacy and digital environment. It is important that an app is not simply recommended as an afterthought at the end of a consultation but recorded in the patient's notes and updated when needed. Some apps are sustainable only through charging a fee, but the NHS expects healthcare to be free. The Hear Glue Ear app was kept free due to charity partnerships, ensuring that it did not propagate health inequalities: Children in low-income families can have poorer outcomes and therefore needed free access to support.

Despite having multiple assurances around the app, the team sought an award for the Hear Glue Ear app in the hope that it would encourage people to use it. The app won children's app of the year at the UK app awards in 2019 and became "award winning" but unfortunately that did not encourage staff to use it.

When the NHS app library collapsed, ORCHA built an app library; new regulations for apps emerged, such as digital technology assessment criteria (DTAC), and app store updates were needed regularly. Funding became an issue, and no discounts or provisions were awarded for apps that were charity funded or trying to remain free to the general public. Charity partnerships were crucial for the Hear Glue Ear app to succeed: The Cambridge Hearing Trust and the National Deaf Children's Society (NDCS) were critical in keeping the app available to families.

A.5 THE COVID PANDEMIC

During the COVID (coronavirus) pandemic, families were unable to access medical services and most children's hearing services were not considered essential. It was announced nationally that grommet operations were unable to be prioritised. The numbers of people using the app increased quickly as patients sought out a solution by themselves. The Hear Glue Ear app was the only solution for glue ear. Driven by patients using the app, organisations started recommending the app and healthcare staff began asking how to prescribe apps. As the popularity grew, the app began to win awards and was included in digital health recommendations. However, the app was still relying on charity funding.

COVID became an opportunity for another research study to see if families could self-manage glue ear remotely at home, without seeing healthcare professionals. Details of the app and a BC headset were sent to families who consented to be part of the trial. Results showed that families were particularly good at self-managing glue ear at home, and as lockdown lifted, families who were part of the study, felt more empowered to manage future recurrences of glue ear. Lockdown meant many children's glue ear resolved over time, so they could be supported until it cleared up naturally, and well over half never went on to have a grommet operation.

A.5.1 Keeping the App Sustainable

As more patients used the Hear Glue Ear app, larger companies became interested in its reach, and became interested in acquiring the app. Since the costs of keeping the app registered as a medical device, further regulatory costs (such as DTAC), app store updates and app improvements were difficult to maintain using only charity funding, an exit started to look appealing (particularly if an exit agreement included the app being adopted in other countries but being allowed to remain free in the UK).

A.5.2 Maintaining Co-Production with End Users

Having learnt from earlier mistakes, the team kept children and their families engaged in product development and improvement. One child managed to make the headset not just acceptable but "super cool by telling her friends it was the 'extendable ear' from Harry Potter. The team then made an ear-shaped cover for the small microphone component of the BC headset, which added fun to the product and, in fact, helped younger children or those with learning difficulties to better understand how the product worked.

Low-income countries became interested in the low-cost solution for the most common type of childhood hearing loss. The Queen Elizabeth Central Hospital in Malawi was an excellent hospital – forward thinking enough to be interested in whether the hearing BC headset and app could be used to alleviate the problem of poor access to healthcare and the need for affordable ear and hearing care. In many low-income countries, there is a higher burden of ear disease and hearing loss, but much of the population will never access audiology services. Low-income countries also have a higher incidence of chronically discharging ears (known as chronic suppurative otitis media), often impacted by poor nutrition, cooking smoke exposure and lack of access to antibiotics and healthcare procedures. Interestingly, home telephones were so slowly adopted that more people had mobile phones than landlines, and some had smartphones despite extraordinarily low average incomes. There was genuine interest in both the headsets and the app to enable people to self-manage hearing difficulties (Figure A.3).

Boxes of donated behind-the-ear hearing aids often sat unused at Queen Elizabeth Hospital due to the inability to source hearing aid batteries, which need replacing every two weeks and are

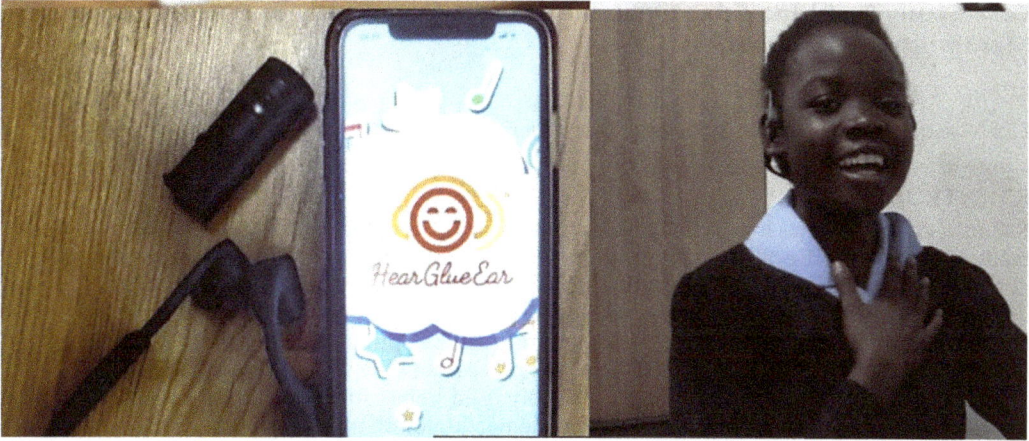

Figure A.3 Self-management of hearing using Hear Glue Ear app and BC headset.

expensive to purchase. Although the BC headset and phone with an app can both be charged, electricity supply is variable across Malawi and many people in 2024 had no electricity in their home. Therefore, the team sourced affordable solar powered chargers locally in Malawi that could charge both the headset and a phone.

The World Health Organisation (WHO) hosts the World Hearing Forum, which prioritises ear and hearing care. Improved hearing can impact education and employment, which in turn can improve the economy of a country. WHO is also supportive of assistive technologies that enable people to self-manage their own hearing without the need for trained audiologists. The team continues to raise money for ongoing work in low-income countries.

Case Study B: AI for Adaptive Learning – A Case Study in Personalising Mammography Education

Ziba Gandomkar, Moayyad Suleiman, Mary Rickard, and Patrick Brennan

B.1 INTRODUCTION

Radiology education has long relied on structured curricula, didactic teaching, and self-assessment modules to train and evaluate diagnostic accuracy. In breast imaging—where early detection of cancer hinges on nuanced interpretation—continued education and feedback are critical. However, despite the availability of self-assessment tools [1], considerable variability remains in individual reader improvement. A standardised approach may not be optimal for all learners, as prior experience, perception of case difficulty, and cognitive processing vary widely among radiologists.

Test set-based assessments have become widely used to measure reader performance outside of the clinical setting. Importantly, research has demonstrated that performance in test set environments can meaningfully reflect real-world diagnostic behaviour. For instance, Soh et al. [2] showed that when prior images are included, test set readings produce a reasonable level of agreement with actual clinical reporting in screening mammography. Using reader-specific test sets derived from clinical cases, the study found statistically significant concordance in group-level performance metrics, such as side-specific sensitivity and ROI-based figures of merit, between laboratory test conditions and clinical outcomes. These findings validate the use of curated test sets as a reliable proxy for clinical performance—especially when used at scale for quality assurance, education, and research.

Nonetheless, the variability in how individual readers respond to test sets—and the limited granularity in how such test sets are currently assembled—presents a missed opportunity for educational optimisation. While test sets provide objective benchmarks, they are often static and lack the responsiveness needed to adapt to each reader's evolving skill level. This case study examines a novel application of *artificial intelligence (AI) to personalise education in mammographic interpretation*, focusing on a system developed at the University of Sydney and Detected-X. This AI-driven framework dynamically adapts test sets based on user profiles, historical interactions, and case complexity, offering a tailored educational experience that addresses the shortcomings of traditional training approaches.

B.2 THE NEED FOR PERSONALISED EDUCATION IN MAMMOGRAPHY

Self-assessment modules in breast imaging—especially mammography—are essential for maintaining diagnostic competence. These modules typically include a mix of normal and abnormal cases with feedback on performance. While effective in principle, empirical studies show that average improvement after such modules varies between 21% and 31% [3], highlighting substantial inter-reader variability.

This variability underscores the limitations of static, one-size-fits-all learning strategies. Artificial intelligence offers the potential to address this gap by modelling individual learning needs and image complexity to deliver personalised, responsive training.

B.3 AI-DRIVEN CUSTOMISATION OF MAMMOGRAPHY EDUCATION

Modern medical education increasingly emphasises personalisation, adaptability, and responsiveness to learner needs. In mammography education, traditional methods—such as fixed curricula or heuristic-based case selection—often fail to account for the diversity of learner backgrounds and the variability in case complexity. To address these gaps, we developed a suite of AI models (Figure B.1) aimed at customising educational pathways in mammographic image interpretation.

Our work brings together a multidisciplinary team of radiologists, computer scientists, and educators to design and implement AI-driven solutions that improve the relevance and effectiveness of self-assessment training modules. Specifically, we focus on three scenarios that reflect distinct learning contexts:

1. **New users without prior engagement,**

2. **Newly uploaded cases requiring difficulty categorisation**, and

3. **Existing users with an evolving interaction history**.

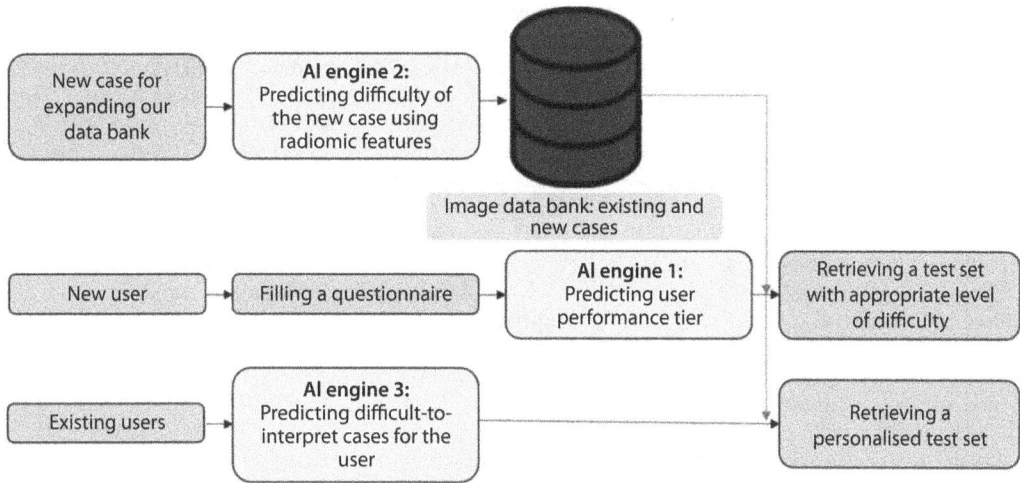

Figure B.1 A Suite of AI models for customisation of mammography education.

Each scenario is supported by a dedicated AI engine designed to enhance the user experience by predicting either reader performance, case difficulty, or reader–case interaction. Together, these engines enable dynamic case allocation—advancing mammography education beyond conventional approaches.

B.3.1 Scenario 1: Predicting Performance of New Users

A critical challenge in customising education for new users is the lack of performance history upon initial entry. Current guidelines for assigning reading tasks are generally heuristic-based and offer only limited predictive value. For example, a systematic review by our group [4] found that individual characteristics such as years of experience or training background are not consistently associated with diagnostic efficacy in screening mammography. While high reading volume and subspecialisation in breast imaging were correlated with better performance, these attributes alone do not provide a comprehensive basis for tailored learning pathways.

To overcome this, we developed an AI engine that estimates a new user's diagnostic performance using machine learning techniques applied to their demographic and professional background. The model was trained on data from 905 radiologists and breast physicians, incorporating variables such as age, gender, fellowship training, job role, weekly reading volume, and time spent in breast imaging. An ensemble of regression trees was used to predict a user's likely accuracy in interpreting screening mammograms, measured by the area under the ROC curve (AUC) [5].

The model achieved a Pearson correlation of 0.60 ($p < 0.001$) between predicted and actual AUCs and an AUC of 0.86 (95% CI: 0.83–0.89) for distinguishing users in the top and bottom performance quartiles. Based on these predictions, the system automatically assigns an initial test set with an appropriate level of difficulty. Moreover, by identifying the user's cohort, the system retrieves historically difficult cases for similar users, providing both challenge and relevance from the outset.

This data-driven approach enables immediate, meaningful engagement for new learners.

B.3.2 Scenario 2: Predicting Case Difficulty for New Materials

The integration of new cases into an adaptive learning platform presents a unique challenge: without any prior reader interaction, it is difficult to determine how challenging a new case will be. Conventional proxies such as breast density or expert consensus are often used, but these are subjective and, as our analyses have shown, fail to reliably capture actual case difficulty. Our approach leverages artificial intelligence—particularly radiomic and deep learning methods—to automatically assess the difficulty of new mammographic cases, enabling real-time triage and targeted allocation of educational content.

Our investigations began with handcrafted global radiomic features (GRFs)—quantitative descriptors capturing the shape, texture, and intensity distribution of mammographic images. We first explored how these features could explain cohort-specific error patterns in a study involving 36 radiologists from China and Australia [6, 7]. Each participant interpreted the same 60 dense mammograms, and global radiomic features were extracted using three spatial sampling methods: a central square region, the retroareolar region, and the whole breast. Using random forest models trained separately for each cohort, we assessed the ability of GRFs to predict three types of diagnostic errors: false positives, false negatives, and incorrect lesion localisation. The results were striking. For Chinese readers (cohort A), average AUCs for detecting false positives, false negatives, and location errors were 0.90, 0.66, and 0.45, respectively. For Australian readers (cohort B), the corresponding AUCs were 0.75, 0.73, and 0.60. These findings not only confirmed that global radiomic features can predict error-prone cases but also highlighted systematic variation in error types across cohorts. In both cohorts, regions with higher Gabor filter responses and maximum response filter outputs were more prone to false positives, while coarse textures and abrupt intensity changes were more predictive of false negatives. This cohort-specific radiomic profiling revealed that reader errors are influenced by training background and perceptual tendencies, reinforcing the value of localised educational strategies that target each group's diagnostic weaknesses.

To include non-dense mammograms and a broader sample of readers, we expanded our analysis to a larger cohort of 537 radiologists and breast physicians from Australia and New Zealand [8, 9]. Participants interpreted 239 normal mammograms, which were categorised as either easy or difficult based on collective error rates. Global radiomic features were extracted from both the craniocaudal (CC) and mediolateral oblique (MLO) views, and a combined CC+MLO model achieved an AUC of 0.71 in distinguishing difficult from easy cases. Of the 34 extracted features, 20 differed significantly between case groups. In contrast, breast density showed no significant association with interpretive difficulty, confirming that global radiomic features provide a more robust and discriminative metric.

Building on these results, we investigated whether global radiomic features could also predict which cases were most challenging for early-career readers. In a study [10] involving 137 radiology trainees interpreting normal mammographic cases, we used reader accuracy to classify cases as hardest or easiest. A machine learning model trained on global radiomic features achieved an AUC of 0.75, with features such as cluster prominence and intensity range emerging as strong predictors of difficulty. Once again, breast density failed to show significant discriminative value. These findings reinforced the ability of global radiomic features to capture image characteristics that impact interpretive complexity—particularly for novice readers who are more vulnerable to subtle visual traps.

To understand why global radiomic features perform so well in predicting interpretive difficulty, we investigated their relationship with radiologists' perceptual processing—specifically, the "gist" signal [11, 12]. Gist refers to the initial, rapid impression a radiologist forms within seconds of viewing a mammogram, and it has been linked to diagnostic accuracy in prior work [13–16]. In this study, experienced readers rated the perceptual gist strength of various mammograms. Radiomic features extracted from these images were then analysed, revealing strong correlations between global radiomic features and perceived gist. A classifier trained to distinguish high- from low-gist images achieved AUCs up to 0.84, suggesting that radiomic features encode the same global cues radiologists use during their intuitive, pre-attentive image assessment. This finding lends theoretical support to the use of global radiomic features in AI-driven education systems: not only do these features correlate with error rates, but they also align with the cognitive processes that underpin expert image interpretation.

With the predictive value of global radiomic features established, we advanced towards building a dedicated AI engine to evaluate new cases at scale. This model [17] integrated both global and local radiomic features to classify cases by difficulty prior to any user interaction. Validated using ten-fold cross validation, the engine achieved an AUC of 0.87 for difficult normal cases and 0.70 for difficult cancer cases. The hybrid approach allowed the model to capture both large-scale parenchymal complexity and fine-grained regional irregularities, offering more comprehensive case assessment. Crucially, this enabled the platform to incorporate new materials into test sets dynamically, providing users with appropriately challenging content regardless of when the case was added. Combining local and global radiomic features has also proven effective in predicting cohort-specific difficult cancer and normal cases [18].

We further refined our models using deep learning techniques. One study [19, 20] employed a convolutional neural network (CNN) with a ResNet-50 backbone to classify small image patches based on their likelihood of generating false positives. The model achieved excellent performance (AUCs of 0.93 and 0.97 across two reader cohorts), demonstrating that even subtle local features could be linked to systematic diagnostic mistakes. This study mapped likely false-positive regions (image patches) in a data-driven way by retrospectively identifying them from reader data. While effective as proof of concept, this approach is not scalable in practice, as it requires manual delineation of false-positive areas before they can be used to train a CNN.

To scale the identification of difficult normal cases, we developed a second deep learning pipeline designed specifically to detect challenging false-positive regions in cancer-free mammograms **in a fully automated way**. This study [21] addressed two key goals: first, to evaluate the extent to which current publicly available AI models can propose regions of interest (ROIs) that overlap with the actual false-positive areas (based on the actual mammogram interpretation by users); and second, to refine a deep learning model—based on the EfficientNet-B1 architecture—to distinguish between challenging and easy-to-interpret false-positive ROIs.

We used a dataset of 441 mammograms, all confirmed cancer-free through at least two years of follow-up, and each interpreted by an average of 142 radiologists or trainees. False-positive annotations were extracted and categorised as challenging if ≥10% of readers incorrectly identified the region, and as easy otherwise. To test the first aim, we submitted all 441 cases to three publicly available AI models, aggregating their ROI proposals and evaluating their coverage of the challenging false-positive regions. Impressively, this ensemble of AI-generated proposals achieved 99.56% coverage of the challenging false-positives and 98.00% of easy false-positives.

For the second aim, we fine-tuned an EfficientNet-B1 model using transfer learning and data augmentation, training it to distinguish challenging-from easy-to-interpret false-positive patches (resized to 250×250 pixels at 0.1 mm resolution). The model demonstrated strong discriminative performance, achieving an AUC of 0.85 (95% CI: 0.84–0.86) in ten-fold cross-validation. This outcome demonstrates that combining coarse ROI suggestions from general-purpose AI with fine-tuned deep learning enables highly accurate identification of interpretively difficult regions—without the need for manual annotation.

By leveraging automated ROI detection, this pipeline offers a scalable and objective method for selecting difficult normal cases. It effectively overcomes a major limitation in current educational practice: the reliance on expert-determined difficulty, which has been shown to diverge from real-world interpretive error patterns. With this approach, educational test sets can be curated in a way that focuses training on the most problematic regions, optimising both efficiency and learning impact.

Together, these studies provide a comprehensive and coherent framework for predicting case difficulty in mammography education. Beginning with handcrafted global radiomic features, expanding to cohort-specific models and perceptual theory, and culminating in region-level radiomic features and deep learning models, this work lays the foundation for a fully adaptive educational platform. By anticipating how a case will be perceived—before it is even read—these AI engines ensure that every user receives a personalised, appropriately challenging learning experience, tailored not only to their performance history but also to their perceptual profile and cohort characteristics.

B.3.3 Scenario 3: AI for Existing Users

In the third scenario, the AI system addresses the case where an existing user encounters a set of previously unseen cases. The system uses prior performance data from the user and interaction data from other users to predict how the individual will perform on new cases [17]. The model utilises matrix factorisation, a collaborative filtering technique commonly employed in recommendation systems. It compares the reader's behavior with that of others by identifying latent (unobserved) features. Unlike traditional image-based approaches that rely on expert annotations or radiomics, this model infers difficulty based on implicit user interactions with the cases.

For example, if User A has shown a particular pattern of performance across cases with specific latent features, and Case X shares those features, the model can estimate how User A is likely to perform on Case X. This approach allows the system to tailor subsequent test sets to the user's ability level, enhancing both engagement and learning outcomes.

Evaluation of this model on cancer and normal cases showed promising results, with area under the curve (AUC) metrics indicating high predictive accuracy. The system not only improved personalisation but also reduced redundancy by avoiding exposure to cases that are either too easy or too difficult for the learner.

B.4 CONCLUSION

The work presented in this case study demonstrates the potential of AI to revolutionise educational strategies in mammography. By combining user-level modelling, radiomic analysis of case difficulty, and predictive algorithms for reader–case interactions, the proposed framework enables a fully adaptive learning environment. This system not only addresses long-standing limitations in traditional self-assessment methods but also enhances educational equity by tailoring content to the needs of individual learners and reader cohorts.

From a clinical perspective, such personalisation holds significant promise. Radiologists vary in training background, exposure to pathology, and perceptual styles—all of which influence diagnostic efficacy. Our AI-driven approach enables a more nuanced and data-driven assessment of these differences, translating them into targeted feedback and optimally challenging test sets. This has the potential to improve diagnostic consistency, accelerate learning curves, and ultimately enhance patient outcomes by reducing interpretive error in screening programs.

Beyond education, the methodologies developed in this project offer transferable value for quality assurance. In particular, the automated identification of difficult-to-interpret normal cases—often the source of elevated false-positive recall—can inform both training and audit systems. As AI continues to integrate into the clinical workflow, maintaining radiologist competence through responsive, intelligent education will become increasingly critical.

Importantly, the principles developed for mammographic education have already been extended to other imaging modalities. A similar AI-driven framework has been adapted for use in Chest CT, initially deployed to support interpretation in the context of COVID-19 pneumonia and subsequently tailored to detect patterns consistent with dust diseases and silicosis. These applications further validate the versatility and scalability of the core AI engines—demonstrating that educational personalisation through AI is not only achievable but broadly applicable across diverse imaging domains.

As radiology continues to evolve, aligning education with both individual reader needs and the complexity of real-world cases will be essential. The integration of AI into education is not merely an enhancement—it is an imperative for future-ready clinical practice.

REFERENCES

1. Suleiman, M.A., Hooshmand, S., Reed, W.M. et al. (2022) Optimising Breast Screen Reading Efficacy. In Digital Mammography: A Holistic Approach (pp. 3–9). Cham: Springer International Publishing. https://doi.org/10.1007/978-3-031-10898-3_1
2. Soh, B.P., Lee, W., McEntee, M.F. et al. (2013) Screening Mammography: Test Set Data Can Reasonably Describe Actual Clinical Reporting. Radiology. 268(1):46–53. https://doi.org/10.1148/radiol.13122399
3. Trieu, P.D., Tapia, K., Frazer, H. et al. (2019) Improvement of Cancer Detection on Mammograms via BREAST Test Sets. Academic Radiology. 26(12):e341–e347. https://doi.org/10.1016/j.acra.2018.12.017
4. Wong, D.J., Gandomkar, Z., Wu, W.J. et al. (2020) Artificial Intelligence and Convolution Neural Networks Assessing Mammographic Images: A Narrative Literature Review. Journal of Medical Radiation Sciences. 67(2):134–142. https://doi.org/10.1002/jmrs.385
5. Gandomkar, Z., Lewis, S.J., Li, T. et al. (2022) A Machine Learning Model Based on Readers' Characteristics to Predict Their Performances in Reading Screening Mammograms. BreastCancer. 29(4):589–598. https://doi.org/10.1007/s12282-022-01335-3
6. Tao, X., Gandomkar, Z., Li, T. et al. (2023) Using Radiomics-Based Machine Learning to Create Targeted Test Sets to Improve Specific Mammography Reader Cohort Performance: A Feasibility Study. Journal of Personalized Medicine. 13(6):888. https://doi.org/10.3390/jpm13060888
7. Tao, X., Gandomkar, Z., Li, T. et al. (2022) Varying Performance Levels for Diagnosing Mammographic Images Depending on Reader Nationality Have AI and Educational Implications. In Medical Imaging 2022: Image Perception, Observer Performance, and Technology Assessment. SPIE. https://doi.org/10.1117/12.2611342
8. Siviengphanom, S., Gandomkar, Z., Lewis, S.J. et al. (2023) Global Radiomic Features from Mammography for Predicting Difficult-to-Interpret Normal Cases. Journal of Digital Imaging. 36(4):1541–1552. https://doi.org/10.1007/s10278-023-00836-7
9. Siviengphanom, S., Gandomkar, Z., Lewis, S.J. et al. (2023) Global Mammographic Radiomic Signature can Predict Radiologists' Difficult-to-Interpret Normal Cases. In Medical Imaging 2023: Image Perception, Observer Performance, and Technology Assessment. SPIE. https://doi.org/10.1117/12.2645377
10. Siviengphanom, S., Brennan, P.C., Lewis, S.J. et al. (2024) A Machine Learning Model Based on Global Mammographic Radiomic Features Can Predict Which Normal Mammographic Cases Radiology Trainees Find Most Difficult. Journal of Imaging Informatics in Medicine. 1–10. https://doi.org/10.1007/s10278-024-01291-8
11. Siviengphanom, S., Lewis, S.J., Brennan, P.C. et al. (2024) Computer-Extracted Global Radiomic Features can Predict the radiologists' First Impression About the Abnormality of a Screening Mammogram. British Journal of Radiology. 97(1153):168–179. https://doi.org/10.1093/bjr/tqad025
12. Siviengphanom, S., Lewis, S.J., Brennan, P.C. et al. (2024) Predicting the Gist of Breast Cancer on a Screening Mammogram using Global Radiomic Features. In Medical Imaging 2024: Image Perception, Observer Performance, and Technology Assessment. SPIE. https://doi.org/10.1117/12.3005470
13. Brennan, P.C., Gandomkar, Z., Ekpo, E.U. et al. (2018) Radiologists can Detect the 'gist' of Breast Cancer Before Any Overt Signs of Cancer Appear. Scientific Reports. 8(1):8717. https://doi.org/10.1038/s41598-018-26100-5
14. Gandomkar, Z., Siviengphanom, S., Ekpo, E.U. et al. (2021) Global Processing Provides Malignancy Evidence Complementary to the Information Captured by Humans or Machines Following Detailed Mammogram Inspection. Scientific Reports, 2021. 11(1):20122. https://doi.org/10.1038/s41598-021-99582-5

15. Gandomkar, Z., Siviengphanom, S., Ekpo, E.U. et al. (2021) To Trust or not to Trust: Radiologist's First Impression Interpreting a Screening Mammogram. In The Royal Australian and New Zealand College of Radiologists (RANZCR) Conference.

16. Gandomkar, Z., Siviengphanom, S., Ekpo, E.U. et al. (2021) The Gist Signal Appears to Capture Malignancy Clues Complementary to the Information Collected During the Localized Mammogram Inspection by Radiologists or Computer. In The Royal Australian and New Zealand College of Radiologists (RANZCR) Conference.

17. Gandomkar, Z., Rickard, M., Jones, C. et al. (2025) Personalising Education for Radiologists Using AI: A Breast Imaging Case Study. The Royal College of Radiologists Open. 3:100166.

18. Tao, X., Gandomkar, Z., Li, T. et al. (2025) Radiomic Analysis of Cohort-Specific Diagnostic Errors in Reading Dense Mammograms Using Artificial Intelligence. British Journal of Radiology. 98(1165):75–88. https://doi.org/10.1093/bjr/tqae195

19. Tao, X., Gandomkar, Z., Li, T. et al. (2024) CNN-Based Transfer Learning with 10-Fold Cross-Validation: A Novel Approach for Customized Education of Mammography Training. In Medical Imaging 2024: Image Perception, Observer Performance, and Technology Assessment. SPIE. https://doi.org/10.1117/12.3006659

20. Tao, X., Reed, W.M., Li, T. et al. (2024) Optimizing Mammography Interpretation Education: Leveraging Deep Learning for Cohort-Specific Error Detection to Enhance Radiologist Training. Journal of Medical Imaging. 11(5):055502–055502. https://doi.org/10.1117/1.JMI.11.5.055502

21. Gandomkar, Z., et al. (2024) Automated Identification of Challenging Mammographic Cases Using Artificial Intelligence: A Novel Approach for Educational Test Set Curation. In Radiological Society of North America (RSNA) Annual Meeting, RSNA: Chicago, IL.

Case Study C: Integrating Artificial Intelligence into Healthcare – The Patient's Perspective

Felix Busch, Lisa A. Adams, and Keno K. Bressem

C.1 INTRODUCTION

An ageing population, rising rates of chronic disease, increasing global healthcare costs, and a shortage of healthcare professionals are expected to place growing pressure on healthcare systems worldwide in the coming decades [1–6]. Consequently, healthcare services that maximise resource efficiency while maintaining patient safety, autonomy, and quality of care will become increasingly important.

In recent years, artificial intelligence (AI) has emerged as a powerful tool to help bridge the gap between healthcare supply and demand [7]. AI applications have shown potential in enhancing diagnostics, personalising treatments, streamlining administrative tasks, and predicting patient outcomes, even outperforming human experts [8–10].

The implementation of AI in healthcare is a multifaceted process involving a wide range of stakeholders, including AI developers, providers, patients, and healthcare professionals [11]. While each of these groups plays a critical role in shaping how AI technologies are designed, regulated, and ultimately implemented in clinical practice, understanding how patients perceive and engage with these technologies is a critical component of successful AI adoption, as they will be the primary beneficiaries of its integration. This chapter provides an overview of what we know so far about patients' attitudes towards AI in healthcare.

C.2 PATIENTS' PERSPECTIVES ON THE USE OF AI

C.2.1 Perceived Benefits

Many studies have shown that patients widely recognise the potential of AI to improve healthcare [12–16]. For example, in a global survey of 13,806 hospital patients from 43 countries, Busch et al. reported that 57.6% of respondents expressed a generally positive attitude towards the use of AI in healthcare [12].

One benefit that patients associate with AI is its ability to improve diagnostic accuracy [12, 17, 18]. In addition, patients see AI as a key enabler of faster diagnostic processes, which is critical in time-sensitive conditions where rapid identification of disease can improve outcomes [12–16]. AI's potential to streamline diagnostic workflows is also associated with improved triage capabilities and more efficient use of human resources [19–22]. In addition, AI's ability to reduce unnecessary medical procedures and doctor visits is seen as a valuable benefit, leading to cost savings for both patients and healthcare systems [13, 23]. Patients also recognise the role of AI in improving remote access to care; for example, AI-enabled telehealth solutions offer greater accessibility to people in areas with limited physical infrastructure or mobility challenges [17, 23, 24].

Furthermore, AI is seen as a tool for patient empowerment. Patients particularly appreciate that AI-based applications improve communication by simplifying complex medical information, thereby increasing their understanding [23–24]. Receiving medical information in plain language may increase patient autonomy and reduce the need for other sources to understand their conditions or medical procedures. Thus, by facilitating access to information and providing decision support, AI could promote a greater sense of control for patients over their health outcomes.

C.2.2 Trust in AI

Trust can play an important role in patient acceptance. Previous studies have shown that patient trust can affect certain healthcare outcomes, such as diabetes management, and may reduce patient adherence [25–26]. Even if the AI tool is highly effective, patients who do not trust the hospital, the AI provider, or the algorithms may avoid seeking care from providers using AI, thus also missing out on the potential benefits of AI-assisted care.

For example, a study from Germany showed that when AI technologies are perceived as reliable, patients are more likely to accept and adopt them in clinical settings, with up to 94% (n=280/298) of dermatology patients willing to use AI to differentiate between benign and malignant skin lesions if the AI demonstrated a high level of diagnostic accuracy [14].

Notably, patients with a history of diagnostic errors, such as missed or delayed diagnoses, and those with chronic health conditions were more likely to engage with AI tools [27]. These patients also perceived AI systems as providing valuable insights into their diagnoses and were more likely to use AI-based symptom checkers to guide their decisions about seeking medical care [27].

C.2.3 Human Oversight

Despite generally positive attitudes towards AI, there is notable scepticism when AI is perceived as a stand-alone system. Concerns about AI's ability to make independent clinical judgements and the potential for algorithmic error raise questions about accountability in healthcare decision-making. Numerous studies suggest that patients are significantly more comfortable with AI when it functions as an assistive tool rather than a stand-alone system [12, 28–30]. For example, a survey conducted in Germany shows that a majority of 96% (n=434/452) of patients prefer that healthcare decisions remain in the hands of human doctors, especially in cases where AI and human experts disagree [31]. In contrast to shared decision-making, which promotes collaboration between humans and AI in patient care, human oversight emphasises the authority of healthcare professionals over AI-generated recommendations as a critical element at both the regulatory and system levels, which is crucial to building and maintaining patient trust in AI systems [32].

C.2.4 Diagnostic Errors

One of the main concerns of patients is that AI may lead to inaccurate diagnoses, potentially leading to inappropriate treatment or even physical harm [18, 24]. In this context, patients also worry that AI systems may lack the contextual understanding and experiential knowledge that human doctors bring to clinical decision-making [20–23]. In addition, studies have shown that patients are concerned about the ability of AI to accurately diagnose rare or atypical conditions [16, 18]. In particular, there is concern that AI systems that rely heavily on algorithmic patterns and datasets may fail to identify less-common conditions, leading to missed or delayed diagnoses with potentially serious consequences. For example, a UK study highlighted participants' concerns about the ability of AI to capture the complexity of clinical presentations, particularly in cases where symptoms deviate from the norm and atypical disease presentations are involved [18].

C.2.5 Doctor–Patient Relationship

Another key concern is the potential for AI to depersonalise the doctor–patient relationship. Fears that AI could reduce face-to-face interaction with healthcare providers are widespread, with many patients expressing concern that the use of AI could diminish the empathy and compassion that are critical components of care [16, 33]. The perceived inability of AI to convey nonverbal communication, express emotion, or demonstrate empathy raises concerns that its integration could reduce the quality of interpersonal interactions [13, 17, 23]. Patients value the emotional and communicative aspects of healthcare, which they believe AI cannot replicate.

C.2.6 Replacement of Human Physicians

Closely related to concerns about depersonalisation is the fear that AI will eventually replace human physicians [13, 14, 20]. This fear is particularly pronounced when AI is applied in areas traditionally confined to human intelligence, such as clinical decision-making and patient management [17, 28]. In this context, patients express concern that AI may not be able to replace human judgement, particularly in complex care scenarios [23, 28]. There is also concern about the risk of overreliance on AI, which could lead to the deskilling of healthcare providers [20, 23]. Patients worry that if doctors become too dependent on AI, they may lose the ability to detect errors or malfunctioning systems, which could compromise patient safety [14].

C.2.7 Risks to Data Security and Privacy

The security and privacy of personal health information are also among the main concerns patients have regarding the use of AI in healthcare. Several studies have reported that patients are concerned about the potential misuse of their data, ranging from 40% to 70.8% of respondents [13, 23, 24, 33]. The sensitive nature of health data heightens the perceived risk, as breaches or inappropriate use of information could have serious personal and legal consequences.

To mitigate these concerns, robust data security measures such as encryption, secure data storage and compliance with regulatory and legal frameworks such as the General Data Protection Regulation in Europe, the Health Insurance Portability and Accountability Act in the USA or the recently adopted European Union AI Act are essential and are also likely to reinforce patient trust [34, 35].

C.2.8 Increased Healthcare Costs

Economic concerns also shape patients' perceptions of AI in healthcare. Patients worry that the implementation of AI technologies could increase healthcare costs, potentially exacerbating existing healthcare inequalities [12–14, 30]. There is particular concern that AI-driven innovations could disproportionately benefit those with higher socioeconomic status, further limiting access to care for disadvantaged populations [23].

Efforts to make AI-enabled healthcare more affordable and accessible will be critical to addressing patient concerns about cost and access. Ultimately, all stakeholders must work together to ensure that AI technologies are implemented in a way that reduces, rather than increases, inequalities in healthcare.

C.3 CONCLUSION

While AI promises to advance diagnostics, personalise treatments and streamline administrative tasks in healthcare, its successful implementation depends on the acceptance of key stakeholders. Consistent with modern healthcare systems and treatment philosophies, promoting patient autonomy and dignity is essential for sustaining health and well-being. Adhering to the concept of patient-centred care, it is imperative to adopt a biopsychosocial perspective that acknowledges each patient's unique experiences, beliefs, and values when integrating AI into healthcare. This approach fosters patient engagement, self-management, and a positive experience with AI. Therefore, there is still a substantial demand for research investigating attitudes across diverse regional and sociodemographic contexts to guide and optimise patient-centred AI adoption.

While patients acknowledge the potential of AI, they also voice concerns about diagnostic errors, depersonalisation of care, job displacement, and issues related to privacy, security, and cost. Maintaining human oversight is essential for preserving trust, as patients prefer AI to serve as an assistive tool rather than an independent authority in clinical decisions. By creating well-structured education strategies and transparently communicating both the benefits and limitations of AI, healthcare systems can cultivate a well-informed patient base and ensure the responsible and successful integration of AI into global healthcare.

REFERENCES

1. Figueroa, C.A., Harrison, R., Chauhan, A. et al. (2019). Priorities and Challenges for Health Leadership and Workforce Management Globally: A Rapid Review. BMC Health Services Research, 19(1). https://doi.org/10.1186/s12913-019-4080-7
2. Roncarolo, F., Boivin, A., Denis, J.L. et al. (2017). What Do We Know About the Needs and Challenges of Health Systems? A Scoping Review of the International Literature. BMC Health Services Research. 17(1):636. https://doi.org/10.1186/s12913-017-2585-5
3. Marchildon, G.P., Allin, S., Merkur, S. (2020). Canada: Health System Review. Health Systems in Transition. 22(3):1–194.
4. World Health Organization. (2016). Health Workforce Requirements for Universal Health Coverage and the Sustainable Development Goals [accessed 30th June 2025]
5. Sinsky, C.A. (2017). Designing and Regulating Wisely: Removing Barriers to Joy in Practice. Annals of Internal Medicine. 166(9):677. https://doi.org/10.7326/m17-0524
6. Drossman, D.A., Ruddy, J. (2020). Improving Patient-Provider Relationships to Improve Health Care. Clinical Gastroenterology and Hepatology. 18(7):1417–1426. https://doi.org/10.1016/j.cgh.2019.12.007
7. Wang, F., Preininger, A. (2019). AI in Health: State of the Art, Challenges, and Future Directions. Yearbook Of Medical Informatics. 28(01):016–026. https://doi.org/10.1055/s-0039-1677908
8. Secinaro, S., Calandra, D., Secinaro, A. et al. (2021). The Role of Artificial Intelligence in Healthcare: A Structured Literature Review. BMC Medical Informatics and Decision Making, 21(1). https://doi.org/10.1186/s12911-021-01488-9
9. Sharma, M., Savage, C., Nair, M. et al. (2022). Artificial Intelligence Applications in Health Care Practice: Scoping Review. Journal of Medical Internet Research. 24(10):e40238. https://doi.org/10.2196/40238
10. Cabral, S., Restrepo, D., Kanjee, Z. et al. (2024). Clinical Reasoning of a Generative Artificial Intelligence Model Compared With Physicians. JAMA Internal Medicine. 184(5):581–583. https://doi.org/10.1001/jamainternmed.2024.0295
11. Razzaki, S., Baker, A., Perov, Y. et al. (2018). A Comparative Study of Artificial Intelligence and Human Doctors for the Purpose of Triage and Diagnosis. *arXiv (Cornell University)*. https://doi.org/10.48550/arxiv.1806.10698
12. Busch, F., Hoffmann, L., Xu, L.et al. (2024). Multinational Attitudes Towards AI in Healthcare and Diagnostics among Hospital Patients. medRxiv. https://doi.org/10.1101/2024.09.01.24312016
13. Gao, S., He, L., Chen, Y. et al. (2020). Public Perception of Artificial Intelligence in Medical Care: Content Analysis of Social Media. Journal Of Medical Internet Research. 22(7):e16649. https://doi.org/10.2196/16649
14. Jutzi, T.B., Krieghoff-Henning, E.I., Holland-Letz, T. et al. (2020) Artificial Intelligence in Skin Cancer Diagnostics: The Patients' Perspective. Frontiers in Medicine. 7:233. https://doi.org/10.3389/fmed.2020.00233
15. Keel, S., Lee, P.Y., Scheetz, J. et al. (2018) Feasibility and Patient Acceptability of a Novel Artificial Intelligence-Based Screening Model for Diabetic Retinopathy at Endocrinology Outpatient Services: A Pilot Study. Scientific Reports. 8(1):4330. https://doi.org/10.1038/s41598-018-22612-2

16. Young, A., Amara, D., Bhattacharya, A. et al. (2021). Patient and General Public Attitudes Towards Clinical Artificial Intelligence: A Mixed Methods Systematic Review. The Lancet Digital Health. 3(9):e599–e611. https://doi.org/10.1016/S2589-7500(21)00132-1

17. Adams, S.J., Tang, R., Babyn, P. (2020). Patient Perspectives and Priorities Regarding Artificial Intelligence in Radiology: Opportunities for Patient-Centered Radiology. Journal of the American College of Radiology: JACR. 17(8):1034–1036. https://doi.org/10.1016/j.jacr.2020.01.007

18. Nadarzynski, T., Miles, O., Cowie, A. et al. (2019). Acceptability of Artificial Intelligence (AI)-Led Chatbot Services in Healthcare: A Mixed-Methods Study. Digital Health. 5. https://doi.org/10.1177/2055207619871808

19. Rawson, T.M., Ming, D., Gowers, S.A. et al. (2019). Public Acceptability of Computer-Controlled Antibiotic Management: An Exploration of Automated Dosing and Opportunities for Implementation. The Journal of Infection. 78(1):75–86. https://doi.org/10.1016/j.jinf.2018.08.005

20. Ongena, Y.P., Haan, M., Yakar, D. et al. (2020). Patients' Views on the Implementation of Artificial Intelligence in Radiology: Development and Validation of a Standardized Questionnaire. European Radiology. 30(2):1033–1040. https://doi.org/10.1007/s00330-019-06486-0

21. Palmisciano, P., Jamjoom, A.A.B., Taylor, D. et al. (2020). Attitudes of Patients and Their Relatives Toward Artificial Intelligence in Neurosurgery. World Neurosurgery. 138:e627–e633. https://doi.org/10.1016/j.wneu.2020.03.029

22. Haan, M., Ongena, Y.P., Hommes, S. et al. (2019). A Qualitative Study to Understand Patient Perspective on the Use of Artificial Intelligence in Radiology. Journal of the American College of Radiology: JACR. 16(10):1416–1419. https://doi.org/10.1016/j.jacr.2018.12.043

23. Nelson, C.A., Pérez-Chada, L.M., Creadore, A. et al. (2020). Patient Perspectives on the Use of Artificial Intelligence for Skin Cancer Screening: A Qualitative Study. JAMA Dermatology. 156(5):501–512. https://doi.org/10.1001/jamadermatol.2019.5014

24. Tran, V.T., Riveros, C., Ravaud, P. (2019). Patients' Views of Wearable Devices and AI in Healthcare: Findings from the ComPaRe e-Cohort. NPJ Digital Medicine. 2:53. https://doi.org/10.1038/s41746-019-0132-y

25. Martin, L.R., Williams, S.L., Haskard, K.B. et al.(2005). The Challenge of Patient Adherence. Ther Clin Risk Manag. 1(3):189–99.

26. Lee, Y.Y., Lin, J.L. (2011). How Much Does Trust Really Matter? A Study of the Longitudinal Effects of Trust and Decision-Making Preferences on Diabetic Patient Outcomes. Patient Education and Counseling. 85(3):406–12. https://doi.org/10.1016/j.pec.2010.12.005

27. Meyer, A.N.D., Giardina, T.D., Spitzmueller, C. et al. (2020). Patient Perspectives on the Usefulness of an Artificial Intelligence-Assisted Symptom Checker: Cross-Sectional Survey Study. Journal of Medical Internet Research. 22(1):e14679. https://doi.org/10.2196/14679

28. Lennartz, S., Dratsch, T., Zopfs, D. et al. (2021). Use and Control of Artificial Intelligence in Patients Across the Medical Workflow: Single-Center Questionnaire Study of Patient Perspectives. Journal of Medical Internet Research. 23(2):e24221. https://doi.org/10.2196/24221

29. Yap, A., Wilkinson, B., Chen, E. et al. (2022). Patients Perceptions of Artificial Intelligence in Diabetic Eye Screening. Asia-Pacific Journal of Ophthalmology (Philadelphia, Pa.). 11(3):287–293. https://doi.org/10.1097/APO.0000000000000525

30. Yang, K., Zeng, Z., Peng, H. et al. (2019). Attitudes of Chinese Cancer Patients Toward the Clinical Use of Artificial Intelligence. Patient Preference and Adherence. 13:1867–1875. https://doi.org/10.2147/PPA.S225952

31. Fritsch, S.J., Blankenheim, A., Wahl, A. et al. (2022). Attitudes and perception of artificial intelligence in healthcare: A cross-sectional survey among patients. Digital Health. 8. https://doi.org/10.1177/20552076221116772

32. Gama, F., Tyskbo, D., Nygren, J. et al. (2022). Implementation Frameworks for Artificial Intelligence Translation into Health Care Practice: Scoping Review. Journal of Medical Internet Research. 24(1):e32215. https://doi.org/10.2196/32215

33. Khullar, D., Casalino, L.P., Qian, Y. et al. (2022). Perspectives of Patients About Artificial Intelligence in Health Care. JAMA Network Open. 5(5):e2210309. https://doi.org/10.1001/jamanetworkopen.2022.10309

34. Murdoch, B. (2021). Privacy and Artificial Intelligence: Challenges for Protecting Health Information in a New Era. BMC Medical Ethics. 22. https://doi.org/10.1186/s12910-021-00687-3

35. Busch, F., Kather, J.N., Johner, C. et al. (2024). Navigating the European Union Artificial Intelligence Act for Healthcare. NPJ Digital Medicine. 7(1):210. https://doi.org/10.1038/s41746-024-01213-6

Case Study D: Transforming Radiology Workflows at Leiden University Medical Centre (LUMC) – A Case Study in the Clinical Integration of AI for Chest X-Ray Interpretation

Milda Shams and Willem Grootjans

D.1 INTRODUCTION

Radiology services across the UK and Europe are under increasing pressure with increasing demand and decreasing resources. According to the Royal College of Radiologists (RCR), the UK has a shortage of over 30% of consultant radiologists, a figure projected to rise to 40% by 2027 if current trends continue [1]. The RCR reports that annual radiology workloads have grown by more than 30% over the past five years, while workforce expansion has failed to keep pace [1]. In 2022 alone, National Health Service (NHS) hospitals in England and Wales reported over 45 million imaging examinations, of which chest radiographs remain the most commonly requested examination, with 22.0 million procedures [2].

These systemic pressures have driven interest in practical artificial intelligence (AI) applications to support diagnostic workflows, alleviate human resource burdens, and enhance consistency in reporting. Particularly in examinations such as chest radiography, where a high percentage of images show no findings, the use of autonomous AI tools presents a scalable and clinically relevant opportunity.

As AI technologies continue to evolve, their clinical application in healthcare is moving from theoretical promise to demonstrable impact. Within radiology, AI has shown particular value in addressing longstanding challenges related to growing diagnostic workloads, radiologist shortages, and variable reporting quality.

This case study contributes to an evolving body of evidence demonstrating real-world AI integration in radiology. It documents how Leiden University Medical Center (LUMC), an academic teaching hospital in the Netherlands, adopted and implemented Oxipit's CE-certified AI solutions, particularly Oxipit ChestLink and Oxipit Quality, to improve workflow efficiency and diagnostic reliability. LUMC serves a regional population of approximately 1,983,700 residents and has an annual workload of 137,000 radiological examinations per year; ~23,000 are specifically chest radiographs [3].

Oxipit is a Lithuanian-based radiology AI company (www.oxipit.ai) and is focused on delivering clinically validated, workflow-centric solutions. Notably, it became the first developer globally to secure Conformité Européenne (CE) Class IIb certification for autonomous radiology reporting of normal chest X- radiographs. The company's approach to AI adoption emphasises full picture archiving and communication systems (PACS) integration, clinician collaboration, and scalability across diverse healthcare environments, from academic hospitals to smaller community sites.

This case study is designed to inform a multidisciplinary readership spanning clinical professionals, educators, data scientists, and health policy stakeholders and offers an in-depth exploration of the practical, legal, and organisational dimensions of AI implementation. It provides a replicable roadmap for future deployments and serves as a reference for discussions on safe, effective, and equitable AI integration in medical imaging.

D.2 THE PROBLEM AND THE SOLUTION

Radiology departments across Europe are navigating increasing imaging volumes in parallel with constrained staffing capacities. This imbalance has led to mounting workloads, prolonged turn-around times, and significant stress on diagnostic resources. Among these, chest radiography stands out as a high-volume, low-pathology modality, making it a prime candidate for targeted workflow innovation.

At Leiden University Medical Center, an academic tertiary hospital in the Netherlands, approximately half of all chest radiographs are ultimately deemed normal. This observation catalysed a strategic exploration into AI applications to streamline reporting, reallocate radiologist effort, and uphold diagnostic quality standards.

While AI in radiology has advanced rapidly from experimental algorithms to CE-certified clinical tools, the transformative potential depends significantly on how it is operationalised within real-world settings. This case study outlines the phased implementation, integration, and impact of Oxipit's AI solutions within LUMC's radiology department, offering insight into the clinical, technical, and organisational dynamics involved.

D.3 BASELINE WORKFLOW AND IDENTIFIED CHALLENGES

Prior to AI deployment, chest radiographs were interpreted manually by radiologists or residents, requiring a consistent investment of approximately three to four minutes per case. Given the high proportion of normal studies and daily volumes of 80 to 100 exams, a substantial portion of clinical capacity was expended on reviewing unremarkable findings.

Medical residents, particularly during overnight or weekend shifts, bore the brunt of this task. Limited senior oversight during these periods further heightened the cognitive load and diagnostic pressure on less experienced practitioners. The cumulative effect was workflow inefficiency and increased risk of interpretive fatigue. In addition to personnel fatigue, the lack of case prioritisation meant that complex or urgent studies could be queued alongside routine normal exams. This could have led to a suboptimal allocation of diagnostic expertise and could have contributed to variability in turnaround times, especially for cases requiring expedited attention.

D.4 INITIAL ENGAGEMENT AND TECHNICAL INTEGRATION

LUMC initiated collaboration with Oxipit in 2018 through the Medical Delta innovation network (https://www.medicaldelta.nl/en). The early focus was on evaluating the performance and feasibility of AI-generated automated chest radiograph reports. However, full diagnostic automation proved premature due to the complexity of integrating relevant clinical context into algorithmic decision-making.

Subsequently, the partnership evolved toward a more pragmatic and clinically tractable use case: automated binary triage (normal vs. abnormal). This shift led to the introduction of Oxipit ChestLink, a CE-certified solution designed to autonomously identify normal chest radiographs with high sensitivity [4].

A critical element in clinical adoption was seamless integration with the hospital's PACS. Oxipit's engineering team collaborated with LUMC IT personnel to embed AI outputs directly into the radiologist's worklist. This eliminated reliance on external portals and preserved existing clinical workflows, significantly enhancing user acceptance. (See Figure D.1.)

D.5 CLINICAL UTILITY AND WORKFLOW IMPACT

Through retrospective and prospective validation involving approximately 20,000 chest radiographs, ChestLink demonstrated the capacity to autonomously report 15–20% of studies as normal,

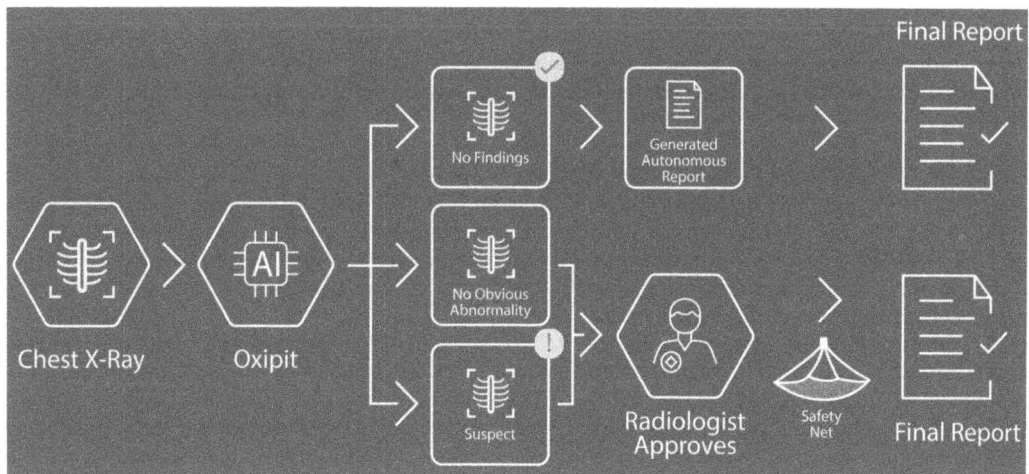

Figure D.1 Clinical workflow with Oxipit integration.

with 99.9% sensitivity. This translated into time savings, particularly in high-volume reporting blocks.

From a clinical operations perspective, this reduction in reporting burden facilitated

- reallocation of radiologist time to complex or urgent cases

- reduced cognitive load on night-shift residents

- enhanced throughput even with a decrease in staffing over time

- prioritisation of cases with likely findings, accelerating diagnostic pathways for higher-risk patients

These changes produced noticeable improvements in departmental efficiency and also contributed to greater consistency in turnaround times. For example, studies triaged as abnormal by the AI system could be surfaced earlier in the worklist, supporting faster intervention.

Parallel implementation of Oxipit Quality, a secondary-read quality assurance tool, further contributed to the quality of radiological services. Occasionally it flagged instances where radiological reports did not align with AI findings, incidentally prompting several clinically relevant reassessments (including a missed pulmonary nodule and subtle fractures). These real-world interventions strengthened confidence in the system's reliability.

AI also has the potential to help refine intra-day workflows. It is planned to use this application In the future, during peak hours, whereby staff will be able to strategically batch or defer confirmed normal studies, enabling radiologists to better manage variable caseloads and unexpected surges.

D.6 PROFESSIONAL CULTURE AND CHANGE MANAGEMENT

Technological adoption required more than technical validation; it demanded cultural alignment. Initial scepticism among radiologists, particularly regarding autonomy and liability was addressed through structured dialogue and collaborative planning. LUMC's leadership emphasised transparency, hosted regular briefings, and positioned AI as an augmentation rather than a threat to clinical judgement.

Crucially, concerns were addressed not solely through empirical evidence but by acknowledging the emotional and ethical dimensions of diagnostic responsibility. Radiologists were included in discussions on deployment strategy, incorporation of AI into daily clinical routine including error management and patient safety protocols.

D.7 LEGAL CONSIDERATIONS AND LIABILITY FRAMEWORKS

Autonomous diagnostic support raises complex questions related to liability, data governance, and clinical oversight. Under Dutch medical law and the European AI act [5], a physician is currently required to validate diagnostic output before it is communicated to patients or referring clinicians. Accordingly, LUMC has not yet transitioned to fully autonomous reporting, though it is actively working with legal and regulatory stakeholders to explore frameworks for shared responsibility.

To that end, LUMC is developing operational protocols in collaboration with clinicians and legal teams and as well as national regulatory bodies. These include models for clinician override, audit logging, and insurance coverage, particularly in edge cases where AI and human interpretations diverge.

D.8 EDUCATIONAL APPLICATIONS AND AI LITERACY

The implementation of AI has also yielded benefits for clinical education. There is potential to integrate AI into the curriculum, but currently there is no consensus on how best to achieve this. It is possible that AI-flagged studies may be used to improve pattern recognition and develop an understanding of normal anatomical variance. Annotated studies and disagreement cases have become valuable learning tools in teaching rounds.

Furthermore, LUMC, together with the Vrije Universiteit Amsterdam (VU), has resurrected a national AI learning lab, focusing on cross-community learning of algorithmic technologies in radiology, an initiative supported by the Dutch Research Council. This platform allows for shared review of AI-generated cases, collaborative annotation, and cross-institutional benchmarking. Several learning modules were created teaching end users of AI systems to responsibly use AI results for their own clinical practice using real clinical cases. The goal is to provide responsible, informed adoption of AI tools through clinician-led peer learning.

D.9 PATIENT-CENTRIC BENEFITS AND COMMUNICATION PATHWAYS

One significant, if indirect, outcome of AI integration is accelerated patient communication. For normal cases flagged with high confidence, referring clinicians can potentially receive rapid clearance when automated reporting is used, sometimes before the patient has left the department. This reduction in turnaround time supports timely reassurance and alleviates anxiety for patients awaiting results.

LUMC is exploring standardised communication templates and automated messaging systems to further streamline this aspect. With the ability to view their own data, patients will be able to see their AI results. This means that there needs to be a clear indication of which results have been obtained using AI and where human interactions did take place and what changes were made. Future iterations of this workflow could enable automated delivery of normal findings to patients directly, with appropriate safeguards and clinician oversight.

D.10 REGIONAL STRATEGY AND SCALABLE SERVICE MODELS

LUMC envisions AI-enabled radiology as a cornerstone of regional diagnostic services. By deploying ChestLink in satellite hospitals, where it can assist radiologists with high-volume chest X-rays exams. This model ensures consistent quality while enabling radiologists in the satellite hospitals to focus on exams that demand advanced expertise.

Furthermore, early pilots are exploring the feasibility of involving radiographers or physician assistants in preliminary validation of AI-cleared studies. Such role redistribution has the potential to enhance system efficiency without compromising diagnostic integrity.

D.11 FUTURE DIRECTIONS: SENSITIVITY TUNING AND REAL-TIME FEEDBACK

To further optimise workflow gains, LUMC is experimenting with sensitivity threshold calibration. A slight reduction in sensitivity could substantially increase the number of studies categorised as normal, albeit with a controlled trade-off in specificity. The team is conducting retrospective analyses to model the impact of these adjustments and to establish acceptable clinical risk boundaries.

A complementary area of development involves real-time quality control. Current quality checks are performed post hoc, but integrating immediate feedback mechanisms such as real-time alerts upon report sign-off could enhance safety and responsiveness.

D.12 CONCLUSION

The deployment of Oxipit's AI solution at LUMC exemplifies how radiology departments can meaningfully incorporate deep learning tools into routine clinical care. Success hinged not merely on algorithmic accuracy, but on thoughtful integration, user engagement, and clear alignment with clinical priorities.

LUMC's experience suggests that AI can serve as a viable mechanism to address resource constraints, support clinical training, and maintain diagnostic quality at scale. However, the broader adoption of such systems requires continued dialogue around regulation, professional accountability, and patient-centred design.

By taking a measured, collaborative approach, LUMC offers a replicable model for institutions seeking to navigate the complex landscape of AI in medical imaging.

"Autonomous AI lets us stop doing tasks we no longer need to do. It's not about the technology, it's about solving real problems, improving care, and using our expertise where it matters most," said Dr. Willem Grootjans, assistant professor and head of imaging services, LUMC.

REFERENCES

1. Clinical Radiology Workforce Census. (2023). rcr-census-clinical-radiology-workforce-census-2023.pdf [accessed June 2025]
2. https://www.england.nhs.uk/statistics/wp-content/uploads/sites/2/2022/07/Statistical-Release-21st-July-2022-PDF-875KB.pdf?utm_source=chatgpt.com [accessed June 2025]
3. https://www.england.nhs.uk/statistics/wp-content/uploads/sites/2/2023/11/Annual-Statistical-Release-2022-23-PDF-1.3MB-1.pdf [accessed June 2025]
4. Grootjans, W., Krainska, U., Rezazade Mehrizi, M.H. (2025). How Do Medical Institutions Co-Create Artificial Intelligence Solutions with Commercial Startups? Eur Radiol. https://doi.org/10.1007/s00330-025-11672-4
5. The European AI Act. (2024). Document 32024R1689 Regulation (EU) 2024/1689 of the European Parliament and of the Council of 13 June 2024 http://data.europa.eu/eli/reg/2024/1689/oj [accessed June 2025]

Index

Note: Page references with *Italics* refer to figures, **bold** refer to tables.

For Product Safety Concerns and Information please contact our EU
representative GPSR@taylorandfrancis.com
Taylor & Francis Verlag GmbH, Kaufingerstraße 24, 80331 München, Germany